ENVIRONMENTALLY AND SOCIALLY
SUSTAINABLE DEVELOPMENT

Biotechnology
and Biosafety

A forum cosponsored by
American Association for the Advancement of Science
The Conservation Fund
Consultative Group on International Agricultural Research
Food and Agriculture Organization of the United Nations
Government of Norway
Government of Sweden
International Council of Scientific Unions
Smithsonian Institution
Third World Academy of Sciences
Union of Concerned Scientists
United Nations Development Programme
United Nations Educational, Scientific and Cultural Organisation
United Nations Environment Programme
United Nations Industrial Development Organization
U. S. National Academy of Sciences
The World Conservation Union
The World Bank Group

Biotechnology and Biosafety was a forum associated with
The Fifth Annual World Bank Conference on
Environmentally and Socially Sustainable Development,
held at the World Bank, October 9–10, 1997

Ismail Serageldin and Wanda Collins, Editors

The World Bank
Washington, D.C.

This report has been prepared by the staff of the World Bank. The judgments expressed do not necessarily reflect the views of the Board of Executive Directors or of the governments they represent.

Cover photographs. Top: A peasant farmer in a northern volcanic area of Rwanda weeds potatoes grown on elevated beds. Bottom: A molecular virologist at the International Potato Center (CIP), Lima, loads an acrylamide "sequencing gel" to sequence the RNA of a potato virus; the resulting genetic fingerprint is in the background. Both photos by permission of CIP, one of the centers of the Consultative Group on International Agricultural Research (CGIAR).

Ismail Serageldin is vice president, Special Programs, at the World Bank. Wanda Collins is deputy director general for research, International Potato Center (CIP), Lima, Peru, one of the 16 research centers of the Consultative Group on International Agricultural Research (CGIAR).

Library of Congress Cataloging-in-Publication Data

International Conference on Environmentally Sustainable Development
    (5th : 1997 : World Bank)
    Biotechnology and biosafety : proceedings of an associated event
of the fifth annual World Bank Conference on Environmentally and
Socially Sustainable Development / Ismail Serageldin and Wanda
Collins, editors.
        p.   cm. — (Environmentally and socially sustainable
development)
    ISBN 0-8213-4242-8
    1. Biotechnology—Environmental aspects—Congresses.   2. Health
risk assessment—Congresses.   3. Agricultural biotechnology—
Congresses.   I. Serageldin, Ismail, 1944– .   II. Collins, Wanda
Williams.   III. Title.   IV. Series: Environmentally and socially
sustainable development series.
TP248.2.I579   1997
660.6—dc21   98-23586
                                                                    CIP

Contents

Preface

Biotechnology—the technique of using living organisms or their parts to make or modify products, improve plants or animals, or develop microorganisms for specific use—comprises an important and powerful set of enabling technologies with which to solve an array of problems. The power of these technologies is unlike any the scientific world of biology has yet seen, and they are responsible for a true biological revolution. The ability to move genes and groups of genes at will, to decipher, to "see," and to manipulate the molecular codes that make us individuals, as well as to "demystify" the genetic makeup of organisms in nature—these tools are now spread before us.

The potential risks of biotechnology go well beyond those we face directly as humans. They go to the very heart of what makes our world survive: the ecosystems in which we live and the organisms, both plant and animal, that make those ecosystems function. New technologies as powerful as those of biotechnology carry with them the burden of making wise and informed decisions of how to use them by asking and answering questions about their safety and assessing what risks are acceptable to human society. It is up to all of us as scientists, policymakers, and concerned members of civil society to make those decisions.

How to maximize the potential of biotechnology while minimizing risk is a critical issue facing scientists and policymakers and was the topic of an intensive, two-day conference at the World Bank in October 1997. The event took as its starting point the findings of a panel of experts commissioned by the World Bank Group and led by Nobel laureate for physics Henry W. Kendall. These findings, published by the World Bank in 1997 under the title *Bioengineering of Crops: Report of the World Bank Panel on Transgenic Crops*, are also presented in Part III of this report to provide the reader with essential background.

The "Biotechnology and Biosafety" conference, an Associated Event of the Fifth Annual World Bank Conference on Environmentally and Socially Sustainable Development, was open to the public. Participants represented a wide cross-section of stakeholders—academics, scientists, international and national research organizations, and representatives from the private sector and civil society. The special focus of debate was on how the promises of biotechnology can be realized for the benefit of the world's poor, the environment, and the safe management of biotechnology products and processes. Because of the significant role of ethics and values in determining choices affecting environmental conditions, an Associated Event on this topic was held prior to the Conference. The proceedings of this Event, *Ethics and Values: A Global Perspective*, include the chapter, "Ethics and Biotechnology: Realities and Uncertainties," which has been reprinted in Part II of this book as an easy reference to the readers.

This publication summarizes the wide-ranging, stimulating, and provocative presentations and discussions that took place during the meeting. While there are still dissenting opinions on some issues, there was surprisingly broad agreement on many others. In areas of divergent opinion this frank and open public discussion served to more clearly focus the debate and—just possibly—point the way forward.

Acknowledgments

Cosponsors

American Association for the Advancement of Science (AAAS)
The Conservation Fund
Consultative Group on International Agricultural Research (CGIAR)
Food and Agriculture Organization of the United Nations (FAO)
Government of Norway
Government of Sweden
International Council of Scientific Unions (ICSU)
Smithsonian Institution
Third World Academy of Sciences (TWAS)
Union of Concerned Scientists (UCS)
United Nations Development Programme (UNDP)
United Nations Educational, Scientific and Cultural Organisation (UNESCO)
United Nations Environment Programme (UNEP)
United Nations Industrial Development Organization (UNIDO)
U.S. National Academy of Sciences (NAS)
The World Bank Group
The World Conservation Union (IUCN)

This conference on Biotechnology and Biosafety was held as an Associated Event of the Fifth Annual World Bank Conference on Environmentally and Socially Sustainable Development (ESSD) and was hosted by the World Bank Group under the auspices of the ESSD vice presidency. In recognition of biotechnology's critical importance to science and society, the event was cosponsored by 17 organizations. The cosponsors, listed above, deserve a special expression of gratitude, having contributed to the organization of an outstanding event that brought together many of the world's most distinguished specialists.

The governments of Norway and Sweden deserve a very special expression of appreciation for their financial support, without which the conference would not have occurred.

The World Bank Group also wishes to express gratitude to all who participated in this event by making presentations or by taking part in the debate. Special thanks are due to Wanda Collins and Sarwat Hussain, who organized the event; Joan Martin-Brown, who oversaw day-to-day organi-

zation of the entire ESSD Conference and affili-
ated events; and Lisa Carlson and other staff of
the World Bank Group, the CGIAR Secretariat,
the International Food Policy Research Institute
(IFPRI), and all the others whose contributions
made this event possible.

The background document for this conference
was *Bioengineering of Crops: Report of the World
Bank Panel on Transgenic Crops*, which was prepared by a panel of experts chaired by Professor
Henry W. Kendall, Nobel laureate for physics
and chairman of the board of the Union of Concerned Scientists. Dr. Kendall and the entire
panel deserve special acknowledgment for their
outstanding contribution to the success of the
conference. The panel's report, which includes a
list of the panel members, is reprinted in this
volume as Part III.

This proceedings was copyedited by Alison
Raphael, desktopped by Gaudencio Dizon, and
coordinated by Lisa Carlson, Alicia Hetzner, and
Virginia Hitchcock.

Abbreviations and Acronyms

AGERI	Agricultural Genetic Engineering Research Institute (Egypt)
AIDS	Acquired immunodeficiency syndrome
APHIS	U.S. Animal and Plant Inspection Service
ARC	Agricultural research center
BSE	Bovine spongiform encephalopathy
BSO	Biological safety officer
Bt	*Bacillus thuringiensis*
CBD	Convention on Biological Diversity
CGIAR	Consultative Group on International Agricultural Research
CIAT	Centro Internacional de Agricultura Tropical
CIMMYT	International Maize and Wheat Improvement Center
CIRAD	Centre de Cooperation Internationale en Recherche Agronomique pour le Developpement
COLCIENCIAS	[Colombia Sciences]
CONABIA	National Biotechnology Commission
CORPOICA	Colombian National Research Corporation
CTNBio	National Technical Biosafety Committee
DNA	Deoxyribonucleic acid
EMBRAPA	Brazilian Agricultural Research Corporation
EPA	U.S. Environmental Protection Agency
EU	European Union
FAO	Food and Agriculture Organization of the United Nations
FBEC	French Biomolecular Engineering Commission
FDA	U.S. Food and Drug Administration
GATT	General Agreement on Trade and Tariffs
GDP	Gross domestic product
GMO	Genetically modified organism
HRC	Herbicide-resistant crop
IARCS	International agricultural research centers
IBC	Institutional Biosafety Committees
ICRISAT	International Crops Research Institute for the Semi-Arid Tropics
ICSU	International Council of Scientific Unions
ICT	Information and communication technology
IFPRI	International Food Policy Research Institute

IITA	International Institute on Tropical Agriculture
IP	Intellectual property
IPM	Integrated pest management
IPR	Intellectual property rights
ISNAR	International Service on National Agricultural Research
IUCN	World Conservation Union
KARI	Kenyan Agricultural Research Institute
LMO	Living modified organism
MAI	Multilateral Agreement on Investment
MVs	Modern varieties
NAGEL	National Agricultural Genetic Engineering Laboratory (Egypt), now AGERI
NARS	National Agricultural Research Systems
NBC	National Biosafety Committee (Egypt)
NGO	Nongovernmental organization
OECD	Organisation for Economic Co-operation and Development
ORSTOM	French National Research Institute for Development Cooperation
R&D	Research and development
r-DNA	Recombinant deoxyribonucleic acid
RNA	Ribonucleic acid
TAC	Technical Advisory Committee
TRIPS	Trade-Related Aspects of International Property Rights
UNCED	United Nations Conference on Environment and Development
UNDP	United Nations Development Programme
UNEP	United Nations Environment Programme
UNIDO	United Nations Industrial Development Organization
UPOV	Union for the Protection of Varieties
USAID	U.S. Agency for International Development
USDA	U.S. Department of Agriculture
WHO	World Health Organization
WTO	World Trade Organization

Part I. Biotechnology and Biosafety

Setting the Stage

Introductory Remarks and Stating the Problem
Ismail Serageldin

February 22, 1997 was the day on which the international community was compelled to come to terms with the spectacular progress of biotechnology: Dolly the sheep was introduced to the world. Dolly's creation immediately focused attention on a branch of science that is little known and less understood by the public at large.

The promise and perils of biotechnology have developed a mystique of their own, and the world was soon buffeted by conflicting stories of the possible benefits of scientifically created superabundance and possible disasters that raised fears from Frankenstein's monster to Jurassic Park. More thoughtful concerns were expressed about the possible health or environmental effects of genetically modified organisms (GMOs), in addition to the ethical concerns of tinkering with nature.

We need to be more dispassionate. Let us disentangle the issues.

Biotechnology could help us to pursue the mission of environmental protection, poverty reduction, and food security by helping to promote a sustainable agriculture centered around smallholder farmers in developing countries. Although the first fruits of the new technology are already benefiting the commercial crops of the industrialized countries, there is no inherent reason why the tools of biotechnology could not be employed in pursuing the mission of environmentally and socially sustainable development.

Biotechnology could be used to introduce environmentally friendly resistance to disease and pests. It could help develop hardier plants with resistance or tolerance to drought, salt, and herbicides. Plant characteristics could be genetically altered to adjust maturation speed, increase transportability, reduce post-harvest losses (such as shelf-life), water content, and stem size. All of these aspects are of great relevance to poor farmers in low-potential environments.

Biotechnology is also relevant to the poor because it is seen to be scale-neutral. Unlike mechanization, for example, it has no intrinsic bias against the smallholder farmer. But the complexity of managing refuge areas in Bt transgenic crop plantings shows that it is not as easy to transfer as might appear at first blush, unless seed mixes prove adequate to the task.

In the case of livestock, so essential for the smallholder farmer, biotechnology provides the most important defense against disease, such as vaccines for east coast fever in east Africa.

The biotechnology revolution is here. It is relevant to the problems of the world and to the work of the World Bank Group and the Consultative Group on International Agricultural Research (CGIAR). But for many of us it raises important questions relating to ethics, intellectual property rights, and biosafety. Let me say a brief word about each of the two first sets of issues—which are not the topic of this conference—and then try to frame the issues for the remaining discussions on biosafety.

The Ethical Issues

Not everything that is technically feasible is ethically desirable. For some, transgenic tinkering with nature raises fundamental issues, which must be respected. Conversely this must be weighed against the possible benefits that biotechnology, with adequate safeguards, can bring to the poor and the environment.

These issues were scrutinized yesterday at a special session that dealt with ethical issues in development; they were also the topic of a workshop held in Brazil under the auspices of the CGIAR Genetic Resources Policy Committee some months ago. Such discussions constitute a major step forward in disentangling the issues and, hopefully, creating a consensus as to the domains that we should pursue and those that we should eschew. There will always be areas of disagreement on such controversial issues, but to the extent that they are thoroughly debated we should all be wiser for hearing each others' point of view.

Intellectual Property Rights

There is no question that intellectual property should be protected. The results of recognition of IPR are increased rewards to the creative and mobilization of resources for research that would not occur if protection were not there. However proprietary science is beginning to pose some problems of access for some of the poorer countries and for those needing to use processes for the purpose of producing public goods.

Balancing the need of private investors to have IPR to recoup their investments and the needs of the poor and future generations to have access to relevant science and suitable products is the real problem posed by IPR in this new biotechnology revolution, which is not only producing undreamed-of breakthroughs, but also is creating a totally new environment for science—a domain of proprietary science with a whole new set of issues to address. I do not propose to address these here.

Safety Issues

Nobody would argue that we should not be on the lookout for the safety of the public, especially in developing countries where there has been inadequate attention to issues of product safety in the past. But that should not translate into the rejection of all types of activities that are labeled biotechnology out of fear or ignorance. The correct balance has to be established when weighing the benefits against the risks of biotechnology.

Fear exists that transgenic plants will turn into weeds; or that biotechnology will provide paths for new genes to move into wild plants that become weeds; or that it will create new viral strains from virus-containing transgenic crops. In addition there is concern regarding possible health or environmental impacts of these transgenic organisms in food crops.

Such concerns are real. They must be examined dispassionately, and we are gathered here today in this important seminar, cosponsored by the most distinguished scientific bodies in the world and key international bodies, to do just that. We are here to assess scientific evidence on the safety of biotechnology applications in agriculture, which should constitute another step in disentangling the issues.

Possible Actions

I believe that this conference should lead to two types of results.

First, a collective judgment, a consensus, on the range of acceptable approaches to the issues of biosafety for both biotechnology research and application. I look to this gathering to replicate in a small way the achievements of the Asilomar conference a generation ago. At that time the uncertainty surrounding the new science of recombinant DNA research attracted much media attention, which shed more heat than light. Scientists met at Asilomar in California and established a set of guiding principles, based on the best available science, to create appropriate protocols for research and the levels of protection appropriate for different kinds of research. It is interesting to see that this set of voluntary guidelines, based on a scientific consensus and subsequently adopted by many institutions, has served the world well for over a quarter of a century.

Second, a specific set of decisions that each of us intends to pursue in the institutions where we work, which have a role in promoting the adoption of the kind of biosafety measures that this consensus will underline.

For the first, I await the results of your deliberations. For the second, I can say something about the World Bank Group and the CGIAR, subject to modifications that may arise from the deliberations in the coming two days.

The World Bank Group and the CGIAR

For the World Bank Group I am happy to endorse the recommendations of the Kendall Panel Report, entitled *Bioengineering of Crops*. I propose to urge the Bank to act in accordance with its recommendations. In fact, I am happy to note, some of the panel's recommendations are already being implemented.

- *Support of Developing World Science*

The Bank should direct attention to the need for liaison with and support for the developing world's agricultural scientific community.

We will support the newly emerging Global Forum for International Agricultural Research. We will continue to support the regionally based National Agricultural Research Systems (NARS).

- *Research Programs*

The Bank should identify and support high-quality research programs dedicated to exploiting the favorable potential of genetic engineering for improving the lot of the developing world.

The recently approved loan for agricultural research in Brazil is a model of our willingness to move in this direction.

- *Surveillance and Regulation*

The Bank should support the implementation of formal, national regulatory structures in its client nations by seeing to it that these structures retain their vigor and effectiveness through the years and by providing scientific and technical support to the client nations as requested. The Bank should support, in each developing country, the deployment of an early warning system to identify any troubles that may arise and to signal successes and introduce improvements in adapting new strains.

We will look into this.

- *Investment in International Agricultural Research Centers*

The Bank should increase its support for research in biotechnology and related areas at international agricultural research centers, because these centers are in the best position to ensure that high-quality, environmentally sustainable agricultural products and processes are developed and transferred in developing countries.

Our support for the CGIAR will continue.

- *The Agricultural Challenge*

The Bank should continue to give high priority to all aspects of increasing agricultural productivity in the developing world, while encouraging the necessary transition to sustainable methods.

This is at the heart of our new rural development strategy and the new emphasis that President James D. Wolfensohn has placed on rural development.

For the CGIAR I am happy to report that the Technical Advisory Committee has just appointed two panels, one to look at biosafety issues and one to look at IPR and the practice of proprietary science. We await their views for a debate on the topic at the annual meetings of the CGIAR later this month. Yet one can still advance some thoughts for consideration. The principles that should guide the actions of the CGIAR can be articulated, fully recognizing that the devil is in the details and that the application of the principles is where the difficulties will lie.

The CGIAR must play a role in ensuring that:
- Access to the potential benefits is guaranteed for the poor and the environment
- The risks of biotechnology are appropriately addressed and adequate biosafety provisions are made for developing countries that want to benefit from this additional tool.

This means intensifying certain things we have been doing. It means adding to our critical mass of scientific effort in the area of biotechnology, but not at the expense of the heartland issues of people-centered policies, inclusion of the farm community, natural resource management, and biodiversity. Let us always remember, too, that biotechnology is a tool to be used in conjunction with other tools, not an end in itself.

Envoi

We often speak of partnerships, of the complementary roles played by the public and the private, the national and the international, the formal and the informal, the farmer and the scientist, nongovernmental organizations and NARS, and the synergies that we have to capture for the benefit of creating a better world—free of hunger and misery, dedicated to the dignity of people, especially the poor and the future generations from whom we have borrowed this planet. Can we define ways in which this can be accomplished in the domain of biotechnology? Can we create adequate safeguards for use of this powerful new technology? Can we find ways to marry the interests of all these actors? I think that we can. I think that this conference will be a major step in that direction.

The time for action is now. Let us move forward with all the deliberate speed that practical wisdom would dictate.

The Scientific Scene
Werner Arber

My intention is to provide background information that could serve to facilitate the debate on biosafety. Advance in scientific research depends on a number of factors, of which I would like to briefly mention three: the introduction of novel technologies, the application of new research strategies, and an essential widening of the knowledge basis, which often involves new conceptual views on natural phenomena. For biotechnology all of these factors are relevant, and are in part also interconnected. In order to render their influence on scientific advance more visible, it might be good to trace important steps in the history of genetics and its applications, paying particular attention to biosafety issues.

Background Information on Genes and Genomes

A few definitions might be helpful for a better understanding. Genetic information is inscribed on long filamentous molecules of deoxyribonucleic acid, or DNA. Its building blocks are four different nucleotides, which are symbolized by the letters A, T, C, and G. The linear sequences of nucleotides encode the genetic information, similar to the information that I provide to the reader by arranging letters in specific sequences to form words and sentences. The unit of genetic information is the gene. The two essential parts of a gene are an *open reading frame*, with the information becoming expressed if the gene gets activated, and the *signals serving to control* time and efficiency of gene expression. We may recall here that gene expression usually results in the synthesis of a specific protein, the function of which is often to act as an enzyme; that is, to catalyze specific molecular interactions.

Each gene has a specific length, which may range from between about 100 to more than 10,000 nucleotides. On DNA molecules the genes are linearly arranged, often with space-filling nucleotides between individual genes. Interestingly, the genetically well-studied bacterium *E. coli* carries all of its 4,288 genes on a single DNA molecule, the bacterial chromosome, which contains 4,639,221 nucleotides. Higher organisms carry much more genetic information, which is found on a number of chromosomes. In each human cell, for example, the nucleus carries two sets of 23 chromosomes representing two sets of about 3×10^9 nucleotides. The entire set of cellular genetic information is called the genome.

Of particular interest to genetic engineering are small, autonomously propagating DNA molecules called plasmids. In some cases their size offers space for just a few genes, while in others there is space for up to 100 genes. This span of sizes happens to coincide with the size of viral genomes, some of which can be carried for periods of time as plasmids in their host cells.

In classical genetics a mutation is defined by a change in the phenotypic appearance of the organism, if such change is transmitted to the progeny. In contrast, the molecular geneticist calls any alteration in the sequence of nucleotides of the genome a mutation. Many, but certainly not all, changes in nucleotide sequences also cause a change in the phenotypic appearance of the organisms.

Roots of Molecular Genetics

During the 1940s scientists realized that bacteria have genes that can mutate similarly to those of higher organisms. Between 1943 and 1953 they discovered three basic natural strategies by which DNA becomes transferred from one bacterium (the donor cell) to another bacterium (the recipient cell): First, donor DNA can become liberated into the ambient medium and later penetrate into a recipient cell. This process is called "transformation." Second, donor and recipient cells can enter into direct contact, a phase during which donor DNA can be transferred directly into the recipient cell. This is called bacterial "conjugation." Third, a virus replicating in the donor cell may enwrap some donor DNA into a viral particle, which may later infect a recipient cell with the donor DNA in a process called "transduction." All three processes of DNA transfer can be followed by a recombinational integration of all or part of the transferred donor DNA into the recipient genome. In these cases the acquired foreign DNA is inherited by the progeny of the recipient cell, to which the acquisition of foreign genetic information represents a mutation.

The experimental demonstration of transformation clearly identified DNA as the carrier of genetic information. Indeed, if donor and recipient had different genetic traits, a donor trait could be acquired by the recipient upon uptake of donor DNA, even if the DNA had been purified from associated proteins. This discovery was made almost 10 years before the double-helical structure of filamentous DNA molecules was described in 1953. However, the roots of molecular genetics reside in both microbial genetics and structural analysis of biological macromolecules.

At about the same time it became clear that some viruses can incorporate their genome in a recombinational process into the host chromosome. The process is reversible, so that at a later date the virus can again assume the virulent phase of its life cycle and produce infectious viral particles. It is during this process that some particles may incorporate host genes and later give rise to transduction. Interestingly, the transducing particles of some bacterial viruses contain hybrid DNA molecules composed of part of the viral genome into which a number of host genes had become inserted. Similar observations were made with some plasmids, in particular those involved in promoting bacterial conjugation. Knowledge of these phenomena was firmly established in 1960 and, 10 years later, played the role of a model for vector DNA molecules in genetic engineering.

During the pioneering phase of bacterial genetics it had already become clear that natural gene transfer by the three processes described above is relatively widespread among bacteria, but that various factors contribute toward seriously limiting the efficiency of gene acquisition, particularly if donor and recipient cells belong to different strains of bacteria. These limitations reside in three areas: the requirement of appropriate surface compatibilities for the uptake of external DNA; the action of restriction enzymes, which can distinguish foreign DNA from the cell's own DNA and subsequently cut incoming foreign DNA into fragments; and the need for functional compatibilities, both for the successful propagation of acquired genes and the biological functions exerted by the acquired genes.

Intracellular DNA fragments resulting from restriction cleavage usually become degraded within minutes by exonucleolytic enzymes. However as long as they are still present, they are an efficient substrate for recombinational integration into the host genome, provided that they find an opportunity to do so. Thus restriction seriously limits DNA acquisition to tolerable levels, but it also stimulates the acquisition of genetic information in small steps; that is, of a small DNA segment at a time. This gives to the resulting complex a good chance not to lose functional compatibility, and thus to survive.

Many restriction enzymes cleave foreign DNA reproducibly at the sites serving for their recognition as foreign. This type of enzyme is widely used in gene technology for cutting long filamentous DNA into shorter fragments, which can be separated according to size by gel electrophoresis.

Major Components of Gene Technology

Around 1970 scientists, aware of the results of microbial genetics outlined above, considered applying this knowledge to develop strategies to analyze the giant molecules of DNA that form the chromosomes of all organisms. The essential components of gene technology include:

1. Site-specific cleavage of filamentous DNA molecules by restriction endonucleases into shorter fragments. The sites of recognition and cleavage are often determined by enzyme-specific sequences of four to six nucleotides. Wherever such a recognition site is found by chance in the genetic message, the DNA filament is cut. Several hundred different restriction enzymes were isolated from different bacteria and are now available for genetic analysis.

2. Gel electrophoresis is an excellent method to separate DNA fragments of different sizes. It also serves to determine the size of each DNA fragment resulting from a cleavage reaction.

3. Following the model presented by viral DNA and plasmids as natural gene vectors, DNA fragments can be spliced at will into such vectors. When the resulting recombinant DNA molecules are introduced by transformation, or other means, into appropriate host cells, the vector can undergo autonomous replication. In this process the inserted foreign DNA fragment also becomes replicated. This is thus a good method to prepare large quantities of a selected DNA fragment, which can later serve for further studies. Depending on the particular structure of recombinant DNA molecules, the inserted genes may also become expressed. In these cases biotechnological uses of the resulting gene products can be considered.

4. In the 1980s an alternative method of amplifying specific DNA segments was developed on the basis of knowledge of DNA replication. This is the polymerase chain reaction, which can be used if some short DNA sequences located in the neighborhood of genes to be studied are known.

5. In the late 1970s efficient chemical methods were developed for the analysis of nucleotide sequences. These methods allow the scientist to read nucleotide sequences starting from the end of a DNA fragment and extending through several hundred positions. Longer DNA sequences can then be composed from individual analyses, like a puzzle.

6. Bioinformatic programs of sequence comparison represent an efficient tool to search for sequence similarities and novel DNA sequences, as well as potential expression control signals and open reading frames, which can give rise to gene expression. Sequence similarities can suggest functional relatedness.

7. For experimental studies on the nature of biological functions, molecular geneticists often place specific mutations at appropriately chosen sites in DNA sequences; for example, at strategic locations in open reading frames or in expression control signals. This strategy is called "site-directed mutagenesis," and was developed in the late 1970s. The mutagenized DNA sequences are then introduced into living cells, either as additions to the genome or, more often, as substitutes for the analogous segment in the genome. The resulting genetically modified organism is then analyzed for functional alterations, which can provide relevant information with regard to the biological functions of the genetic information in question.

Comparison of Classical and New Strategies of Genetic Research

Molecular genetics, including gene technology, has revolutionized genetic studies over the last 20 years. The new approach, also called "reverse genetics," is in many respects much more precise, and thus safer, than classical genetic experimentation.

In classical genetics scientists start to look for mutant organisms with an altered phenotypic appearance. If this alteration is inherited by the progeny, the change is likely to be caused by a genetic alteration. From the affected phenotype, the scientists can often draw conclusions about biological function. Recombination between differently affected individuals allows the scientist to localize on the chromosomes the genetic information responsible for the observed phenotypic alterations, which leads to the establishment of genetic maps. However classical genetics is an abstract approach, and does not require knowledge of which kind of biological molecules carry the genetic information. Hence classical genetics begins with observed functional alterations and eventually localizes genes on an abstract linear map. In order to dispose of enough individual mutants, classical genetics often uses chemical or radiation mutagenesis acting randomly on the entire genome.

In contrast, in new or "reverse" genetics the scientist knows that genetic information is carried on filamentous DNA molecules. Investigations start with DNA, which is purified and relevant segments of which are amplified. The subsequent sequence analysis can reveal potential genes by identifying open reading frames and potential expression control signals. Mutations are then placed at expected strategic sites by site-directed mutagenesis. The resulting mutants are reintroduced into the genome of living cells. Such introduction into the germline can result in genetically altered organisms. Their phenotypes may show specific alterations, as compared to the original organism. This can indicate which specific biological function is encoded by the gene under study. Hence reverse genetics starts from DNA as carrier of genetic information and investigates the biological functions expressed by the studied DNA segment.

The strategies involved are very purposeful. The researcher knows which kind of mutations are placed at which specific sites in the genome and is also able to verify the result of the intervention. This contributes strongly to the minimization of biohazards in the experimentation process. The new genetics contrasts with the old habits of random mutagenesis practiced in classical genetics by the application of mutagens to entire genomes without an efficient way to verify the outcome of the manipulation.

Gene Technology Benefits Biotechnology

Biotechnology applies acquired knowledge on biological functions by the strategic use of such functions for the benefit of mankind and also, more and more, to sustain ecosystems. The development of biotechnology is very similar to that of genetics.

In classical biotechnology, appropriately selected organisms were used as they were found in nature. Improvements of quantity and quality of useful products were sometimes reached by breeding strategies often using random mutagenesis and appropriate screening techniques at the selection stage.

Modern biotechnology proceeds quite differently. It benefits from the exploration of molecular mechanisms of biological functions. In view of a targeted use of such functions, it is possible

to improve yield and quality of the specific products by site-directed mutagenesis of open reading frames and expression control signals. In addition the specific genetic information to be used can be introduced into the most appropriate organism for reliable mass production. However it must clearly be said that not all strategic plans designed by scientists lead to success. New genomic combinations are always submitted to the force of natural selection. Some genetic alterations may affect the functional harmony of a cell to a degree that the cell may lose its viability or may not be able to yield the expected product in useful quantities. The risk of obtaining such negative responses grows substantially depending on the extent of the introduced genetic alteration.

These considerations imply that a careful molecular genetic approach toward developing beneficial uses of biological functions by biotechnology can largely ensure the biosafety of the productive organism. This statement can be substantiated as follows. Let us relate the genetic information of genomes with the information contained in books by comparing the number of nucleotides of a genome with the number of letters and open spaces in our written language. The genome of *E. coli* bacteria roughly corresponds to the contents of a book the size of the Bible. Higher organisms, such as human beings and certain plants, have genomes with information that would fill up an encyclopedia of about 1,000 volumes! A single gene may correspond to between a few lines and one-to-two pages. In site-specific mutagenesis, usually one or relatively few letters are substituted by others, or they are deleted or added by insertion. Alternatively, in the production of a transgenic organism, one or a few pages containing one or a few genes are isolated from the encyclopedia of a given organism and transferred into a volume belonging to the genetic encyclopedia of another organism. In any of these manipulations the researcher can clearly verify the result of the modification both at the level of the genome and at the gene products. As expected such genetic alteration normally does not affect the basic nature of the concerned organism. A mouse is still a mouse, a bacterium is still a bacterium, and a rice plant is still a rice plant. The genetically altered organisms may simply display changes in one or a few of their phenotypic properties, which can easily be monitored. Again we see that advanced technology ensures not only more efficiency but also a considerable reduction of biohazards, if the appropriate controls are carried out responsibly and conscientiously.

Genetic Engineering Involves Steps in Biological Evolution

Site-directed mutagenesis and the deliberate transfer of genetic information from a donor organism into a recipient organism, resulting in a transgenic organism, represent alterations in the genome of the concerned cells and organisms. These alterations may or may not lead to phenotypic changes in the concerned organisms, just as is the case with spontaneous mutagenesis.

Let us recall that mutations are the driving force of biological evolution, but that only a small proportion of spontaneously occurring genetic alterations result in better fit organisms. The term "better fit" in this context means that the mutant experiences an advantage under the encountered living conditions, as compared to its parent that did not suffer a genetic change. This process, called natural selection, occurs based on the effects of all the gene products present in the living organism. One can thus state that the direction of biological evolution is determined by the process of natural selection, although it also depends on the chance availability of better fit mutants. In order to complete the inventory of factors influencing biological evolution, we should also mention that reproductive and geographic isolation can affect the evolutionary process.

Spontaneously occurring genetic alterations are usually more or less random in time and with regard to the location on the genome involved. In contrast the genetic engineer introduces deliberate changes at well-chosen genome locations. However, as is the case under natural conditions, the products of genetic engineering are also submitted to the force of natural selection. The only interference that the scientist may apply at this stage is to choose particular living conditions to be offered under containment. This may play a role in biotechnological applications. These considerations suggest that a good understanding of the basic mechanisms of biological evolution can be essential for the assessment of biohazards related to genetic engineering.

Involvement of Evolutionary Genes in Microbial Evolution

Fifty years of intensive research in microbial genetics with bacteria and their plasmids and viruses yielded a large amount of experimental data, allowing researchers to develop an accurate picture of the molecular evolution of these organisms (see figure). Bacterial evolution depends on three natural strategies of genetic variation. The first of these strategies brings about small local sequence changes such as a nucleotide substitution, a small deletion, a small insertion, or a small sequence duplication. These changes often result from replication infidelities that occur spontaneously with low probability. Efficient DNA repair systems considerably limit the frequency of mutations produced by this route. The same is true for local sequence changes due to the action exerted on DNA by internal or environmental mutagens.

The second strategy of genetic variation involves the rearrangement of the genetic information of the genome. This may be initiated by a mutagen such as ultraviolet or ionic radiation, but more often it depends on the activities of mobile genetic elements or of site-specific or other recombination systems. These are very widespread in bacteria, and they occasionally bring about a recombinational reshuffling of the genomic DNA. These processes are mediated by specific enzymes encoded by genes forming the essential parts of mobile genetic elements and other recombination systems.

The third natural strategy to increase genetic diversity is DNA acquisition. As noted earlier this process involves horizontal transfer of DNA, which is normally also mediated by enzymes.

In natural mixtures of bacterial populations any of these three strategies steadily yields new genetic variants. With modern molecular genetic techniques it is possible, although labor-intensive, to determine the contribution of any single mechanism producing genetic alterations at the genome level. The three strategies are not mutually exclusive; they work in parallel to each other and each makes qualitatively different contributions to the overall genetic variation.

Local sequence changes represent a major source of new biological functions and play an important role in the step-by-step improvement

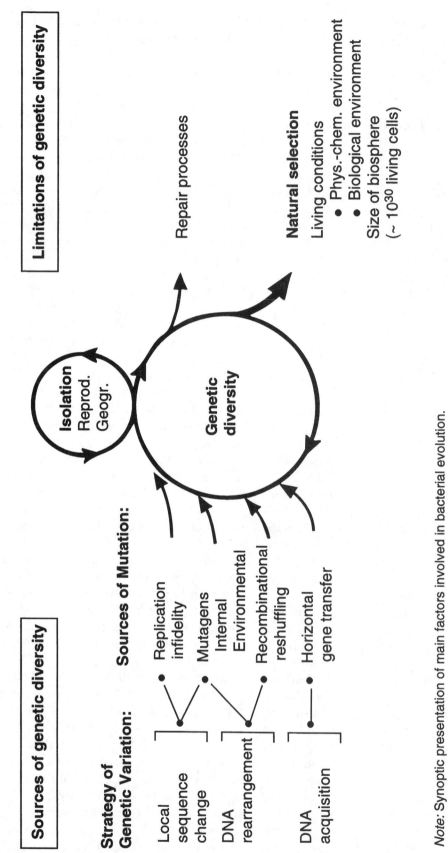

Sources of genetic diversity

Strategy of Genetic Variation:

Sources of Mutation:

Local sequence change
- Replication infidelity
- Mutagens Internal Environmental

DNA rearrangement
- Recombinational reshuffling

DNA acquisition
- Horizontal gene transfer

Isolation Reprod. Geogr.

Genetic diversity

Limitations of genetic diversity

Repair processes

Natural selection

Living conditions
- Phys.-chem. environment
- Biological environment

Size of biosphere
($\sim 10^{30}$ living cells)

Note: Synoptic presentation of main factors involved in bacterial evolution.
Source: Author.

of available biological functions. One can assume that, in general, many consecutive steps of mutagenesis are required before a properly functioning novel gene is obtained. Thus, per step of mutagenesis, this strategy is relatively inefficient.

In contrast DNA acquisition is, from an evolutionary perspective, a very efficient strategy. The acquisition of a gene for a function that had rendered service in a donor organism often brings an advantage to the recipient organism. The acquisition strategy may have its main relevance for accessory genes of use under particular living conditions, such as genes providing resistance to antibiotics. But acquisition may also provide means to modify housekeeping genes by conversion. Thus DNA acquisition can be seen as a sharing of successful developments made by others.

DNA rearrangements can bring about an improvement of available capacities. The recombinational fusion of gene segments representing different functional domains can bring about new gene activity, and the fusion of an expression control signal with a specific open reading frame can bring the latter under a different control element.

At this point it should be reiterated that there is no experimental evidence that any of these processes would be principally adaptive; that is, that they will respond specifically to a perceived need under an encountered living condition. Rather the genetic variations are nondirected, and it is natural selection that favors the rare "better fit" mutants and disfavors a majority of the novel mutants, which as a result will more or less rapidly disappear from the mixed populations of genetic variants.

Enzymes are involved in all of the molecular processes bringing about occasional genetic variations. Many of these enzymes are not needed for the life of individual bacteria from one generation to the next. We therefore postulate that the enzymes contributing in one way or another to increase genetic diversity in microbial populations may primarily serve the purpose of biological evolution. The genes encoding these enzymes are thus called evolutionary genes. In a crude way these genes can be grouped into two classes: those which generate genetic variations (by DNA reshuffling), and those which modulate the frequency of genetic variation (by DNA repair). According to this view the bacterial genome carries not only genes working to the benefit of each individual cell, such as housekeeping genes and accessory genes of use under particular life conditions, but also carries evolutionary genes, the products of which act to the benefit of the evolutionary development of populations. Obviously the products of some bacterial genes may serve both purposes, but a good number of evolutionary genes make no essential contributions to individual life.

A potential generalization of the theory of molecular evolution, as presented here along main lines, has not yet been seriously discussed by the scientific community. It is feasible that higher organisms also carry evolutionary genes. It might, however, be more difficult to identify them because of the higher complexity of the life cycle of higher organisms, including differentiation, for which still other specific genes play important roles.

Uniqueness of DNA Sequences Longer than 80 Nucleotides

In principle gene technology can aim to introduce any possible DNA sequence into a given genome. In reality, however, the proportion of possibilities that can be explored through experimentation is extremely small. This has to do with the fact that with the four-letter genetic alphabet, tremendous numbers of different sequences can be written. For a sequence with only ten letters there are $4^{10} = 10^6$ (one million) different ways to arrange the four letters. A row of 100 letters can be arranged in 10^{60} different ways and a row of 1,000 letters (corresponding to a gene of medium size) in 10^{600} different ways.

In this context it may be of interest to estimate how often a given DNA sequence may reappear in the course of the evolutionary process. To do so we can roughly estimate the biosphere of the planet Earth to accommodate about 10^{30} living cells at any time. This number results from the estimated volume of the condensed biosphere and from the known average volume of living cells. Let us further assume that, on average, each living cell carries in its genome 10^5 different standard genes. We know that life on Earth has existed for about three billion years, or about 10^{15} minutes. If we assume that in each of these genes one new sequence had been explored per minute (which is far more than corresponds to today's known mutation rates), we can calculate the total number of sequences already explored in nature to amount to $10^{30} \times 10^5 \times 10^{15} = 10^{50}$ sequences, which may be unique if none of the sequences had been tested more than once. With these simple considerations we can locate the threshold of sequence lengths to uniqueness to be at about 80 linearly arranged letters. Indeed, a sequence of 80 letters can be written in 10^{48} different ways. We are aware that a sequence of 80 nucleotides may roughly correspond to a functional domain or to a very small gene, while most genes are much longer than this and thus must be unique from the evolutionary standpoint. This implies that genomes have a high degree of uniqueness even in haploid clonal organisms such as bacteria, which is a stringent consequence of steadily exerted spontaneous mutagenesis.

What do such considerations have to do with biotechnology and biosafety? They can help us to bring natural biohazard and biohazard-related objections to genetic engineering into the right perspective, if we also are aware of the knowledge on the mechanisms of molecular evolution outlined above.

At present no theoretical basis for allowing scientists to devise a new kind of gene expressing a novel function is available. All that can be done is to start from existing genes (the functions of which have already been explored) and to try to change these functions to satisfy possible needs for biotechnological applications. Even for such minor interventions we still lack general theoretical rules, and predictability is accordingly low. However as was already said, gene technology offers a good means to experimentally test properties of organisms with engineered genetic alterations. In this sense molecular genetic strategies are much more precise, more reliable, and thus less hazardous than classical breeding methods. Still, the tremendous richness of different potential DNA sequences, and the fact that nature does not always precisely follow the plans designed by genetic engineers, justifies the call for caution and responsibility in any work done with genetic information, to minimize biohazards.

The Special Case of Agricultural and Food Biotechnology
Henry W. Kendall

I am grateful for the chance to speak today on some of the problems and opportunities presented by the emerging technology of genetic engineering of crops. I am grateful to Ismail Serageldin for his initiation and support of the report that is the focus of this meeting and for his warm reception of its recommendation.

What I would like to stress in my remarks has not so much to do with the science involved in biotechnology. A particle physicist by trade, I have been, over 25 years, involved in numerous controversies in the public domain in which science and technology have played a major role. These technologies have not always been carefully managed, a root cause of difficulties and consequent controversy. As you know, the great power of science and technology can bring with it both benefits and, in some cases, trouble. Thus the introduction of technical advances must be thoughtfully managed in order to maximize the benefits and minimize the side effects. Matters of this sort have received much of my attention over many years. My remarks will be directed at the means of introducing this new technology as well as other problems that must be addressed in the agricultural sector.

The biotechnology issue arises as one part of the solution to a great nest of problems that the human race faces at the present time—problems of environmental pressures, many of them adverse and some quite damaging, as well as resource mismanagement problems, all of which occur in the context of a continuing swell of the world's population.

The industrial world's population is hardly growing at all, but in the developing world growth rates are quite high. At the present time there are roughly 1 billion people living in conditions that the World Bank Group describes as utter poverty and another half-billion people who do not get enough to eat and suffer continued malnutrition. The group of half billion people that I mention, in aggregate, is growing at a rate of about 2.8 percent per year, which, if continued, will result in a doubling in the size of this group in 24 years—an extraordinarily short time.

The challenge is to ensure that the world's expanding population has enough food to eat, to avoid the continuing infliction of misery upon a fraction of them. A number of groups have studied prospective food demand, and there is a general agreement that, because of improving circumstances in much of the world, food demand will double in roughly 30 years; that is, demand will grow faster than population growth over the next decades.

This doubling of demand comes at a point when there is very little additional potentially arable land for expansion, and what land there is to expand into is generally of much lower quality than that which is already in use.

Water is in short supply in the world. Forty percent of the world's present population lives in areas that are chronically short of water, and the scale of human activity is so large that at the present time we already use more than one-half of all of the fresh water that is potentially available to us. Provision of adequate water supplies represents a daunting challenge.

I think it is clear that the industrial world is not going to suffer food shortages. No matter what happens, they will always have the economic resources, the strength and power, to feed themselves adequately in any manner they wish. It is in the developing world that hardships will be inflicted if there is an incapacity or failure to meet the growing demand for food. I want to emphasize that in the face of the challenges in the food sector, 30 years is no time at all.

If demand is not met, there will be grave difficulties in the future—not the distant future, but soon. One can see pieces of these difficulties arising at the present time, such as the production of migrants from environmentally injurious activities in the host countries; migrants that stream within countries and across national borders. Such displaced people are already becoming a challenge to the developing world and to industrial nations, and their numbers are increasing.

Thus while the industrial nations will remain well fed into the indefinite future, the difficulties that arise from food shortages will not be restricted to the developing nations where they are most troubling, but will affect all nations in our interdependent world. It is not true that one end of a boat can sink. We will all feel troubled and bear a heavy burden if the industrial nations do not help to expand world food supplies.

It is necessary to exploit every avenue that may potentially benefit the expansion of food supplies. Biotechnology is one element that can aid in such an expansion. It is a powerful technology. Its full potential has not yet been explored (much less exploited) and like all powerful technologies it must be guided carefully so that unexpected harm does not accompany its utilization. In addition biotechnology must be exploited in such a way as to maximize the benefits.

Much of the incentive to develop biotechnology improvements in crops arises in the industrial nations. It is the industrial nations that have the resources, both intellectual and economic, to push the research necessary to exploit the technology and bring the results to widespread adoption.

The incentives that drive these improvements are those of the industrial world. But for the developing world the needs are different, and so some of the incentives drive developments that

are inappropriate, such as the improved appearance of fruits or vegetables. We do not have the mechanisms fully in place to get the necessary and important research and development carried out that will benefit developing world agriculture. Here the World Bank Group can play a leading role in expanding the horizons of helpful research and can aid in guiding it.

Biotechnology may prove to be a helpful factor in meeting the pressing need for expansion of food supplies. But by itself, it clearly cannot suffice. Far more will be required. There is a list in the report of other actions that must be taken and avenues that must be explored. We call attention to them because they are very important. The list includes such things as a continued emphasis on improvements by conventional genetic techniques, integrated pest management, and the control of a very troubling difficulty in agriculture, which is agricultural activities that are damaging arable land and harming sources of water for irrigation.

These damaging activities are numerous and very serious. Erosion continues to be a major problem in many parts of the world. There are substantial uncertainties in estimates of the rate at which soil is being washed away, eroded, and lost to agriculture. But they suggest that this loss may be in the vicinity of 0.7 percent per year. That sounds very small, a loss which might be easily accommodated, almost negligible. Indeed the consequences over a few years can go unnoticed, easily masked by improvements in agricultural techniques. For a short period increases in pesticide or fertilizer use will conceal the consequences of soil loss. But if the loss rate persists over half a century or a century, very substantial fractions of the world's soil will be lost. By the year 2100, at the current rate, we will have lost over 30 percent of the world's soil, an irreversible loss, nearly impossible to make up and with a major impact on agricultural productivity. One can see the consequences of harsh erosion, for example, in Haiti, where large sections of former agricultural land have been reduced to barren fields, where no further erosion is even possible. So there is much to do.

There are also difficulties in water management: over-pumping from fossil water supplies, which are only very slowly recharged; intrusions of salt water in coastal fresh water aquifers that are being pumped for irrigation; and over-irrigation and resulting buildup of salt in the soil. Thus water management is another problem area that needs more attention than it is currently getting.

One additional difficulty is very likely to be damaging in the future: disruption of the climate from greenhouse gas warming. These gases are largely, although not entirely, the consequence of fossil fuel use. Possible climatic change has claimed the attention of climate experts for many years. Indeed, warming of the climate from fossil fuel use was identified as a possibility in the last century, although scientists' warnings have been neglected until recently.

From the scientific information now on hand it appears that human activities already have had a discernible effect on the climate. I have concluded that the most damaging and widespread consequence of climatic change is going to be felt in agriculture, because agriculture is a system that is already coming under stress and experiencing daunting pressures that will continue in the decades ahead.

What should be done about possible climate disruption? The broad conclusion of the scientific community is that the human race must diminish greatly its use of fossil fuels, substituting energy sources that are benign, renewable, and do not put heavy pressure on the global environment. This includes energy captured from the sun, the winds, the oceans, and if possible from biomass—so-called energy crops. Nuclear power might contribute, provided its difficulties related to safety, economics, waste disposal, and public acceptance can be resolved. It is both technically and economically feasible to make such an energy transition, although the scale of energy use worldwide makes it an enormous enterprise.

Implementing the transition is thus a daunting challenge in its own right. The industrial nations so far have been the greatest emitters of carbon dioxide, the principal greenhouse gas. But emissions in the developing world are increasing rapidly. At present China is the second largest emitter of carbon dioxide in the world, after the United States; emissions in other developing nations are growing as well. Many of them contribute not only through fossil fuel use, but also by the cutting and burning of forests, both tropical rain and temperate forests. The need to start the transition away from fossil fuels is immediate, in no small measure because avoiding disruption of agriculture is of such great importance.

There is suddenly, and I may say happily, very much increased attention to this issue throughout the world. In the United States President Clinton has, within the past few months, seized it as a major topic and a high priority for him and his Administration. The hope is that the first binding agreements between nations on schedules and goals for the reduction of global carbon dioxide emissions will soon come into being.

In order to carry out the changes I have mentioned, plus a number that I have not mentioned, there is a great need for competent science in the developing world. This issue is mentioned in the recommendations of our report. One recommendation calls for an outreach that fosters the education of scientists in developing nations; gives them links to scientists in the industrial world; and allows them to be part of their government's planning, organization, and control not only of biotechnology, but of the great changes in energy use which will have to accompany all of these changes.

The World Bank Group has a critical role to play in all of these matters—biotechnology as a piece of the food problem; the World Bank Group as a helper with the greater problems of energy change and energy use in the developing world; and with the development of scientific liaison, the scientific networks that are so important to the developing world; and the proper use (and control of misuse) of biotechnology and other technologies.

Over the years I have been on a number of panels of one sort or another and every now and then I chair one. It is uncommon that the reports are carefully read by the host organization. It is even more rare that the recommendations are embraced as warmly as the ones in this report, and for that the panel is extremely grateful. Again, my thanks to Ismail Serageldin.

Discussion
Moderator: Peter J. Matlon

Peter Matlon: The Kendall Report sets out a uniquely accessible and thoughtful set of perspectives and recommendations on the issue of biosafety. Over the next two days we will be trying to move toward a consensus as to what the institutional responses to the opportunities and challenges of biosafety should be. We will address the question of how to work together more effectively in regard to biosafety issues, and we will work toward the creation of regulatory mechanisms and stimulation of greater awareness among decisionmakers in developing countries so that they can address these issues in a thoughtful and responsible way.

Mae-Wan Ho: I am here representing the Third World Network as a scientific adviser. What Werner Arber might have also mentioned in his presentation is that the viruses and plasmids used in horizontal gene transfer also carry antibiotic resistance genes, which are routinely used as selectable markers for genetic engineering. A main concern is the possibility that horizontal gene transfer might inadvertently generate new viruses, new pathogens, which in this case which are also antibiotic-resistant.

I would like to ask Werner Arber whether there is a need to reexamine this very large-scale commercial genetic engineering biotechnology that we are engaged in, because the whole orientation of industry is to facilitate and enhance horizontal gene transfer between unrelated species. I also want to ask whether, if we do not have adequate regulations, it is a good idea to proceed

as though there are potential benefits, but only hypothetical risks.

Werner Arber: The historical development of antibiotic resistance in enterobacteria is a very interesting case. I think we must be aware that thanks to this development, microbial genetics has made more rapid and larger advances toward better understanding the evolutionary process, because in around 1960 this became a serious medical problem and many investigations were devoted to understanding what has happened.

This horizontal transfer is a normal process. It usually occurs at low rates; but if it occurs in large populations, and these large populations are then exposed to more than one antibiotic, only the few lucky bacterial cells that recently have acquired such genes will survive and very quickly overgrow the previous population.

The measures taken beginning early in the 1950s and particularly in the early 1970s were first, to be quite careful and not prescribe antibiotic treatment if it is not really needed. Second, you may be aware that in the first enthusiasm about the action of antibiotics, they were mixed into cattle feed in order to prevent infectious diseases and improve their health. But when this antibiotic resistance came up, an agreement was rapidly reached between the medical and agricultural world to use diffrent antibiotics for human medicine and animal feed additives.

We have to live with these resistances, and the industry has undertaken to look for new antibiotics. I think this is a good example of the need to be aware that we have no absolute security. Evolution goes on and fills gaps that all of a sudden open up. We have to live with that. The only message I can give you is that it is quite important that the knowledge of the evolutionary process at the molecular level become better understood. I think one can also learn from behavior, particularly with regard to measures for biosafety, if one understands the natural evolutionary process.

What can we do about it? I do not think that we have any way to change the course of natural evolution, but we can learn. Once we understand, we can be aware and watch it more closely.

Michel Petit: I am with the World Bank Group. I would like to ask the two panelists, particularly Werner Arber, who was not a member of the Kendall panel, to comment on the following.

In the Kendall Report four risks are identified, and my understanding is that these are indeed the risks that biosafety should be concerned with: gene flows to wild plants; development of new viruses; the effect of plant-produced insecticides; and more broadly, ecosystem damage.

My question is: Are these really the four risks? Are there others that we should be concerned with? And does he have any advice for us to pass on to governments about what they should be doing to develop biosafety regulations?

Audience question: My main question is about long-term impact. When you discuss issues of genetics, you are discussing issues that may have impact at this very point or maybe within five years. But sometimes impact will only be felt after 25 or 30 years, and by then it may be irreversible.

The Green Revolution in India is a classic example, which leads me to the second question. We worked on the study of Green Revolution, which supposedly brought bountiful food to India. We are told by the government that India is food self-sufficient. In reality, it is not.

Today, according to the government of India, one out of five Indians are malnourished; there is insufficient food available to them. That is the case practically all over the developing world. So the question of this bountiful food that may come due to all these kind of changes, I think, should be examined more carefully.

Henry Kendall: I find it both interesting and pleasing that all of the questioners are raising issues that go beyond biotechnology itself to touch on either closely or distantly related problems. It is important to do that in general, to take a look at the breadth and depth of difficulties. This is becoming increasingly important in our society.

Let me come to the remark that may have been misunderstood with respect to the industrial world and the developing world and the capacity of those groups to feed their people now and in the future. There is hunger in the industrial world. There is hunger and malnutrition in the United States; this has been a growing problem, especially since the 1980s. The way this was stated in the biotechnology report is as follows: "The wealthy nations have high levels of nutrition and will have little problem supplying all their citizens with adequate food when they wish to do so." The resources are certainly there to do so in the wealthy nations. This is not necessarily true in the developing world.

Ismail Serageldin: I have one brief comment, because there is an implication that sometimes things have to be mutually exclusive. When you talk about India being food self-sufficient or not, the fact is that right now India has some 33 million tons of surplus grain; surplus in the sense that it is available in storage. The big problem is access and distribution, which is associated with extreme poverty. This is not to say that if it were just a matter of production there would not be a single hungry person in the United States, but that is not the issue.

Production is extremely important, because if there is not sufficient production, prices will increase and those who do not have access will be even greater in number. So production is a necessary, but not sufficient, condition to deal with the issue of world hunger. I think this is an absolutely essential point. It is not an either/or issue; but if you do not have production, then you will have hunger because there will be greater rationing of available resources.

Having plentiful resources does not mean that everybody has access. The operative words in the Kendall Report is that the industrialized countries can feed everybody in their societies if they so wish, if they have the political will to ensure that there is access to the poor and the marginalized and the excluded in society.

The issue of increasing production within the available parameters of land and water requires that we make use of all the tools that we can, but taking care of two things: safety, and ensuring that we do not rush blindly into things, while at the same time being fully aware that the production side is only one half of the equation.

The recommendation of the Report, which the World Bank Group certainly adopts, is that production is only one piece of the problem. Biotechnology is only one piece of production; it is not a silver bullet, but rather one piece of the whole picture.

Henry Kendall: There is a widely believed, but mistaken, idea that turns up in public opinion polls in the United States that science and technology will in some way rescue us from these difficulties that we have been discussing. The senior scientific community in the world does not believe that, because the problems are at root human problems, not purely technical problems.

That is not to say that science and technology are not important. They are critically important and, in fact, science and technology have become a life-support system for the human race as it currently carries out its activities. Science and technology will play extremely important roles—biotechnology is one example—in securing a decent future. But many profound changes have to be made in the human approach to these problems before we will really be in a position to solve them.

Sivramiah Shantaram: First and foremost, gene escape is only possible in the plant kingdom through vertical gene transfer, which is through sexual transmission among sexually compatible species. It is not very clearly known whether there is horizontal gene transfer from plants to other organisms, such as animals and microorganisms.

Second, fear of the antibiotic-resistant marker genes that are in use comes from the examples that people have now gotten from clinical environments. I think it is mostly due to the misuse or overuse of antibiotics and chemotherapy, as opposed to the resistance gene itself. In fact, the resistance gene has already spread.

There is a well-documented study from the School of Microbial Ecology at Michigan State University that shows that even organisms from virgin soils already have antibiotic-resistant marker genes, where no one in the recorded history of that piece of land or soil had ever even stepped.

The other important technological advance coming on the horizon is that once a marker gene is put into transgenic plants, once a selection is already done, there are mechanisms by which you can get rid of these marker genes. These things are coming along, and hopefully in the very near future we will have technologies that would completely get rid of these so-called marker genes. Then the transgenic crop lines or organisms that will be eventually field-tested may not have these genes at all.

Jeremy Wright: I am from the Wellness Foundation and I would like to ask a question about what we do if something goes wrong and how is that handled. I would like to ask the panel questions about liability, about responsibility, and how individual citizens, and indeed governments, will deal in the future not just with the containment issue if something goes wrong, but with public health issues, and also with the issue of liability and responsibility for global health issues that can arise from a major mistake.

Henry Kendall: I would like to respond to the very interesting and important questions concerning what to do if something goes wrong. This is clearly the other side of the question that our Report addresses in detail, which is how to make sure that everything goes right. But that is never guaranteed.

Because the important biotechnology improvements that will be needed prospectively have not yet been carried through and deployed widely in the developing world, any answer I give as to what to do—what will get done, as opposed to what should get done should something go wrong—has to be answered hypothetically. We have recourse only to historical, idiosyncratic data, which unfortunately is scattered.

Various sorts of things that have gone wrong in the past in other technologies have been dealt with in a variety of ways, some of them good, but by no means all of them. In the area of biotechnology our panel has attempted to set out the circumstances that would lead to controls before widespread injury is visited on somebody as a result of something going wrong. Such controls would require support by the World Bank Group and other people of appropriate regulatory structures in each nation that will be exploiting biotechnology advances. It would not be the World Bank Group's responsibility, but many of us believe that this is needed badly in the United States, as well. Maybe the World Bank Group can help there.

So in most cases it is possible, in principle, to identify who should be responsible if something goes wrong. The challenge is to get the mechanisms in place to make that identification, set up the guidelines, make sure that everybody knows who would be responsible, and have obvious mechanisms for redress so that there is some caution in the marketplace. That is what one hopes will happen.

The sad alternative would be not to do that adequately. Then other mechanisms come into play, and if there is overt damage there will be a response. But one must live with the damage, and it might be in some measure irreversible, which no one wants.

Kathy McAfee: I am from Grass Roots International and the University of California at Berkeley. This discussion of the health and safety risks leaves me wondering whether or not we might expect—given the current, increasingly market-oriented structure of incentives that determine scientific research priorities—adequate or proportional research going into the safety risks.

I want to ask a parallel question that might broaden the issue a little bit. Werner Arber gave us a mind-boggling figure of the numbers of genetic combinations that have never been experimented with in either nature or science, leaving us with the suggestion that there is so much more that science might be able to create.

But I wonder whether or not this focus on the technological possibilities may cause us to move forward at the expense of adequate attention to an equally mind-boggling number of possibilities that nature has already created and that nature, interacting with human beings, has already created. I am thinking of the hundreds of thousands of existing landraces of important food crops, the tremendous multiplicity of food systems that farmers all over the world have devised over the centuries.

Ismail Serageldin mentioned that biotechnology does not discriminate against the small farmer. Theoretically, scientifically, that is true; but institutionally, socially, and economically, the way things are organized now, it may not be true. I would like to invite people to address that in this session and in the sessions that follow.

Ismail Serageldin: I think there is a major set of issues that deal with socioeconomic organization—governance issues, marginalization of the poor and particular constituencies, discrimination against women farmers, in particular—in many of the parts of the world. For example, in Africa women produce 80 percent of the food, yet they receive 10 percent of the wage labor and 1 percent of the land. There are many such issues.

Biotechnology does not discriminate against the poor farmer or the smallholder farmer to the extent that the delivery mechanism does not assume an organizational structure such as mechanization, for example, which inherently favors larger land parcels over smaller land parcels in order to be able to work; that is, it does not inherently have a bias against the poor.

That does not mean that whether it is vaccines for children or seeds for new varieties or credit that is available, there may not be other discriminatory barriers. All I was saying is that inherently biotechnology does not seem to discriminate. That is why I flagged that. I simply pointed out that inherently there were some possibilities there that seemed to be scale-neutral.

It is difficult, but I think we should try to disentangle the issues and really focus on the issue of safety, because the access and discrimination issues are there. They require a different kind of discussion, but they are there in a wide range of issues. They are there in access to credit, titling of land, and many other issues, from vaccination of children to nutritional content. You can have surplus grain sitting in silos in India and still have malnourished children. There are many other issues involved.

But can we at least reach a consensus on some of the safety issues and liability questions that emerge. We need to continue to try to disentangle the issues.

Audience comment: Regarding the Kendall Report and the increase of food demand, we do realize that increasing production is not going to solve the problem, because 60 to 70 percent of our production is lost after harvest. So implementing and developing biological technologies or biotechnology for preservation is really a critical element in the strategy to respond to food demand.

Audience comment: With regard to this question of responsibility, are we not in a situation in which, if there is a risk, it puts a terrible burden on the initiators of experiments if the risk is not shared? That is why I think that the involvement of the Consultative Group on International Agricultural Research, the World Bank Group, and others is so fundamental. We are talking about potential risks of a magnitude that we cannot predict. We operate in an area fraught with substantial limits, and we should not forget it. We should give all the support we can to multilateral involvement in this responsibility.

Ricarda Steinbrecher: I am a genetic scientist and consultant to the Women's Environmental Network and the Third World Network. I would like to address a point concerning the benefits, or so-called benefits, especially in relation to whether smallholder farmers benefit as well, or whether they have a problem with this new technology.

For example, if we look at the herbicide-resistant plants currently being genetically engineered for wide use, we find two major herbicides, Roundup® and Buster. These are being used because there is a single gene available for this resistance, so it is easy to genetically engineer and one can put it in all different kinds of plants very quickly.

The situation we hear about with respect to the benefit is difficult, because there is no proof of the benefit. We keep talking about proof for the risk. We should have a proof for the risk as well, obviously, but most of all we should have a proof of the benefit. I have asked different companies, including Monsanto, for proofs of the benefits. I have not seen any yet.

If we look, for example, to the promises and the future, there will be crops which are resistant to salinity, drought-resistant; these are multigene traits. Therefore, it will take a long, long time to create that, if ever. So I feel one thing we really

will have to address is to prove the benefit, and when we can prove it and prove that it will not pose additional serious risks, then we can look further. But the proof of the benefit really is necessary.

Ismail Serageldin: When you talk about private sector research, the proof of the benefit is very simple. It is whether people will buy the product, and whether the farmers who buy the product find that there is value in paying for it. Since the private sector is not giving products away, but rather selling them, there is a real market test. They can go out of business if that product does not deliver the presumed benefit.

It is important to focus on the risks, because there may be hidden risks that are not sufficiently understood by the public and must be flushed out into the open. Farmers may buy because there is a short-term gain, but may not be fully aware of the longer-term risk. That is why the discussion should focus on safety issues.

Shifting discussion to the safety side, the focused side, the risk side seems to me to be the right way to go. That would really educate the public and make us better understand what the tradeoffs are and whether, in fact, the prices really reflect the full environmental and social costs.

Henry Kendall: One questioner mentioned correctly that the testing of some of these biotechnology activities is different in the developing world than in the industrial world. That is correct, and this matter is addressed in the report that we have prepared. Biotechnology needs in the developing world are quite different than what will be occurring here.

In the United States, for example, the commercial ethic and the various drives are in quite different directions than they would be in a developing nation; for example, in a tropical area. This is something that the panel identified very clearly, felt was a significant problem, and to which a number of the recommendations were addressed. But they were addressed in the direction of supporting science and technology and scientists in the developing world so that these different needs can be identified.

We specifically asked the World Bank Group to pay attention to these priorities and support those that need support. Many of them will need support, unlike, for example, decreased blemishes on foods sold in the United States, which will naturally bubble to the top in the commercial sector.

Werner Arber: I have given much thought to risk. It is eventually the involved people and the larger society that together should have that responsibility. In our world of democratic governments it is not easy. And we should be aware that it was also said today that there is no zero risk; there is always some remaining risk.

We should try to minimize that, and I think the measures proposed up to now, which have largely been followed, contribute to that. That does not mean that we should not always make efforts to improve. This is a very important question about which we scientists are always concerned. My organization, the International Council of Scientific Unions, has made quite a number of contributions during the past 20 years toward harmonizing guidelines and conduct worldwide, because our nongovernmental organization spans all the countries that carry out activities. I think we have been successful, at least to some extent, but new problems always come up. You never are actually at the end, and we are willing to continue in this way.

The Promise and the Perils

Overview
Christopher R. Somerville

By the year 2003 we will have the fully sequenced genomes of at least 20 bacteria, two fungi, one nematode, one insect, and one plant. I suspect it will be at least two plants and 50 bacteria. We already have the full sequence of ten bacteria, one fungus, and about half a nematode.

The plant that is going to be sequenced is the *Arabidopsis.* We already have about 20 percent of this plant sequenced, and I suspect we will have it completely finished by 2001. This plant is a model for all higher plants. By "fully sequenced," I mean the complete chemical structure of all the DNA in this organism has been analyzed.

The second plant will almost certainly be rice, which I suspect will probably be finished by 2003 or 2004. The Japanese government just provided a grant for US$100 million to one laboratory, and a bill is currently working its way through the U.S. Congress that would allocate a large portion of a US$40 million-a-year grant to study of the rice genome.

There are 100,000 base pairs of *Arabidopsis* genome; we already know the function of many genes, and we plan to literally work our way through the whole genome, assigning function to every gene.

At this point we can assign general function to nearly 60 percent of all the genes that we encounter in a plant; about 44 percent we cannot yet assign function to at present. One of the things that the full sequencing of these genomes allows is the assignment of function to every gene. During the next 10 to 15 years, researchers will actually go in and determine the function of every gene in *Arabidopsis* and probably in rice. It is the significance of that effort in this context that I wanted to convey, to stress that biotechnology is not some sort of dabbling approach. We are building agricultural biotechnology on a very solid base of knowledge.

We do not have complete knowledge yet, but it is within sight. Certainly in the timeframe by which innovations will arrive in the developing world, we will have a very profound knowledge of what we are doing at some level, so that when we make a modification of a plant we will know very clearly what the significance of such an action is.

One of the tools that will facilitate this work is new technologies, such as a newly developed gene chip that allows introduction of a sample of DNA into a small hole in its center and can subsequently be used to simultaneously read the expression of thousands of genes at a time.

This kind of technology will allow us to look at the expression of all the genes in an organism simultaneously, in response to any changes that we make, changes in environmental conditions, and anything that might affect the expression.

My point is that biotechnology is being built on a much larger base of basic knowledge, which will allow us to proceed in a real engineering context. Most of us think of engineers as people who, when they build a bridge, have a very good idea of what they are doing. I hope that because of this kind of work, in the foreseeable future the directed manipulations we make will be built on a similarly deep biological base.

The opportunities are obvious: we can alter nutritional quality and feed efficiency; decrease losses to pests and pathogens, and increase stress tolerance. I think there is a possibility for intrinsic yield increases as well. We can adapt plants through agricultural practices and facilitate hybridization, presumably realizing large gains in productivity by extending hybrid vigor.

Another possibility, which is not talked about very much, is that we could also accelerate domestication. Many of us would like to expand the number of plants that are used, and I believe that biotechnology offers certain tools that may be useful in this respect. Most of these things are discussed at length in the Kendall Report, so I thought I would mention a few things that may have been overlooked and that have consequences for this discussion.

The kinds of gains that we might realize by actually solving or understanding pest and pathogen resistance are tremendous. A large proportion of plant productivity is lost to pests and pathogens; in Africa and Asia it is estimated that about 40 percent of total productivity is lost.

Such targets are rather well-suited to the application of biotechnology, because plants can be engineered for very specific resistance; it is not accidental that the some of the first applications have been in this domain.

In addition, however, biotechnology could have implications for yield. Research indicates that that the record yield for all the important plants greatly exceeds the average yield. This indicates that the architecture, the intrinsic productivity, of plants has a long way to go. This is in some respect what the long-term targets of biotechnology are—to learn how to engineer plants to more regularly achieve record yields rather than their current average yields. Generally this is going to be achieved by adaptation to various nonbiotic stresses.

I think this is very hopeful in that it shows that the limitations are not intrinsic to the plants, but rather related to the circumstances under which we are growing them, or their adaptation to those circumstances.

I want to move now to the kind of applications that received far less discussion, and which I think raise some important issues. One of the most important discoveries of the last several years was reported in *Nature*. A poplar tree, an aspen, was induced to flower within three months by the introduction of a gene, making it a transgenic aspen tree. As you probably know, poplar and many other trees normally flower in the timeframe of 12-to-15 years. As a result very little breeding has been done on these species, so that we actually do not know what their yield potential is in comparison to vegetative species on which a great deal of breeding is done because of the annual cycles.

I think this is a very exciting discovery because it raises the possibility of breeding in a rapid cycle on very important tree species and, at the last stage, after some rounds of breeding, crossing out the gene and producing an improved fiber species. Man does not live from food alone; a significant proportion of our resources are used to produce fiber, both for fuel and other purposes.

There is a wide range of other products that are relevant. Because a large proportion of the surface of the Earth is used for fiber production, there are many opportunities to use biotechnology to improve the efficiency with which we use it. It is a very dirty industry, and I think that by modifying trees we will be able to improve that.

There have been many opportunities to produce specialty chemicals; I will give you a few examples. There are also many opportunities to produce polymers and to alter plant architecture for efficiency. For example, a plant like kapok, which is a tropical species that used to be widely used as a fiber crop, has gone out of production—displaced by synthetics—partially because it has to be harvested at fairly high expense.

There is a reasonable possibility that the tools of biotechnology can alter the architecture of kapok so that it could be more easily harvested. But there are many applications like this and I do not think in the short time I have I can go through them, other than to raise them as examples.

Perhaps one of the most dramatic examples that will illustrate the point I want to make is a plant that is 15 percent, by weight, plastic! Through electron micrograph photographs, grains of biodegradable thermoplastic in the leaf sections of plants can be seen.

This plastic has the following properties: it is truly biodegradable, so it is renewable because it can be grown. Perhaps equally important is the fact that it sells for many, many times the price of food on a per-pound basis. This particular material currently sells for around US$4 a pound. Cornstarch sells for around US$0.05 a pound, and this is a problem.

Higher plants also make a wide variety of what I would call technical materials. Several lipids with interesting chemical groups on them might lend themselves to industrial applications. One, for example, is ricinoleic acid, the most useful natural material in the world. It has 400 nonfood uses and sells for approximately twice as much per pound as edible oil, just because of the presence of the hydroxyl group there.[1]

Almost all the genes that make these chemical modifications are now available and can be used to make transgenic plants that produce variants of these technical oils. These are things that should not be eaten, as anyone knows who has had castor oil. The utility of these things in one context is that they have high unit value. Making a transgenic plant that produces castor oil will add considerable value to that plant because of its industrial uses.

It is possible to produce environmentally benign, renewable, biodegradable materials. Developing countries can use these as domestic sources of materials with industrial uses. Malaysia, for example, is developing an oleochemical industry based on palm. The ability to diversify the chemical industry can pay obvious dividends by increasing the value of that oil. It displaces the dependency on petroleum. Particularly over the long term, that is going to be an issue. Palm is an excellent example of a plant that will benefit by the application of this technology—if you consider making technical materials a benefit.

However this is an area where there are genuine risks. One obvious risk is that these technical materials will be placed in plants that are otherwise used as food and confused with food crops. A second risk is that they might be placed in plants susceptible to being eaten by wildlife.

I think such problems can probably be solved; there are many conceivable solutions. One that comes to mind is that we only produce technical materials in plants that are already poisonous, such as the castor plant, which is certainly one of the most poisonous plants around but is still grown widely in the tropical world, in Brazil, India, and Thailand. This plant is fairly productive and could be engineered to produce other technical materials. I do not think anyone would confuse it with something that might be eaten.

There are other consequences that need to be thought about, and they are probably the most serious. The first is that because these materials have higher value than food, a situation might evolve in which acreage is used to produce nonfood cash crops. The value of these things can be sufficiently high and the demand very large. Let me put it this way: the entire U.S. corn crop could not satisfy world demand for polyethylene if it were converted quantitatively. So the demand for technical materials is very high, and as these things become available they will pose a threat.

It will undoubtedly create the growth of private markets, I do not know the full extent of that, but it is an inevitable consequence. Because these things will be created by people with access to technology, various traits may be bundled together that impose restrictions on how these materials can be used.

I want to conclude with one final point. Introducing the Rambo gene for total resistance may have been a mistake. This is the scenario that many people are apparently concerned about in regard to transgenic plants. But there are other concerns that are probably more significant, which are the sociological, rather than the directly biological, consequences.

Note

1. For example, castor oil is obtained from the seeds of the *Ricinus communis* plant. It consists principally of the triglyceride of ricinoleic acid (hydroxyoleic acid).

The Opportunities and the Risks

Biotechnology and Sustainable Development
Robert B. Horsch

Green plants are the primary renewable source of energy and biomaterials on Earth and one of the key recyclers of air, water, and bioavailable minerals. Agriculture is the foundation of human economies and peoples' well being. As crop yields have increased, the cost of food has dropped, allowing simultaneous increase in the food supply and available income to be invested in better healthcare, education, cultural pursuits, and other facets of an improved standard of living. Agriculture is also responsible for humankind's biggest impact on nature, because it is the largest source of competition for land and water between humans and nature.

Opportunities

In agriculture the challenge and the opportunity is to simultaneously increase the productivity of agriculture per unit of land, resources consumed, and negative impact on the environment without systematically reducing the sustainability of agriculture. Just as increasing economic productivity is the key to economic growth, so increasing resource productivity is the key to sustainable growth, waste reduction, and environmental protection. Biotechnology provides huge breakthroughs on all of these fronts by substituting "information for stuff" and by doing so in cyclic, photosynthetic, and nonpolluting ways.

The key contributions of biotechnology will be severalfold.

- Producing more food on the same area of land, thereby reducing pressure to expand into wilderness, rain forest, or marginal lands that support biodiversity and vital ecosystem services
- Reducing post–harvest loss of food and improving the quality of fresh and processed foods, thus boosting the "realized nutritional yield" per acre (1 acre = 0.405 hectares)
- Displacing resource– and energy–intensive inputs, such as fuel, fertilizers, or pesticides, thus reducing unintended impacts on the environment and freeing those resources to be used for other purposes or conserved for the future
- Encouraging reduction of environmentally damaging agricultural practices and adoption of more sustainable practices, such as conservation tillage, precision agriculture, and integrated crop management
- Stimulating a new kind of economic growth— more benefit with less throughput and harm.

Plant breeders have been introgressing genes into crops for a wide range of beneficial traits for millennia. Most of our major food plants do not even resemble their original wild relatives. Genes for improved resistance to pests, tolerance to environmental stresses, ability to take up nitrogen and other soil nutrients, growth habit, yield, quality of proteins, oils, and starches have all been intensely concentrated in modern varieties from sources as distantly related as possible. Using biotechnology, we now have the ability to more broadly introgress genes from virtually any other organism and to directly engineer those genes before introduction into the crop. Our experience over the past 20 years supports the assertion that biotechnology will be just as powerful as plant breeding for continuing to improve all aspects of crop growth and development for the benefit of humans. Biotechnology must be combined with the best that breeding has to offer so that it amplifies the importance and contribution that breeding continues to make. Biotechnology also meshes well with integrated crop management and precision agriculture technologies. The biotechnology pipeline is full of traits for resistance to fungi, insects, viruses, nematodes, and other pests; tolerance to a host of environmental stresses; improved utilization of nitrogen; improved quantities of oils, proteins, starches, and other compounds; and even improved yields.

Examples

I would like to use as an example the New Leaf® potato, a Monsanto product. Using actual figures for insecticide use on the leading variety of potatoes in the United States, I calculated what it would take to manufacture, distribute, and apply those products for one year. Since the same chemistry is often used to control Colorado potato beetle and potato leaf roll virus vector insects, I made a projection for the amount of pesticide that could be replaced by genetic resistance for both pests. The main point from this analysis is the environmental load conventional Russett Burbank potatoes carry compared to New Leaf Plus™ potatoes genetically improved to resist Colorado potato beetle and leaf roll virus. This load includes 4 million pounds of raw materials to make conventional insecticides, resulting in 2.5 million pounds of manufacturing waste, 180,000 containers, and 150,000 gallons of fuel to transport and apply the pesticides. Most of the insecticide never reaches the target pest and contributes further to the environmental load of pest control.

Compare this to the New Leaf® potato, where you teach the plant how to use sunshine, air, and nutrients to make a biodegradable protein that affects one specific insect pest and only those individual insects that actually take a bite of the plants. The genetically improved potato costs the farmer less to grow, works better at controlling the pest, is better for the environment, and is more ecoefficient. We do not yet know how significant the benefit will be from sparing the lives of beneficial insects in the potatoes fields,

which previously were killed by a broadspectrum insecticide.

One more illustration of the power of biotechnology is provided by Roundup Ready® soybeans, another Monsanto product that was introduced last year in the United States. Weeds are the most serious pest of cultivated crops, including soybeans. Some herbicides used on soybeans are persistent enough to control weeds for the full growing season, and may even present a carry-over problem for crop rotation the next year. Roundup® herbicide is nonpersistent. It biodegrades within a few weeks and is highly unlikely to migrate into ground water, since it binds tightly to soil particles. Glyphosate, the active ingredient in Roundup®, has the most favorable toxicological property rating that the U.S. Environmental Protection Agency (EPA) gives; it works by inhibiting an essential pathway in plants that animals, including people, do not have. It is also very effective at killing weeds—so effective that it will control soybeans as well as weeds. Thus it cannot be used to control weeds growing within a soybean crop. Or rather it could not be used until we developed Roundup Ready® soybeans, which are "substantially equivalent" to ordinary soybeans after processing. Roundup Ready® soybeans have an added protein, which is able to overcome the inhibitory property of glyphosate. Thus Roundup Ready® soybeans will thrive even when sprayed with typical doses of Roundup® that effectively eliminate weeds interspersed with the soybean plants.

Let us compare three situations: a soybean farm without weed control; a soybean farm with a typical spectrum of herbicides and plowing for weed control; and a soybean farm with No-till, Roundup® herbicide and Roundup Ready® soybeans. In the first scenario (no weed control) weeds would steal the sunlight, water, and nutrients from the soybeans, and the harvest would be contaminated with weed seeds. The magnitude of the problem varies by year and location but is sufficiently bad that virtually all soybeans grown in the U.S. today are treated with herbicides, and most are also plowed every year.

In the second scenario a typical Iowa farmer growing soybeans would: (a) burn fuel for plowing, (b) spray or soil-incorporate a variety of herbicides, (c) lose several tons of topsoil per acre from wind and water erosion, (d) lose some of the soil nitrate due to runoff and leaching, and (e) lose valuable carbon from the soil due to more rapid oxidation after plowing.

In the third scenario, combining no-till with Roundup® herbicide and Roundup Ready® soybeans, the same Iowa farmer would save fuel, reduce CO_2 emissions, and reduce machinery wear by avoiding plowing. The farmer would also conserve almost all of his or her topsoil, increase soil organic matter, reduce nitrate runoff, and cut loss of soil carbon. In some soil types carbon would actually be accumulated in the soil rather than lost to the atmosphere on a net basis. The increase in use of Roundup® herbicide would be offset by a reduction in the use of more persistent herbicides, in many cases decreasing the total amount of herbicide-active ingredient used on the crop.

In addition the farmer who decides to plant Roundup Ready® soybeans while using conservation tillage techniques and Roundup® herbicide typically can reduce production costs, compared with use of traditional practices. The lower herbicide cost more than offsets the higher Roundup Ready® seed costs. Better weed control can lead to higher yields, especially under intense weed pressure, which also can increase economic returns. Thus farmers will not need to compromise price and performance to improve their efficiency and sustainability, while reducing environmental impact. A study commissioned by Monsanto last year surveyed more than 1,000 Roundup Ready® soybean growers and found that an overwhelming majority expressed satisfaction with the performance of the soybeans, as well as with weed control and crop yields. Acreage of Roundup Ready® soybeans has been limited by availability of seed, but nonetheless increased from about 1 million acres in 1996 to about 9 million acres in 1997 in the United States.

Fulfilling the Opportunities

Because biotechnology reduces the need for resource consumption in agriculture, it is urgent to explore the potential of biotechnology to help resource-poor farmers around the world. A number of public and nongovernmental organizations have targeted biotechnology as a key to solving food production problems in developing countries. However while resource costs are dramatically reduced with biotechnology, and there are often less expensive research and registration costs than for agricultural chemicals, biotechnology is more expensive than traditional breeding and will require more education of growers to capture maximum benefit. It will also be even more important to deliver top quality seeds of the best adapted varieties for each region. Thus for most effective transfer of biotechnology, we must do a better job with the more traditional technologies as well. Risk management issues have a regional component that should be addressed locally.

To gain maximum advantage from biotechnology in resource-poor areas it will be even more important than in industrial countries to make sound choices that target the greatest opportunities first and minimize both cost and risk. Agricultural research and development, both public and private, is underfunded in comparison to its benefit and the need for improvements. A fundamental policy issue facing developing countries and international institutions is the degree to which private investment is fostered, both locally and globally, for research and development, seed production and distribution, other inputs, and on-farm services. This will be determined largely by choices about intellectual property rights, contract law, predictable and science-based regulation, and international trade practices.

Even if a very favorable climate is created for private investment and business development, there will still be a large underserved constituency of resource-poor farmers who do not have access to the funds, information, or markets necessary to make investments or obtain returns in their own "businesses." There will also be a number of important crops and traits that will not attract investment, even under favorable conditions, which will need to be improved in public sector or nonprofit programs. There are a number of examples of public-private partnerships to transfer technology for some of these "orphan applications," which provide paradigms for trying to help resource-poor farmers without discouraging private investment and business development. In the United States, with its long history of private investment in agricultural products, technologies, and services, public institutions play a vital role in education; basic scientific discovery; extension services; and comprehensive, unbiased local testing of competing products and technologies. Thus the public sector will play a necessary role even in a flourishing market economy, and public-sector funding needs to be fostered and increased as well.

One project that we have been pursuing in partnership with the Kenyan Agricultural Research Institute (KARI) since 1991 is the development of genes for resistance to a devastating virus of sweet potatoes. Beginning with Dr. Florence Wambugu's work on the tissue culture and transformation of Kenyan varieties during 1991-94, her work has been continued by Daniel Maingi, Charity Macharia, and now, Dr. Duncan Kirubu. The director of KARI, Dr. Cyrus Ndiritu, has been instrumental in supporting the project with some of his best scientists. Dr. Maud Hinchee of Monsanto has provided tireless leadership and support for the project. Despite facing an unexpectedly difficult technical problem, the team now has in hand more than 200 independent transgenic lines of sweet potato, which are being prepared for shipment to Kenya for testing, hopefully next year. Early testing in growth chambers indicates a number of very promising lines that are not infectable with the virus. Because sweet potato produces enough calories globally to feed 400 million people, but is devastated by chronic virus diseases in Africa, our hope is that this single target will have a large impact on food security in Africa. The project involved several strategies that I believe are important.

1. The choice of target and technology was made by KARI and Dr. Wambugu.

2. The project involves training of local scientists.

3. The work has led to development of technological infrastructure for a vital "orphan crop."

4. The program has fostered broad cooperation among public, private, and nongovernmental organizations for the benefit of resource-poor farmers. Participants include Monsanto, KARI, the U.S. Agency for International Development, the International Service for the Acquisition of Agri-biotech Applications, and several universities.

Risks

Risk is the degree of possibility of loss or injury. A hazard is something that is able or likely to inflict injury. Injury occurs only when a hazard coincides with exposure to circumstances under which the hazard inflicts injury. Thus risk equals the degree of hazard times the degree of exposure to the hazard. We manage risk by the decisions we make about hazardous substances or situations and exposure to the circumstances under which injury could occur. A decision is a determination or choice arrived at after consideration. We make decisions to gain benefit as well as to manage risk.

For example, electricity is a serious hazard at 110 or 220 volts. We could drop the voltage entering our homes to 12 volts to reduce the hazard. Why don't we? One reason is that it would cost a fortune to replace everything with 12-volt appliances. But even more importantly, 12 volts would required huge currents of electrons to deliver the equivalent power. The thickness of the wires would have to be greatly increased and we would need much more copper and stronger poles. The loss of power over transmission lines would be much larger; more coal would have to be burned for the same benefit. So instead of reducing the hazard by reducing the voltage, we use circuit breakers, insulation, recessed outlets, and sealed appliances to effectively reduce exposure to the hazard. Thus we make the risk low and the benefit high. One more point with this example: electricity is less hazardous and exposure to its hazard can be managed better than is the case with most alternative sources of power. For example, the risk of fire and lung ailments from the use of electric light bulbs is much lower than from the use of oil lamps. The implication is that many key decisions are based on comparing risk to risk in proportion to benefit—not by looking narrowly at absolute risk.

What are the potential risks of biotechnology, and how do we make decisions to manage those risks? Over the past decade an elaborate system of checks and balances has been developed by government regulatory agencies, scientific expert panels, and industry working groups to look for potential risks and make appropriate decisions to identify and address issues of risk—both hypothetical and real. A number of science-based regulations, reviews, and decision trees have been developed, discussed, debated, and deployed regarding these key issues.

The most important issue is food safety. Plants commonly contain toxic compounds that we must either avoid eating or consume only in quantities that our bodies can tolerate. Breeding can cause unintended changes in nutritional content or toxicants in foods, but since the probability of these changes is low, centuries of ignoring the potential risk in classical breeding has not yet resulted in a serious problem. However, crops improved with biotechnology methods are comprehensively analyzed for changes in the composition of key nutrients and toxicants that may occur before regulatory approvals are granted.

Another key issue is the safety of the newly added gene and the protein it encodes. Requests to regulatory agencies for approval of new products include results of a variety of studies or tests to evaluate the digestive fate, toxicity, allergenicity, and animal-feeding effects of the new protein. Other studies examine the environmental effects of the gene in the recipient crop, as well as the potential for outcrossing to a wild relative species that might coexist with the crop. These studies are not conducted for traditional breeding, even though modern food crops contain dozens of intended genes and hundreds or thousands of unintended genes. None of these new genes introduced by breeding or their corresponding proteins are usually characterized for toxicity, allergenicity, or environmental impacts, despite the fact that they have been genetically introgressed from wild species collected around the world.

Companies involved with agricultural biotechnology have examined these issues early and made choices not to develop specific products that may carry a risk. For example, one company stopped development of a nutritionally enhanced soybean when their tests showed the new protein to be an allergen. My guess is that the cost of managing exposure to that hazard would exceed the value of the product. Thus it was a logical decision to stop the work. Monsanto has decided not to pursue the development of Roundup resistance in sorghum, a crop that outcrosses to johnson grass, which is a weed currently controlled by herbicides such as Roundup.

In the United States all food crops with engineered genes are reviewed by the Food and Drug Administration for human food and animal feed safety and by the Department of Agriculture for safety to agriculture and the environment. Crops with traits for pest resistance are also reviewed by the EPA. The professional staff of these agencies evaluate the safety of proposed new traits and crop varieties, while scientific expert panels review regulatory policy and safety assessment approaches, as appropriate.

The first transgenic plants were precisely engineered in 1982. To date more than 3,600 field trials have been authorized at over 15,000 individual test sites in at least 34 countries and with at least 56 different crops. At least 35 different genetically modified plant products have been approved by at least one country. This year, 1997, represents the second year of large-scale commercial planting of genetically modified crops. Approximately 30 million acres of genetically modified crops were planted globally in 1997, a significant increase from the 4 to 6 million acres planted in 1996. These introductions were preceded by a comprehensive safety analysis and decisionmaking process carried out in science-based ways by companies, government agencies, and scientific expert panels. The bottom line is that every review concluded that there are no new risks inherent in the process itself, and that the products approved so far are substantially equivalent to their traditional counterparts. Moreover, the new proteins added to these genetically modified crops have been shown to pose no significant risks. Review will continue on a case-by-case basis as the science and the technology evolve and expand.

Choices

Critics and proponents of biotechnology alike are creative at spinning scenarios of theoretical risks that biotechnology might cause. No one can guarantee that biotechnology will never cause an unforeseen problem. That is why biotechnology is regulated and scrutinized by a comprehensive system of checks and balances. But the critics dismiss our ability to assess and manage these possible risks and seem to believe that the world is fine the way it is or that we should adopt a low-tech version of agriculture.

I fear that continuing the status quo or returning to low-tech agriculture will lead us to plow, drain, or degrade much of the rest of the planet—rainforests, wetlands, temperate forests, prairies, streams, lakes, and seas. This would be disastrous for other species with which we share the Earth and for ecosystems that provide essential services to the biosphere. But it would be even more disastrous for us. The economic consequences would plunge more people into poverty, malnutrition, and starvation, while reducing the ability and willingness of wealthier people and nations to help those less fortunate. The actual situation is less binary than these simple alternatives. Too little investment or over-regulation will result in foregoing benefits we might otherwise have realized. Too much investment or too little oversight will result in opportunity cost and excessive risk.

The Earth is a large space ship, a closed system. We receive an income of sunlight. We dispose of radiant heat. We are otherwise limited to the resources and energy stores already on Earth, and we are stuck with whatever waste we make. Our population will increase by several billion people in the next 40 to 50 years. Even today we are not caring adequately for many of the world's inhabitants, human or other species. The precautionary principle tells us that even without full certainty about the paths ahead, we should act to avert the serious and irreversible harm that is occurring even as we speak. Failure to move forward with new technology, global trade, business development, and other forms of sustainable development and economic growth is probably the biggest risk we face. Inertia will harm us for sure if we act too slowly.

The complete solution set will span technological, economic, social, and political innovations. No one part of this set can solve the sustainability crisis alone. But working together I believe we can rise to the challenge. I believe increasing global investment in plant science, agricultural science, and agricultural biotechnology is one the best ways to reduce the risk of environmental degradation and economic stagnation. Real gains in productivity, such as those biotechnology brings to agriculture, are the surest way to alleviate poverty. Sustain means to support and nurture, not just to continue. Develop means to grow and change. The industry and economy of the future must grow and change to increase the level of support for people, while decreasing the throughput and the harm—similar to substituting "information for stuff"—as biotechnology does for agriculture. My colleagues and I at Monsanto are eager to work with others who are also determined to meet the challenge of sustainable development.

The Opportunities and the Risks

The Environmental Risks of Transgenic Crops: An Agroecological Assessment
Miguel A. Altieri

Genetic engineering is an application of biotechnology involving the manipulation of DNA and the transfer of gene components between species in order to encourage the replication of desired traits (OTA 1992). Although there are many applications of genetic engineering in agriculture, the current focus of biotechnology is on developing herbicide-tolerant crops and pest- and disease-resistant crops. Transnational corporations such as Monsanto, DuPont, Norvartis, and others, which are the main proponents of biotechnology, view transgenic crops as a way to reduce dependence on inputs such as pesticides and fertilizers. It is ironic that the biorevolution is being brought forward by the same interests that promoted the first wave of agrochemically based agriculture. But this time, by equipping each crop with new "insecticidal genes," they are promising the world safer pesticides, reduction of chemically intensive farming, and more sustainable agriculture.

As long as transgenic crops follow closely the pesticide paradigm, such biotechnological products will do nothing but reinforce the pesticide treadmill in agroecosystems, thus legitimizing the concerns that many scientists have expressed regarding the possible environmental risks of genetically engineered organisms. The most serious ecological risks posed by the commercial-scale use of transgenic crops are listed below. (See Rissler and Mellon 1996; Krimsky and Wrubel 1996.)

- The spread of transgenic crops threatens crop genetic diversity by simplifying cropping systems and promoting genetic erosion.

- The potential transfer of genes from pesticide-resistant crops to wild or semidomesticated relatives, thus creating superweeds.
- Herbicide-resistant crop volunteers become weeds in subsequent crops.
- Vector-mediated horizontal gene transfer and recombination to create new pathogenic bacteria.
- Vector recombination to generate new virulent strains of virus, especially in transgenic plants engineered for viral resistance with viral genes.
- Insect pests will quickly develop resistance to crops with biotechnology toxin.
- Massive use of Bt toxin in crops can unleash potentially negative interactions, affecting ecological processes and nontarget organisms.

The above impacts of agricultural biotechnology are evaluated here in the context of agro- ecological goals aimed at making agriculture more socially just, economically viable, and ecologically sound (Altieri 1996). Such evaluation is timely, given that worldwide there have been over 1,500 approvals for field testing transgenic crops (the private sector has accounted for 87 percent of all field tests since 1987), despite the fact that in most countries stringent procedures are not in place to deal with environmental problems that may develop when engineered plants are released into the environment (Hruska and Lara Pavón 1997). A main concern is that international pressures to gain markets and profits are resulting in a situation in which companies are releasing transgenic crops without proper consideration for the long-term impacts on people or the ecosystem (Mander and Goldsmith 1996).

Actors and Research Directions

Most innovations in agricultural biotechnology are profit-driven rather than need-driven, so that the thrust of the genetic engineering industry is not really to solve agricultural problems, but to create profitability. This statement is supported by the fact that at least 27 corporations have initiated herbicide-tolerant plant research, including the world's eight largest pesticide companies (Bayer, Ciba-Geigy, ICI, Rhone-Poulenc, Dow/Elanco, Monsanto, Hoescht, and DuPont) and virtually all seed companies, many of which have been acquired by chemical companies (Gresshoft 1996).

In the industrialized countries from 1986-92, some 57 percent of all field trials to test transgenic crops involved herbicide tolerance, and 46 percent of all applicants to the U.S. Department of Agriculture (USDA) for field testing were chemical companies. Crops currently targeted for genetically engineered tolerance to one or more herbicides include: alfalfa, canola, cotton, corn, oats, petunia, potato, rice, sorghum, soybean, sugarbeet, sugar cane, sunflower, tobacco, tomato, and wheat. It is clear that by creating crops resistant to its herbicides a company can expand markets for its patented chemicals. The market for herbicide-resistant crops (HRCs) has been estimated at more than US$500 million by the year 2000 (Gresshoft 1996).

Although some testing is being conducted by universities and advanced research organizations, the research agenda of such institutions is being increasingly influenced by the private sector in ways never seen in the past. Some 46 percent of biotechnology firms support biotechnology research at universities, while 33 of the 50 U.S. states have university-industry centers for the transfer of biotechnology. The challenge for such organizations will be not only to ensure that ecologically sound aspects of biotechnology are researched and developed (such as N fixing and drought tolerance), but to carefully monitor and control the provision of applied nonproprietary knowledge to the private sector, to ensure that such knowledge will continue in the public domain for the benefit of all society.

Biotechnology and Agrobiodiversity

Although biotechnology has the capacity to create a greater variety of commercial plants, the trend of transnational corporations is to create broad international markets for a single product, thus creating the conditions for genetic uniformity in rural landscapes. In addition patent protection and intellectual property rights espoused by the General Agreement on Trade and Tariffs (GATT), which inhibit farmers from reusing, sharing, and storing seeds raise the prospect that a limited number of varieties will dominate the seed market. Although a certain degree of crop uniformity may have certain economic advantages, it has two ecological drawbacks. First, history has shown that a huge area planted to a single cultivar is very vulnerable to a new, matching strain of pathogen or pest. Second, the widespread use of a single cultivar leads to a loss of genetic diversity (Robinson 1996).

Evidence from the Green Revolution leaves no doubt that the spread of modern varieties (MVs) has been an important cause of genetic erosion, as massive government campaigns encouraged farmers to adopt MVs and abandon many local varieties (Tripp 1996). The uniformity caused by increasing areas sown to a smaller number of varieties is a source of increased risk for farmers, as the varieties may be more vulnerable to disease and pest attack, and most of them perform poorly in marginal environments (Robinson 1996).

All the above effects are not ubiquitous to MVs, and it is expected that, given their monogenic nature and fast acreage expansion, transgenic crops will only exacerbate such effects.

Environmental Problems of Herbicide-Resistant Crops

According to proponents of HRCs this technology represents an innovation that enables farmers to simplify their weed management requirements by reducing herbicide use to post-emergence situations using a single, broad- spectrum herbicide that breaks down relatively rapidly in the soil. Herbicide candidates with such characteristics include Glyphosate, Bromoxynil, Sulfonylurea, and Imidazolinones among others.

However the use of herbicide-resistant crops is actually likely to increase herbicide use, as well as production costs, and cause serious environmental problems.

Herbicide Resistance

It is well documented that when a single herbicide is used repeatedly on a crop, the chances of herbicide resistance developing in weed populations greatly increases (Holt and others 1993). The sulfonylureas and the imidazolinones are particularly prone to the rapid evolution of resistant weeds, and up to now 14 weed species have become resistant to sulfonylurea herbicides. Cocklebur, an aggressive weed of soybean and corn in the southeastern U.S., has exhibited resistance to imidazolinone herbicides (Goldburg 1992).

The problem is that given industry pressures to increase herbicide sales, acreage treated with these broad-spectrum herbicides will expand, exacerbating the resistance problem. For example, it has been projected that the acreage treated with glyphosate will increase to nearly 150 million acres. Although glyphosate is considered less prone to weed resistance, increased use of the herbicide will result in weed resistance, even if more slowly, as has already been documented with populations of annual ryegrass, quackgrass, birdsfoot trefoil, and *Cirsium arvense* (Gill 1995).

Ecological Impacts of Herbicides

Companies affirm that bromoxynil and glyphosate, when properly applied, degrade rapidly in the soil, do not accumulate in groundwater, have no effects on nontarget organisms, and leave no residues in food. There is, however, evidence that bromoxynil causes birth defects in laboratory animals, is toxic to fish, and may cause cancer in humans. Because bromoxynil is absorbed dermally, and because it causes birth defects in rodents, it is likely to pose hazards to farmers and farmworkers. Similarly, glyphosate has been reported to be toxic to some nontarget species in the soil—both to beneficial predators such as spiders, mites, carabid, and coccinellid beetles and to detritivores such as earthworms, as well as to aquatic organisms, including fish (Pimentel and others 1989). As this herbicide is known to accumulate in fruits and tubers suffering little metabolic degradation in plants, questions about food safety also arise.

Creation of "Superweeds"

Although there is some concern that transgenic crops might themselves become weeds, a major ecological risk is that large-scale releases of transgenic crops may promote transfer of transgenes from crops to other plants, which may then become weeds (Darmency 1994). The biological process of concern here is introgression; that is, hybridization among distinct plant species. Evidence indicates that such genetic exchanges among wild, weed, and crop plants already occur. The incidence of shattercane (*Sorghum bicolor*), a weedy relative of sorghum, and the gene flows between maize and teosinte demonstrate the potential for crop relatives to become serious weeds. This is worrisome given that a number of U.S. crops are grown in close proximity to sexually compatible wild relatives. There are also crops that are grown near wild or weedy plants that are not close relatives but may have some degree of cross compatibility, such as the crosses of *Raphanus raphanistrum X R.. sativus* (radish) and Johnson grass x sorghum (Radosevich and others 1996).

Reduction of Agroecosystem Complexity

Total weed removal via the use of broad-spectrum herbicides may lead to undesirable ecological impacts, given that an acceptable level of weed diversity in and around crop fields has been documented to play important ecological roles, such as enhancement of biological insect pest control, better soil cover, and reducing erosion. (Altieri 1994).

HRCs will probably enhance continuous cropping by inhibiting the use of rotations and polycultures susceptible to the herbicides used with HRCs. Such impoverished, low-plant-diversity agroecosystems provide optimal conditions for unhampered growth of weeds, insects, and diseases because many ecological niches are not filled by other organisms. Moreover HRCs, through increased herbicide effectiveness, could further reduce plant diversity, favoring shifts in weed community composition and abundance, which in turn favors competitive species that adapt to these broad-spectrum, post–emergence treatments (Radosevich and others 1996).

Environmental Risks of Insect-Resistant Crops

Resistance

According to the industry the promise of transgenic crops inserted with Bt genes is the replacement of synthetic insecticides now used to control insect pests. Since most crops have a diversity of insect pests, insecticides will still have to be applied to control pests other than Lepidoptera that are not susceptible to the endotoxin expressed by the crop (Gould 1994).

But several Lepidoptera species have been reported to develop resistance to Bt toxin in both field and laboratory tests, suggesting that major resistance problems are likely to develop in Bt crops, which through the continuous expression of the toxin create a strong selection pressure (Tabashnik 1994). Given that a diversity of different Bt-toxin genes have been isolated, biotechnologists argue that if resistance develops, alternative forms of Bt toxin can be used (Kennedy and Whalon 1995). However, because insects are likely to develop multiple resistance or cross-resistance, such strategy is also doomed to failure (Alstad and Andow 1995).

Others, borrowing from past experience with pesticides, have proposed resistance-management plans with transgenic crops, such as the use of seed mixtures and refuges (Tabashnik 1994). In addition to requiring the difficult goal of regional coordination between farmers, refuges have met with little success for chemical pesticides because insect populations are not constrained within closed systems and incoming insects are exposed to lower doses of the toxin as the pesticide degrades (Leibee and Capinera 1995).

Impact on Nontarget Organisms

By keeping pest populations at extremely low levels Bt crops can starve natural enemies, as these beneficial insects need a small amount of prey to survive in the agroecosystem. Parasites would be most affected, because they are more dependent on live hosts for development and survival, whereas some predators could theoretically thrive on dead or dying prey.

Natural enemies could also be affected directly through intertrophic-level interactions. Evidence from studies conducted in Scotland suggest that aphids were capable of sequestering the toxin from Bt crops and transferring it to its coccinellid predators, thus affecting reproduction and longevity of the beneficial beetles (Birch and others 1997). Sequestration of plant allelochemicals by herbivores, which then affect parasitoid performance, is not uncommon (Campbell and Duffey 1979). The potential of Bt toxins moving through food chains poses serious implications for natural biocontrol in agroecosystems.

Bt toxins can be incorporated into the soil through leaf materials, where they may persist for two-to-three months, resisting degradation by binding to clay particles while maintaining toxin activity (Palm and others 1996). Bt toxins that end up in the soil and water from transgenic leaf litter may have negative impacts on soil and aquatic invertebrates and nutrient cycling processes (James 1997). All of these issues deserve serious further inquiry.

Downstream Effect

A major environmental consequence resulting from the massive use of Bt toxin in cotton or other crops occupying a large area of the agricultural landscape is that neighboring farmers who grow crops other than cotton, but share similar pest complexes, may end up with resistant insect populations colonizing their fields. As Lepidopteran pests that develop resistance to Bt cotton move to adjacent fields where farmers use biotechnology as a microbial insecticide, they may render farmers defenseless against such pests, as they lose their biological control tool (Gould 1994). Who will be accountable for such losses?

Impacts of Disease-Resistant Crops

Scientists have attempted to engineer plants for resistance to pathogenic infection by incorporating genes for viral products into the plant genome. Although the use of viral genes for virus resistance in crops has potential benefits, there are also some risks. Recombination between RNA virus and a viral RNA inside the transgenic crop could produce a new pathogen, leading to more severe disease problems. Some researchers have shown that recombination occurs in transgenic plants, and that under certain conditions it produces a new viral strain with altered host range (Steinbrecher 1996).

The possibility that transgenic, virus-resistant plants may broaden the host range of some viruses or allow the production of new virus strains through recombination and transcapsidation demands careful further experimental investigation (Paoletti and Pimentel 1996).

Performance of Field-Released Transgenic Crops

Thirteen genetically modified crops that were already on the market or in the fields for the first time had been deregulated by the USDA by early 1997. Over 20 percent of U.S. soybean acreage was planted with Roundup®-tolerant soybean, and about 400,000 acres of maximizer Bt corn were planted in 1996. Such acreage expanded considerably in 1997 (transgenic cotton to 3.5 million acres, transgenic corn to 8.1 million acres, and soybean to 9.3 million acres) due to marketing and distribution agreements entered into by corporations and marketers (for example, Ciba Seeds with Growmark and Mycogen Plant Sciences with Cargill).

Given the speed with which products move from laboratory testing to field production, are transgenic crops living up to the expectations of the biotechnology industry? According to evidence presented by the Union of Concerned Scientists, there are already signals that the commercial-scale use of some transgenic crops poses serious ecological risks and does not deliver the promises of industry (see table 1).

The appearance of "behavioral resistance" by bollworms in cotton; that is, when the herbivore was capable of finding plant tissue areas with low Bt concentrations, raises questions not only about the adequacy of the resistance-management plans being adopted, but also about the way biotechnologists underestimate the capacity of insects to overcome genetic resistance in unexpected manners (The Gene Exchange 1996).

Similarly, poor harvests of herbicide-resistant cotton due to phytotoxic effects of Roundup® in

4,000-5,000 acres in the Mississippi Delta (*New York Times* 1997) points to the erratic performance of HRCs when subjected to varying agroclimatic conditions. Monsanto claims that this is a very small, localized incident that is being used by environmentalists to overshadow the benefits that the technology brought to 800,000 acres. From an agroecological standpoint, however, this incident is quite significant and merits further evaluation, since assuming that an homogenizing technology will perform well through a range of heterogeneous conditions is incorrect.

Conclusion

We know from the history of agriculture that plant diseases, insect pests, and weeds become more severe with the development of monoculture, and intensively managed and genetically manipulated crops soon lose genetic diversity (Altieri 1994; Robinson 1996). Given these facts there is no reason to believe that resistance to transgenic crops will not evolve among insects, weeds, and pathogens as has happened with pesticides. No matter what resistance-management strategies may be used, pests will adapt and overcome the agronomic constraints (Green and others 1990). Diseases and pests have always been amplified by changes toward homogeneous agriculture.

The fact that interspecific hybridization and introgression are common to species such as sunflower, maize, sorghum, oilseed rape, rice, wheat, and potatoes provides a basis to expect gene flow between transgenic crops and wild relatives to create new herbicide-resistant weeds. Despite the fact that some scientists argue that genetic engineering is not different from conventional breeding, critics of biotechnology claim that rDNA technology enables new (exotic) genes into transgenic plants. Such gene transfers are mediated by vectors derived from disease-causing viruses or plasmids, which can break down species barriers so that they can shuttle genes between a wide range of species, thus infecting many other organisms in the ecosystem.

But the ecological effects are not limited to pest resistance and creation of new weeds or virus strains. Transgenic crops can produce environmental toxins that move through the food chain and also may end up in the soil and water, af-

Table 1. Field performance of some recently released transgenic crops

Transgenic crop	Performance	Reference
1. Bt transgenic cotton 1996;	Additional insecticide sprays needed due to Bt cotton failing to control bollworms in 20,000 acres in eastern Texas	*The Gene Exchange*, Kaiser 1996
2. Cotton inserted with Roundup Ready™ gene	Bolls deformed and falling off 4,000-5,000 acres in Mississippi Delta	Lappe and Bailey 1997; Myerson 1997
3. Bt corn	27 percent yield reduction and lower Cu foliar levels in Beltsville trial	Hornick 1997
4. Herbicide-resistant oilseed rape	Pollen escaped and fertilized botanically related plants 2.5 km. away in Scotland	Scottish Crop Research Institute 1996
5. Virus-resistant squash	Vertical resistance to two viruses and not to others transmitted by aphids	Rissler, J. (personal communication)
6. Early FLAVR-SAVR tomato varieties	Did not exhibit acceptable yields and disease-resistance performance	*Biotech Reporter* 1996
7. Roundup Ready Canola	Pulled off the market due to contamination with a gene that does not have regulatory approval	Rance 1997
8. Bt potatoes	Aphids sequestered the Bt toxin apparently affecting coccinellid predators in negative ways	Birch and others 1997
9. Herbicide-tolerant crops	Development of resistance by annual ryegrass to Roundup®	Gill 1995

fecting invertebrates and probably ecological processes such as nutrient cycling.

Many people have argued for the creation of suitable regulation to mediate the testing and release of transgenic crops to offset environmental risks, and have demanded a much better assessment and understanding of ecological issues associated with genetic engineering. This is crucial, as many results emerging from the environmental performance of released transgenic crops suggest that in the development of "resistant crops," not only is there a need to test direct effects on the target insect or weed, but that the indirect effects on plants (such as growth, nutrient content, or metabolic changes), soil, and non-target organisms must also be evaluated.

Others demand continued support for ecologically based agricultural research, as all the biological problems that biotechnology aims at can be solved using agroecological approaches. The dramatic effects of rotations and intercropping on crop health and productivity, as well as of the use of biological control agents on pest regulation have been confirmed time after time by scientific research (Altieri 1994; NRC 1996). The problem is that research at public institutions increasingly reflects the interests of private funders at the expense of public-good research, such as biological control, organic production systems, and general agroecological techniques (Busch and others 1990). Civil society must demand a response to the question of who the university and other public organizations are to serve and request more research on alternatives to biotechnology. There is also an urgent need to challenge the patent system and intellectual property rights intrinsic to the GATT, which not only provide multinational corporations with the right to seize and patent genetic resources, but also accelerate the rate at which market forces encourage monocultural cropping with genetically uniform transgenic varieties.

The various recommendations for action that NGOs, farmers' organizations, and citizen groups should bring forward to local, national, and international fora include:

- End publicly funded research on transgenic crops that enhance agrochemical use and pose environmental risks.
- HRCs and other transgenic crops should be regulated as pesticides.
- All transgenic food crops should be labeled as such.
- Increase funding for alternative agricultural technologies.
- Ecological sustainability, alternative low-input technologies, the needs of small farmers, and human health and nutrition should be pursued with greater vigor than biotechnology.
- Trends set by biotechnology must be balanced by public policies and consumer choices in support of sustainability.
- Measures should encourage sustainable and multiple use of biodiversity at the community level, with an emphasis on technologies that promote self-reliance and local control of economic resources as a means to foster a more equitable distribution of benefits.

References

Alstad, D.N., and D.A. Andow. 1995. "Managing the Evolution of Insect Resistance to Transgenic Plants." *Science* 268: 894-6.

Altieri, M.A. 1994. *Biodiversity and Pest Management in Agroecosystems*. Haworth Press: New York.

———. 1996. *Agroecology: The Science of Sustainable Agriculture*. Westview Press: Boulder, Col.

Biotech Reporter. 1996. Financial Section, March 1996, 14.

Birch, A.N.E., and others. 1997. "Interaction between Plant Resistance Genes, Pest Aphid Populations, and Beneficial Aphid Predators." *Scottish Crops Research Institute (SCRI) Annual Report 1996-97*, 70-72.

Busch, L., W.B. Lacey, J. Burkhardt, and L. Lacey. 1990. *Plants, Power, and Profit*. Basil Blackwell: Oxford, U.K.

Campbell, B.C., and S.C. Duffy. 1979. "Tomatine and Parasitic Wasps: Potential Incompatibility of Plant Antibiosis with Biological Control." *Science* 205: 700-2.

Darmency, H. 1994. "The Impact of Hybrids between Genetically Modified Crop Plants and Their Related Species: Introgression and Weediness." *Molecular Ecology* 3: 337-40.

Fowler, C., and P. Mooney. 1990. *Shattering: Food, Politics, and the Loss of Genetic Diversity*. University of Arizona Press: Tucson.

Gill, D.S. 1995. "Development of Herbicide Resistance in Annual Ryegrass Populations in the Cropping Belt of Western Australia." *Australian Journal of Exp. Agriculture* 3: 67-72.

Goldburg, R.J. 1992. "Environmental Concerns with the Development of Herbicide-Tolerant Plants." *Weed Technology* 6: 647-52.

Gould, F. 1994. "Potential and Problems with High-Dose Strategies for Pesticidal Engineered Crops." *Biocontrol Science and Technology* 4: 451-61.

Green, M.B., A.M. LeBaron, and W.K. Moberg, eds. 1990. *Managing Resistance to Agrochemicals*. American Chemical Society: Washington, D.C.

Gresshoft, P.M. 1996. *Technology Transfer of Plant Biotechnology*. CRC Press: Boca Raton, Fla.

Holt, J.S., S.B. Powles, and J.A.M. Holtum. 1993. "Mechanisms and Agronomic Aspects of Herbicide Resistance." Annual Review Plant Physiology. *Plant Molecular Biology* 44: 203-29.

Hormick, S.B. 1997. "Effects of a Genetically Engineered Endophyte on the Yield and Nutrient Content of Corn." (Interpretive summary available through Geocities Homepage: www.geocities.com).

Hruska, A.J., and M. Lara Pavón. 1997. *Transgenic Plants in Mesoamerican Agriculture*. Zamorano Academic Press: Tegucigalpa, Honduras.

James, R.R. 1997. "Utilizing a Social Ethic toward the Environment in Assessing Genetically Engineered Insect-Resistance in Trees." *Agriculture and Human Values* 14: 237-49.

Kaiser, J. 1996. "Pests Overwhelm Bt Cotton Crop." *Science* 273:423.

Kennedy, G.G., and M.E. Whalon. 1995. "Managing Pest Resistance to *Bacillus thuringiensis* Endotoxins: Constraints and Incentives to Implementation." *Journal of Economic Entomology* 88: 454-60.

Krimsky, S., and R.P. Wrubel. 1996. *Agricultural Biotechnology and the Environment: Science, Policy, and Social Issues*. University of Illinois Press: Urbana.

Lappe, M., and B. Bailey. 1997. "Genetic Engineered Cotton in Jeopardy." www2.cetos.org/1/toxalts/bioflop.html

Leibee, G.L., and J.L. Capinera. 1995. "Pesticide Resistance in Florida Insects Limits Management Options." *Florida Entomologist* 78: 386-99.

Lipton, M. 1989. *New Seeds and Poor People*. Johns Hopkins University Press: Baltimore, Md.

Mander, J., and E. Goldsmith. 1996. *The Case against the Global Economy*. Sierra Club Books: San Francisco, Cal.

Mikkelsen, T.R., B. Andersen, and R.B. Jorgensen. 1996. "The Risk of Crop Transgenic Spread." *Nature* 380:31-2.

Myerson, A.R. 1997. "Breeding Seeds of Discontent: Growers Say Strain Cuts Yields." *The New York Times*. Business Section, Nov. 19, 1997.

National Research Council. 1996. *Ecologically Based Pest Management*. National Academy of Sciences: Washington D.C.

Office of Technology Assessment (OTA). 1992. *A New Technological Era for American Agriculture*. U.S. Government Printing Office: Washington D.C.

Palm, C.J., D.L. Schaller, K.K. Donegan, and R.J. Seidler. (In press). "Persistence in Soil of Transgenic Plant-Produced *Bacillus thuringiensis* var. Kustaki-Endotoxin." *Canadian Journal of Microbiology*.

Paoletti, M.G., and D. Pimentel. 1996. "Genetic Engineering in Agriculture and the Environment: Assessing Risks and Benefits." *BioScience* 46: 665-71.

Pimentel, D., and others. 1992. "Environmental and Economic Costs of Pesticide Use." *BioScience* 42: 750-60.

Pimentel, D., M.S. Hunter, J.A. LaGro, R.A. Efroymson, J.C. Landers, F.T. Mervis, C.A. McCarthy, and A.E. Boyd. 1989. "Benefits and Risks of Genetic Engineering in Agriculture." *BioScience* 39: 606-14.

Radosevich, S.R., J.S. Holt, and C.M. Ghersa. 1996. *Weed Ecology: Implications for Weed Management*, 2d ed.. John Wiley and Sons: New York.

Rissler, J., and M. Mellon. 1996. *The Ecological Risks of Engineered Crops*. MIT Press: Cambridge, Mass.

Robinson, R.A. 1996. *Return to Resistance: Breeding Crops to Reduce Pesticide Resistance*. AgAccess: University of California at Davis.

Scottish Crop Research Institute 1996. "Research Notes, Genetic Crops Community Institute." SCRI: Edinburgh, Scotland.

Steinbrecher, R.A. 1996. "From Green to Gene Revolution: The Environmental Risks of Genetically Engineered Crops." *The Ecologist* 26: 273-82.

Tabashnik, B.E. 1994a. "Delaying Insect Adaptation to Transgenic Plants: Seed Mixtures and Refugia Reconsidered." *Proc. R. Soc. London* B255: 7-12.

———. 1994b. "Genetics of Resistance to *Bacillus thuringiensis*." *Annual Review of Entomology* 39: 47-79.

Tripp, R. 1996. "Biodiversity and Modern Crop Varieties: Sharpening the Debate." *Agriculture and Human Values* 13: 48-62.

Union of Concerned Scientists. 1996. "Bt Cotton Fails to Control Bollworm." *The Gene Exchange* 7: 1-8.

Discussion
Moderator: Roger N. Beachy

Roger Beachy: We have heard some examples of serious concerns that natural and native knowledge is being lost, that biotechnology will accelerate that process, and that its applications are much overstated. Robert Horsch and Miguel Altieri have presented very different views on these matters.

The fact is that we have a growing population. We have as many as 20 million people in cities and certain concentrated areas. It is very difficult to feed 20 million in the city, even with family farms that are fully sustainable. We need to produce much more food at relatively low cost.

In the U.S. we have the luxury of living with food costs that are in the range of 10 to 12 percent of take-home income. This is not the case in other parts of the world. Sometimes we in the U.S. speak with the arrogance of plenty, of wealth. It is important to recognize that this wealth is not available in most of the world.*

Judith Chambers: For those who are concerned about biotechnology and the resistance that may be developing because of the deployment of Bt transgenic plants, let me remind you that up until the advent of genetic engineering, Bt had been a fairly useless product. It was very underused in most of the world, with the exception of a few places in Southeast Asia, where it was heavily used. It breaks down in sunlight in its native

form. There were only a few Bts that were of application in agriculture, because we did not have the expertise of biotechnology to explore the variety of strains that are there and develop them into a number of different, highly useful genes and products.

So I think it is a bit disingenuous to make the argument that biotech is going to be the destruction of Bt. I would argue, on the contrary, that biotech has definitely helped Bt in terms of its utility in agriculture.

It is also disingenuous to argue that this technology is not being effectively deployed in addressing developing-country problems, and then to put numerous roadblocks in the way so that the technology cannot get there. USAID decided to put its resources into the development of a genetically engineered, heat-stable version of the rinderpest vaccine. In three years the scientist, an Ethiopian-born professor at the University of California-Davis, developed the vaccine. It took an additional four years to get it through all of the regulatory hoops that it had to jump through to actually get this vaccine to the point where we could test it—even under very contained conditions in Africa. Four years!

As a result there was no more money to carry out the test; it had all been spent on regulatory approvals and licenses—not from the Africans, who were wondering what was taking us so

---

* Following his introductory remarks, Roger N. Beachy asked Judith Chambers of the U.S. Agency for International Development to moderate the discussion.

long—it was the international organizations and nongovernmental organizations (NGOs) that were opposed to the deployment of the technology, and sad to say, to the U.S. government.

What is the upshot? We now have a wonderful vaccine. It is highly effective at controlling the disease and is heat-stable. It is still in development because of the delay. Meanwhile, right now in Africa 70 to 80 percent of the wild buffalo and lesser kudu in the game parks on the Serengeti border between Kenya and Tanzania are being destroyed by a mutant variety of rinderpest. If that is not a threat to biodiversity, I do not know what is.

Michel Petit: I am a little frustrated, frankly, because we have here two camps and, as happened yesterday in the debate on ethics and biotechnology, it is a dialogue of the deaf. So I am going to try to sort out the differences and hopefully see where they are irreconcilable and where there may be some consensus. For the World Bank Group the existence of these two camps is provoking paralysis.

First, there is clearly a philosophical difference that is not going to be reconciled this afternoon. Miguel Altieri expressed it clearly. He criticized biotechnology as being the pursuit of a reductionist approach, opposed to what I think he would call ecological agriculture.

I do not believe that we can get to an agreement on these two different philosophies, but I would be glad to get comments from the two speakers.

Hopefully the problem can be treated in more specific cases, and that is where possibly we can achieve some degree of consensus. One area where we have an agreement is that biotechnology is developed in the private sector and, very properly, the private sector is seeking profits; since we rely on market mechanisms, we know that when this happens the public good is going to be neglected. So we all agree.

In the World Bank Group we are dealing with governments; we advise them, provide support, and therefore we are interested in seeing how we can help them seek the public good in complementarity with what the private sector will do. So I do not believe we have a disagreement on this—that the public good is not necessarily going to be served by profit-seeking firms.

Another area where we could have agreement goes back to my question this morning. The Kendall Report identified four risks. Two or three were touched upon by Miguel Altieri. The threat to the ecosystem, development of new viruses, pesticide-resistance, and the transfer of genes to weeds.

Do we have an agreement that these are the risks? Is there a consensus? I did not hear any difference of view on this, so hopefully we agree. What I heard is disagreement about the magnitude of the risks involved. Can this be reconciled?

A second set of issues about which there might be consensus is that if we accept that risks exist, what can be done to mitigate them? That is the biosafety precaution. And do we get any guidance, because Robert Horsch referred obviously to the U.S. case where the industry is regulated. It is regulated in Organisation for Economic Co-operation and Development member countries, but in many developing countries the question we ask is what kind of regulatory framework should be put in place.

We should have a clear view of what the risks are and how they can be mitigated. Is the recommendation that the regulatory framework that applies in the U.S. be simply transferred to developing countries? Is this feasible? Does it mean that they will not adopt biotechnology because it will not have a proper regulatory framework? These are the questions which I very much would like to see addressed.

Audience comment: What I heard today, especially from Robert Horsch, is that the perception is that private industry is trying to get away from regulation.

I want to remind you that thalidomide, because of the strength and courage of a lady who was heading the U.S. Food and Drug Administration, was not allowed to be used in the United States. It was used outside, and we know the disasters that happened.

I disagree also with the moderator in the sense that she wants to weaken the regulation. We have to find a middle ground. We cannot really deregulate. She said that regulation stopped the progress of that vaccine.

Judith Chambers: My point was not regulation, per se, but excessive regulation, overregulation, in proportion to the risk for doing a contained field test.

Audience comment: That is debatable. You are saying that the risk is one to minus 30. Maybe that is too much safety, but I think Miguel Altieri is correct that we have to be careful.

Christopher Somerville, when he presented the overview of the case, showed that there are risks, and we should talk about them. We should not deregulate it completely. We have to be on the conservative side.

The last point I want to make is that I do not think the World Bank Group is equipped to talk about regulation. We have to discuss this in a more concentrated debate, not in a four- or five-day conference.

Audience comment: I want to make three points. First, six weeks ago Monsanto introduced bovine growth hormone milk in India. Nobody knew about it. Unlike in this country, there are no regulations, and no kind of analysis was carried out in India.

Second, in 1800 we had about 42,000 varieties of rice in India. Today the number hardly reaches 2,800. What happened to the species of rice that existed, developed through millions of years of experiment? We are in a hurry, and there are too many people and everybody wants the same thing. I think it is time to recognize the larger impact on the ecological system, before all these varieties of rice disappear.

The third point: in 1991, the World Health Organization (WHO) told us that in India we have in mother's milk nine times more DDT than is even allowed by WHO. A study on Indian children showed that 12 percent are suffering from neurological disabilities. There are no regulations. Nobody goes to court.

The price for this risk is paid by society. Under these circumstances claims by biotechnology companies that there is a utopia waiting—there will be no ecological problems, there will be no problems to humans, there will be no waste—have to be challenged by people who understand the real nature of crisis we are facing.

Timothy Reeves: I would like speakers to comment on a point that Michel Petit made. This whole question of diversity in sustainable systems is absolutely critical, and I certainly have no argument at all with Miguel Altieri in relation to diversity being key for sustainable systems.

But in order to gain diverse systems in the complex world in which we now exist, we need to think of using the tools of science, biotechnology—all of the advances we can devise to build diverse systems.

We could use a new technology to drive toward monoculture, but I would argue that you could use the same technology to aid diversification of systems. If resource-poor farmers can grow their food needs on half of the small piece of land they have, the other half can be released for more diverse crops, woodlots, agroforestry situations, or livestock.

If we can harness this technology to increase productivity so that those basic needs can be produced on a smaller area, we do not have rifts out there. We have an opportunity to put these technologies together to build diverse systems.

Robert Horsch: The question here is not what has Monsanto claimed biotechnology can do for the people of the developing world. The question is: is there or should there be, can there be, public-private collaboration that can take what is well-established to be a very powerful and very useful technology and transfer it such that it can be of benefit?

To the points on biosafety, I think that there are some intelligent dialogues that we can have on what we can do to make intelligent choices and what can be done to share and transfer technology. If that is a completely wrong world-view, if we want a world that does not have private companies, that does not have products that come from more than 15 miles away from their source, then that is a question I do not even know how to begin addressing.

I think Michel Petit's question is a good one. It is one for which I do not have a final answer today, but it occurs to me that we have a lot of infrastructure and experience in the U.S. that is available to be shared. Europe, Japan, and a number of countries—Mexico and to some extent Costa Rica and, I think, Kenya—have invested effort in this. I am sure there are dozens of other countries that have already begun to question what they are going to do about technologies such as biotechnology.

I would recommend that the answer be logical and science-based, and that it should look at getting benefit at the best-cost equation. I also agree that the World Bank Group is not equipped to answer that question. You need some other source of experts.

Biodiversity is an interesting issue. In a sense diversity is a kind of high information content, and it goes to my point about the importance of information technologies, information densities, that goes to management practices, that goes to crop rotation, that goes to good genotypes, that goes to blending the best genotypes with the best practices.

I think that economic forces alone will drive that in a naturally beneficial direction. My prediction is that the tools of biotechnology, the molecular markers and the coupling with precision agriculture kinds of technologies, will drive us towards a more diverse agriculture in the future. Just the very basic energetics of the system that Christopher Somerville pointed out—we actually waste a huge amount of the sunlight that hits land because our plants are not in full growth until the middle of the summer, and then they senesce and dry down well before the frost in the fall. We are wasting a lot of sunlight; more diverse systems should be able to capture more of that.

This natural drive toward more productivity is going to take us back in the direction of more diversity. I think, though, you have to put this on the table as a question. Who do you want to make grow these diverse genotypes so that they are preserved? And is it a rational choice to say you are forbidden other technologies or you must use this other technology because otherwise the world will lose a resource? And who are you going to insist keep growing the old varieties when other more productive varieties are available? Or is there another mechanism—germplasm banks, preservation programs, wilderness set-aside areas? Is that perhaps another way to do it, and then let growers pick whatever works best in their individual situation?

Miguel Altieri: I have tried to expand the view of the risks to encompass the fact that we cannot allow the complex systems and problems we are facing today to be dominated by solutions that are reductionist and are also profit-driven. We need to take account of much wider visions, because the problems are not only technological. They are also sociological, economic, and political, and therefore we need the participation and partnership of several groups, using the different tools that are available, including biotechnology.

As chairman of the NGO Committee of the Consultative Group on International Agricultural Research, I have pointed out many times that there is a tremendous potential for biotechnology to be utilized for drought resistance, pest resistance, and other challenges that farmers throughout the developing world, and even in the industrial world, are facing.

I think that what is going to be critical here is that somehow these partnerships that we are trying to promote get to the field and do the work together. Otherwise we are going to continue with these arguments. Scientists can express different views, depending on their worldviews and the pressures they are receiving from different sources.

We need to try to come up with the best expertise, including peasants and indigenous people's scientific approaches (ethnoscience), in addition to the scientific expertise of the universities and international centers and the practical knowledge of NGOs working with the poor on concrete projects.

There are tremendous success stories that we can identify throughout the world, but it has been tremendously difficult to obtain the partnerships and funds to scale them up to the level that will show impact.

The South is tired of hearing: "You are going to miss the train." What if the train goes to the wrong station? There has been failure after failure of top-down development. We need now participation by local people in deciding what kind of technology they need, and we need to have different partners, policies, and incentives to support sustainable agriculture.

My main worry about risk is not so much focused on whether Bt transgenic crops are going to become resistant or not. They are going to become resistant. We all know that. The issue is that you can delay the resistance by deploying strategies. Or you can make more combinations of mix varieties and delay that.

If we take only a genetic, deterministic kind of approach, it will undermine the possibilities of a sustainable agriculture that relies on much more holistic approaches and will promote diversity. So I am not saying do not use biotechnology if it is appropriate and the developing countries want it.

Regulatory Framework Issues

Panel Presentation
Hamdallah Zedan

Biotechnology, biodiversity, and biosafety are now household words, thanks to the Convention on Biological Diversity signed at the Rio Earth Summit in 1992. Although the three are closely linked, each has a complex web of issues and stakeholders.

It must be emphasized that biotechnology is a term that has been used broadly and has a variety of meanings in different contexts. It is comprised of a continuum of technologies ranging from long-established and widely used classical technologies (based on the use of microbes and other living organisms) through the more advanced, modern technologies (based on the use of recombinant DNA techniques, cell and tissue culture, cell fusion, and novel bioprocessing methods).

It must also be emphasized that biotechnology is as old as man. Its development could be divided into three parts: (a) the early period, when primitive biological processes were discovered by accident and incorporated into daily life; (b) a middle period, beginning around the 17th century, when scientific explanations for some of these primitive processes began to be established and followed; and (c) the modern period, during which microbes have become the basis of great industries and modern techniques have given us new and far-reaching powers.

The products of biotechnology offered, and will undoubtedly continue to offer, immense benefits to society by increasing the production of food, energy, specialty chemicals, and other raw materials; alleviating or mitigating health prob-

lems; and improving environmental management. However, although biotechnology with its advanced techniques will generate considerable rewards for humanity, its benefits are accompanied by controversy. Like many technologies, modern biotechnology may not be without problems.

Two major issues will, however, affect the transfer and application of modern biotechnology and modern bioproducts for sustainable economic development in developing countries. The biotechnology industry should do more to harness the potential of biotechnology to satisfy the expectations and aspirations not only of developing countries but also the global public.

The first major issue of concern to developing countries is that not enough is being done to harness recent innovations in biotechnology to their needs. The technologies developed in industrial countries are not always suited or easily adaptable to the problems of developing countries. A large share of the products of biotechnology research are not specifically aimed at developing countries. Most of the research and development in this field addresses the pressing issues facing industrial, rather than developing, countries. Two areas deserve high priority, namely drylands agricultural productivity and health problems caused by tropical, vector-borne diseases. There were once great hopes that the biotechnology revolution, with its new techniques and bioproducts, would contribute to the solution of these problems. But to date modern biotechnology is far from being harnessed to assist those living in dryland agricultural areas. Likewise, little has been done to combat tropical, vector-borne diseases.

Many developing countries have substantial areas of their potentially productive land located in drylands. Drylands represent about one-third of the total land area of the world and are inhabited by significant numbers of people—almost one-third of the total population, estimated at 5.77 billion in mid-1996. This contradicts the common belief that drylands are uninhabitable.

Biotechnology can and should play a crucial role in sustainable drylands management. This will require access to the best available knowledge and technologies. Degradation of drylands is severe, posing a threat to the carrying capacities and biological diversity of these lands. It also poses a threat to the stability of the physical landscape and to the almost 2 billion people and their neighbors who live in other ecosystems closely linked to the drylands.

An estimated 10 million square kilometers of Africa is infested by various species of *Glossina*. The habitat of these tsetse flies also happens to be some of the more fertile agricultural soils on the continent, which receive adequate rainfall. Heavy infestation has made these virgin lands inaccessible to human agriculture. It is estimated that 25 to 30 percent of the potential livestock production areas in Africa are not utilized due to livestock trypanosomiasis.

It is often argued that tsetse fly infestation has had positive consequences. Large tracts of land in the heartland of Africa remain ungraded; woodlands, such as those in Tanzania, and forests in Zaire are untouched, thus supporting diversified flora and fauna. This argument, however, does not support the concept of sustainable utilization of resources, now encompassed within conservation.

There is a need to develop partnerships in relevant aspects of biotechnology with the aim of improving the scientific and technical capability of developing countries in this field and responding effectively to their needs. Although many developing countries are reshaping their economic polices to reflect the needs of the agriculture and health sectors, only a few seem to have formulated biotechnology policies, while others have incorporated biotechnology concerns into their national development strategies.

The second major issue is the regulatory climate governing the safe development and application of biotechnology and the safe transfer and use of modern bioproducts.

There are questions about not only the human health, but also the environmental, social, and economic implications of developing and using biotechnology products. The focus of concern in industrial countries in the early days of biotechnology was on human health. Now, however, environmental impacts are becoming the main concern in industrial countries, while the threat to socioeconomic security of many people is surfacing as another focus of considerable concern in developing nations.

Environmental Concerns

There is no consensus between the views of molecular biologists and ecologists on the possible environmentally harmful effects of introducing genetically modified organisms (GMOs) into the environment. There is, however, consensus that risk analysis should be based on the end product designed for release, rather than the method by which it was produced. Questions that arise on the deliberate release of genetically engineered organisms into the environment include:

- Will these organisms survive?
- Will they multiply?
- Will they disturb fundamental ecosystem processes?
- Will they affect nontarget organisms?
- Will they be transported to unintended sites?
- Will they transfer the inserted genetic material to other organisms?
- What are the conditions that encourage transfer or maintenance of the inserted genes?
- If transferred, will the new genetic material be expressed?
- If transferred and expressed, will there be any positive or negative environmental consequences?
- Will seemingly benign forms somehow mutate beyond laboratory and field-testing expectations when they spread in the environment?
- Can quantitative environmental risk assessment be made for comparison of risks and benefits and determination if the risk is "unreasonable?"

What role can the scientific community play, given these concerns?

- Identify scientifically sound general principles and approaches upon which methodologies for field testing and assessment can be developed. This will allow for more accurate extrapolation of laboratory and small-scale testing to predictions of large-scale and commercial application and the reduction of scientific uncertainty associated with risk assessment.
- Define deficiencies in our knowledge regarding various testing parameters that might limit the applicability of the general principles.
- Conduct coordinated research and development programs to correct identified deficiencies.
- Provide a global forum for free information exchange by which a continuous dialogue between scientists, regulators, and policymakers can be maintained.

Socioeconomic Concerns

The socioeconomic impacts of biotechnology are a focus of considerable concern and controversy in developing countries. Questions arise regarding the likely socioeconomic consequences of biotechnology for vulnerable sections of the population. Among these concerns and questions are those listed below:

- Substitution of developing countries' agricultural and/or industrial exports
- Lower commodity and raw material sales and prices due to overproduction
- Increased or decreased agricultural land value
- Relocation of the production of certain materials from developing country farms to industrialized countries' laboratories
- Decreased dependence of industrial countries on developing countries
- Relocation of the production of certain materials from one country to the other
- Fall in employment if conditions necessitate less work
- Increased marginalization of small farmers and strengthening of large-scale farms
- Accelerated migration from rural areas and overcrowding in urban settlements
- Northern and private enterprise domination and foreign control of the technology
- Inequitable conditions for acquiring new biotechnologies

- Abundance of traditional techniques, technologies, and practices already mastered by developing countries
- New types of technological dependence and increased external dependence on industrialized countries
- Direction of biotechnology towards export products rather than products for local needs
- Increased competition among nations and between industrial and developing countries for traditional markets
- Inequitable distribution of biotechnology benefits and income as industrial and developing countries' needs may differ considerably
- Erosion of the genetic diversity required for continuous agricultural and industrial development.

The impact of these changes is likely to be profound and irreversible, particularly on developing countries, since these changes are taking place and most countries have not made policy decisions on how to respond to them.

Regulatory Concerns

There is no consensus on the need for, or scope and nature of, a globally binding regulatory framework for safety in biotechnology, particularly on the release of GMOs. Some feel that modern biotechnology is in the early stages of development, during which advances in techniques and ideas for application are proceeding in the absence of appropriate regulatory control. Over the past decade biotechnology has been perceived as a subject of contained scientific research, and appropriate regulatory measures were accordingly developed and imposed. These measures were not particularly designed to regulate the uncontained applications of biotechnology products and processes developed from basic research, such as the release of GMOs from the laboratory to the environment. It is therefore important that a thorough assessment be undertaken for each development that will make use of biotechnological advances. At the same time the biotechnology industry feels that too much attention is being paid to remote and negligible risks and is expressing great concern about the prospects of excessive restrictions that could limit biotechnology research and application.

Questions arise regarding the capacity of existing regulatory approaches and institutions to address issues related to safety in biotechnology. From a review of existing guidelines and legislation at both the national and international levels, it may be noted that: (a) relative to safety considerations associated with contained applications, little attention has been paid to uncontained applications of biotechnology; (b) a large number of countries have no national safety framework regulating living modified organisms (LMOs) resulting from biotechnology; (c) existing national biosafety regulations address only activities relating to domestic handling and use of LMOs; (d) efforts at promoting international agreements on biosafety often address issues from different perspectives; and (e) relevant international agreements and guidelines currently under consideration are limited in scope. In essence they lack the qualities that would characterize effective biosafety frameworks; that is, they should be flexible, transparent, predictable, focused with clear objectives, cost-effective, and adaptable to accommodate different environmental, socioeconomic, and cultural conditions.

Political and Public Concerns and Perceptions

Also of concern are the risks of biotechnology applications whose environmental or socioeconomic long-term impact, or both, is unknown, and the possible diversion of research in this area to the production of organisms that are hazardous to health or the environment and could be deliberately released in case of war or conflict. The difficulty posed by their detection and monitoring is mobilizing public and political concerns at the national, regional, and international levels.

Another key concern is the limited flow of information and resulting lack of transparency due to the dramatic changes being seen in the area of property rights. The biotechnology industry in industrial countries is "locking up" the new technologies through patents, and this trend is growing. In the past most inventors were satisfied with the product type protection. Under the existing patent systems of industrial countries, biotechnology industries are allowed to protect the product as well as the process, and therefore to limit the flow of technical information. Although advances in basic technology research were made in public academic institutions, the application of research findings is being undertaken by the private sector. Over the years large biotechnology corporations have formed a wide range of institutional arrangements with universities and research institutions to ensure the continuity of innovation, accessibility of scientific findings, and rights to license the resulting technologies. Development and diffusion of any technology would essentially be based on the international exchange of technology through technology-transfer agreements, training, and research collaboration. Procedures and policies that would promote widespread access to these technologies are still lacking. The fact that most biotechnology information is governed by secrecy and intellectual property rights reduces the amount of information available to the scientific and regulatory communities and the public. This increases uncertainty and reduces the capacity of the public to make appropriate decisions about the risks involved.

Strict regulations in some of the industrialized countries on the release of GMOs or their products might encourage some biotechnology industries to conduct their experiments in developing countries without government knowledge or approval, because of lack of regulation, technical information, and public accountability. It is strictly legal, as there are no laws in these countries requiring prior government clearance or consent. Existing guidelines adopted by some industrial countries to govern the release of GMOs do not contain provisions for testing and application of organisms in other countries. This opens the door for the biotechnology industry to enter into bilateral agreements with other countries (where legislation is nonexistent) to test new biotechnology products and probably to locate their production facilities in these countries. The biotechnology industry, while respecting the environmental legislation of their countries, should also comply with this legislation elsewhere.

While biotechnology should address more effectively the needs of sustainable development, some biotechnology research is being directed towards unsustainable development and does not necessarily reflect the long-term interests of the international community. In theory biotechnology would help to make agricultural practices more environmentally sound by eliminating or reducing heavy reliance on potentially polluting agrochemicals. But now biotechnology is being used to extend the agrochemicals era. For example, instead of fusing the technology to make crops resistant to pests and thus reduce the need for pesticides, biotechnology is being used to develop plants resistant to pesticides, thus increasing the use of these chemicals.

Need for an International Framework on Biosafety

Adequate safety mechanisms and international agreements on safety in biotechnology can contribute to the sustainable development of biotechnology and to international trade in biotechnological products. For biotechnology, as with any new technology, the rate of development and level of success are dependent not only upon the scientific and technical capabilities of the country, but also upon a supportive infrastructure and accepting environment in which to introduce and use it. A key component in the formulation of a "biotechnology-accepting" environment is the establishment of adequate national and international regulatory frameworks.

Recently the biosafety issue was considered in two global fora. At the United Nations Conference on Environment and Development (UNCED), Chapter 16 of Agenda 21 on "Environmentally Sound Management of Biotechnology" recognized that the community at large can only benefit maximally from the potential of modern biotechnology if it is developed and applied judiciously, to avoid possible negative side-effects that have diminished the potential of many new technologies in the past. Chapter 16 highlighted the need for internationally agreed-upon principles as a basis for guidelines to be applied for safety in biotechnology.

The issue of safety in biotechnology was also considered within the framework of the Convention on Biological Diversity in Articles 8(g) and 19, paragraphs 3 and 4. In Article 8(g) parties to the Convention are called upon to establish or maintain means to regulate, manage, or control the risks associated with the use and release of LMOs resulting from biotechnology that are likely to have adverse impacts on the conservation and sustainable use of biological diversity.

In Article 19(3) the parties are called upon to consider the need for and modalities of a protocol for the safe transfer, handling, and use of LMOs resulting from biotechnology that may have an adverse effect on the conservation and sustainable use of biological diversity. Article 19(4) states that each party is obliged directly, or by requiring any natural or legal person under its jurisdiction providing the organisms referred to in paragraph 19(3), to provide any available information about the use and safety regulations required by that party in handling such organisms, as well as any available information on the potential adverse impact of the specific organisms concerned, to the party into which those organisms are to be introduced.

As a follow-up to some of the actions called for in Chapter 16 of Agenda 21, and in support of the work undertaken by the Conference of the Parties to the Convention on Biological Diversity on development of a protocol on the safe transfer, handling, and use of LMOs resulting from modern biotechnology that may have adverse effects on the conservation and sustainable use of biological diversity, guidelines have been developed by the United Nations Environment Programme, based on a draft prepared by the Netherlands and U.K. departments of the environment. The guidelines reflect common elements and principles derived from relevant national, regional, and international instruments, regulations, and guidelines, and draw upon experience already gained through their preparation and implementation. They are based on the premise that adequate mechanisms for risk assessment, risk management, and capacity building through—among other things—the exchange of information and the use of these guidelines at the national, regional, and international levels can contribute significantly to safety in biotechnology.

The guidelines address the human health and environmental safety of all types of application of biotechnology, from research and development to commercialization of biotechnological products containing or consisting of organisms with novel trait(s). They recognize that before such biotechnological products are placed on the market they must comply with any specific product requirements, such as food safety, efficacy, and quality; but these matters are not addressed in the guidelines. The guidelines can be implemented by using existing structures and measures or by introducing new ones.

However it must be stressed that neither an international biosafety protocol nor guidelines will, in and of themselves, ensure the safe development and application of biotechnology. There must be a capacity to implement the regulations based on sound scientific principles with consistency, competence, and expedience.

Regulatory Framework Issues

Biosafety Regulations and Processes
Desmond Mahon

This meeting is on biosafety; so far I have heard a great deal about biotechnology, but not very much about biosafety. So I would like to take the discussion back to biosafety by spending a few minutes talking about the Convention on Biological Diversity (CBD), because it addresses a number of the issues that have been talked about here, and then focusing on biosafety under the Convention.

We are talking about international regulatory mechanisms. You can look at this as two separate and independent components or as an international regulatory framework. The international framework could consist of two pieces, a national regulatory framework that is integrated from all the individual states, and an international framework that requires loss of sovereignty, or a combination of both. With the CBD, you come up with both.

What does the Convention say about regulatory frameworks for biotechnology? The Convention's objective is to ensure the conservation and sustainable use of biodiversity. In other words, there are two halves. It does not just say we should keep biodiversity, it is good, and we need it. It is says we must work on mechanisms by which we can safely use biotechnology to increase the wealth of the world, to increase equity and benefits worldwide. So there are three considerations under the CBD: conservation, sustainable use, and equitable sharing of benefits.

The CBD also contains a variety of articles that call upon sovereign states to address specific items, preferably in a consensual mode. Intellec-

tual property is one, indigenous knowledge is another, equitable sharing of wealth and traditional methods are others. Everything we have talked about during this conference is addressed under the CBD, but these issues are not biosafety. They are aspects of biodiversity and the protection and use of biodiversity.

Biosafety is addressed twice in the CBD. It is first addressed in Article 8(g), which says that each Party to the Convention should develop or maintain the procedures required to be able to assess the risks associated with living modified organisms and their release into the environment. The governments that are Parties to the CBD have agreed to this, and are developing national systems.

The second reference to biosafety is in Article 19(3), which says the Parties shall determine the need for, and the structure and modalities of, a protocol on biosafety. That protocol would be an international instrument.

In looking at the proposed protocol the first thing one must consider is the mix-up between policy, science, and legislation. The discussion of whether or not there is a need for such a protocol is past. Eighteen months ago the Parties to the CBD (168 states and one economic region)agreed that we need an international protocol. So there is no longer dispute as to whether or not to have a protocol, because the Parties have decided to have one. This was a policy decision.

The basic premise that we accept is that the governments who made those decisions sought advice from their scientific advisers and either acted upon it or declined to use it. It does not really matter. The decision has been made, so there will be a protocol.

What is the difference between the protocol and the Convention? The Convention lays out policies that governments have agreed to, and then says: "Go away and do it your way." In other words, Article 8(g) does not say: "Here is how you will establish your national regime and this is what it must do." It simply says you must have one.

Under these circumstances the U.N. Environment Programme international technical guidelines on biosafety have been an extremely useful tool. The guidelines lay out, for those countries that do not have a regulatory structure, the steps to follow in developing one, taking into account the flexibility and fluidity of the system. But they do not demand; they simply say: "These can be of benefit."

The protocol, however, is a law, and law is not subject to flexible interpretation. The law will be implemented by Parties that ratify the protocol as a separate instrument to the Convention.

What stage have we reached with the protocol? In the first phase we reached the point of looking at the content of the protocol; that is, the articles. Governments were requested to provide specific ideas and, if they could, possible text for articles under the protocol, and we received many good ideas. The next meeting on the protocol will try to put this material into a form from which the actual articles can be put on paper for negotiation.

In other words we have not yet arrived at a real negotiation process. What we have is rather a need to get to a negotiating text from which everyone can start to negotiate what they want in and want out. It will have to be a concrete discussion focusing on what is wanted from the protocol and what role it should play.

When the Parties to the Convention sit down to draft the protocol, many of the articles will address procedures, but some will address specific issues. Clearly, if the protocol is to address potential risks, both risk assessment and risk management must be addressed. It is absolutely clear that risk assessment is, in general, a scientific issue. There is a consensus, at least in the developed world, that regulation should be based on a science-based risk assessment, and everybody believes it for their own reasons. What you

will get eventually is a science-based methodology of assessment that is as up to date as possible, based on current science.

Risk management is not a science-based approach; it is a pragmatic approach. It may be absolutely perfect in one scenario and absolutely useless in another. You cannot take an international system and say: "Apply this method of risk management in these conditions." If it works in North Dakota, it is highly unlikely to work in the Central African Republic. It is simply not appropriate. You can only provide guidance on risk management.

Another difference between the Convention and the protocol is what the protocol does and does not do. I have constantly heard the terminology "regulation." The protocol would require that an exporting entity provide sufficient information to the competent authority in the importing country to allow the latter to make a risk assessment.

Terminology is incredibly important. I do not consider a requirement to provide information for a risk assessment or the development of a risk assessment to be regulation of either an industry or a product. When the competent authorities in the importing country have made a decision, they may decide to regulate the product, impose conditions, or reject the application. That is regulation. So the protocol does not regulate the industry; it simply requires that a sovereign state be provided with the information it needs to make a decision. The protocol also indicates that it is a sovereign right of the importing country to make that decision.

By definition the protocol also has other consequences. It automatically brings about harmonization, which is a benefit to society and to the industry. It establishes a transparent process because it will be visible to everyone what information, at a minimum, has to be provided for an assessment. What that information is will be determined by the Parties, because they must make these decisions in the design of the protocol. Governments will presumably have sought advice from their scientists, from their own legislators, from any group they felt could provide them with competent advice. I feel that groups here can provide them with competent advice, but they have got to focus on what point the Parties have reached in the process.

There are several other outstanding issues, which I call "generic" issues, that await discussion, such as socioeconomics, liability and compensation, and scope.

The question of socioeconomics was tabled during the process of developing the protocol. It is a significant issue. A basic question being posed by many countries is the inclusion of socio-economics in a protocol, and then subsidiary to that, its inclusion in a risk assessment. Are socioeconomic factors an appropriate item to be included in a risk assessment? And if not in the risk assessment, is it appropriate to include them in the protocol—keeping in mind that the protocol will do more than simply look at risk assessment?

The second items that clearly will come up for discussion are liability and compensation, which are particularly thorny issues. This was touched upon this morning. These two items will be major issues for debate by the Parties over the next week, because they will have to begin to reach consensus on what to include in the protocol.

The third absolutely critical item is scope, and by scope I mean: to what will the protocol apply? The scope is already somewhat limited, in that it is a protocol on living modified organisms, which is wider than genetically modified organisms (GMOs) because there is obviously international debate as to what a GMO is. That differs from country-to-country, and indeed from agency-to-agency within any country. So the Parties wisely elected to use a neutral term and wait to see if the discussion will be resolved.

The terms of reference provided by the Conference of the Parties restricts the scope of the protocol at this point to transboundary movement; in other words, taking an organism and moving it across a border to a receiving country. So the scope of the protocol in terms of its generic application is quite restricted. But the scope of the protocol in terms of what products or organisms would fall under it and the requirement for advanced, informed procedures has not been determined.

It may be useful to bear in mind that for many reasons the international and national instruments, while they may differ in scope, really cannot differ dramatically regarding the procedure used for determining or assessing risk. Because if you have the same product produced inside the country—as opposed to imported into the country—the assessment procedure under a variety of international instruments must be similar.

My last comment is that having done the assessment, the final decision may have absolutely nothing to do with science. The risk assessment may and probably should be science-based, but the decision on regulating or import need not be. Legislators are the people who make decisions, and very few of them are practicing scientists. So do not expect the decision to mirror science. There are many more aspects that go into the making of a decision than, to use a colloquial term, a "science-based risk assessment."

Regulatory Framework Issues

Intellectual Property Rights, the Private Sector, and the Public Good
Timothy W. Roberts

What has intellectual property (IP) to do with biosafety? While the connection is not direct, it was decided that this conference should have some discussion of IP because of the level of interest in the subject. This talk is a rapid survey.

First, why do we have IP at all? Madame Curie was quoted this morning, to the effect that all knowledge is for humanity. That is the general rule: all knowledge should be free and freely available for use. This is a subset of the general principle that people should be free to do as they choose insofar as it does not damage others. IP is an exception to this rule, but it must be kept in balance.

"We must always bear in mind that monopoly legislation is the end result of a balancing act; is the restraint on competition justified by the benefits it gives to society at large?"[1]

What are the objectives of IP? They are of two types:

1. *Societal goals*: To encourage invention, investment in innovation, and disclosure of new technology

2. *Equity goals*: To recognize and reward the innovator.

The patent system makes a bargain with the inventor: in return for disclosure of the invention, the inventor receives the exclusive right to use it for a limited period. I remark in passing that inventors are often highly motivated and need little encouragement. Investors are more cautious. Innovation requires investment as well as invention, and without the protection of a patent such investment will often not be made.

"Traditional" forms of IP are of two types. The first includes copyrights, trademarks, and designs. While some doubt whether it is fair to give monopolies to inventors, few challenge the right of authors or composers to protect against copying. The second type, including patents and plant variety rights, is more relevant to biotechnology.

Traditional safeguards, which are essential to a proper balance of rights include:

- Limited term (except trademarks). Copyright is for the life of the author plus 70 years in Europe; patent rights are generally for 20 years from the date when the patent specification was filed. Note that development can take ten years off this patent life.

- "You cannot stop people from doing what they were doing before." This is a general principle. If it seems to be violated, either there is a misunderstanding or something has gone wrong and needs to be put right. The fundamental principle is that you cannot take existing knowledge out of the public domain by patenting. This means that public goods are protected from expropriation.

How do these principles apply in biotechnology? Biotechnology innovations are expensive to develop, particularly because of essential safety testing, and easy to copy—in fact, they copy themselves. Thus there is a special need for strong protection.

But does this mean allowing people to protect natural genes that they have not invented? We see many patents apparently claiming natural genes; this causes great concern. In Europe, particularly, the law says that you cannot patent discoveries, you can only patent inventions. Genes are discoveries, therefore they cannot be patented. This argument does not apply in America because the law is differently phrased. An invention is defined as an invention or discovery (35 USC 100). But in fact, though different words are used, there is little if any difference on this point between U.S. and European law. I speak as one who has spent most of his working life patenting discoveries, mostly of pesticidal activity in chemicals. The important principle is that patents must not stop people from doing what they were doing before. Thus, a patent related to a natural gene sequence must be limited to the use of something that did not exist before; the isolated sequence, for example, or recombinant DNA containing it. Most U.S. "gene" claims do this explicitly; some European patents do not (which is a pity, as it causes misunderstanding), but they will have the same effect as the U.S. claims.

As well as such "traditional" IP rights we have an emerging area of newer rights, not always considered as intellectual property but nevertheless directly analogous. These include the Convention on Biological Diversity (CBD), "farmers' rights," and traditional resource rights of indigenous peoples.

The CBD asserts sovereignty over genetic resources held within borders and sets norms for the use of those resources by others. "Farmers' rights" is an idea only enunciated in the 1980s, although its roots go much further back. Newer still is the idea of indigenous resource rights. This comprises the rights of indigenous people to their way of life and all that it involves, including the technologies that they practice, which hold considerable promise in some areas. This is an important and contentious issue; I mention it only to introduce a brief discussion of the use by others of traditional knowledge—or its misuse, sometimes called "biopiracy."

Many people are aware of the controversy about patents on the Neem tree. There is a complex of around 40 patents, mostly filed in the U.S. in the names of various patentees, based on uses of the neem extract derived from the Neem tree. This is an Indian tree that has many traditional uses, in particular, as a natural insecticide, and its properties have been known and used in India for thousands of years.

Several questions arise. Is it wrong that industry should monopolize existing traditional knowledge? It is not difficult to answer that question; it is surely contrary to everyone's idea of equity and common sense. It is equally contrary to the fundamental patent principle mentioned above. To be fair, it seems quite doubtful that the Neem tree patents that caused the trouble did, in fact, infringe this principle. What was being claimed was not the traditional uses of the Neem tree extract, but a new, improved formulation of that extract, which allegedly lasted longer. However, there are other patents that may well infringe this principle. There is a U.S. patent on male-sterile plants of the South American cereal quinoa in a form suitable for making hybrids. It is claimed that such plants have been known for many years in Bolivia. There is a U.S. patent on the use of the spice turmeric to heal wounds, a use for turmeric that has apparently been known for centuries in India.

A more difficult question is whether industry should be free to develop and improve traditional knowledge. It has contributed nothing to the production of such knowledge. I suggest that we should apply the principle set out at the beginning of this paper, that is, all knowledge is free unless there is a good reason why it should not be. If traditional knowledge can be developed and improved, then there does not seem to be sufficient reason to prevent such improvements from being patented, provided the original knowledge remains free.

Now some further consideration of farmers' rights. These were defined in the United Nations Food and Agriculture Organization International Undertaking in the 1980s as: "Rights arising from the past, present, and future contributions of farmers in conserving, improving, and making available plant genetic resources." At that time they were vested in the international community, which was seen as a trustee to conserve the rights and distribute benefits arising from their use. However, this formulation does not fit well with the national rights in germplasm now recognized by the CBD. In consequence the International Undertaking is being renegotiated—slowly and with great difficulty. It would be reckless to predict how that will come out.

The CBD has three main objectives: conservation of biodiversity, sustainable use of biodiversity, and equitable sharing of the benefits of such use. What is the relevance of intellectual property rights, in particular, patents, to these objectives? They do not contribute significantly to conservation. They do provide an incentive to develop sustainable uses (and, of course, nonsustainable uses). Their greatest use can be in recovering from ultimate consumers a proportion of the value such uses generate. Such value is then available to be shared with suppliers of the biodiversity.

An important current controversy is whether the Convention should be backdated to earlier than the date on which it entered into force (29 December 1993). If so, how far? Any backdating will amount to retrospective legislation, always difficult to administer and often unfair. A modest backdating (10 years or so) hardly seems to meet the perceived problem, while a back- dating of several centuries or more would raise all sorts of difficult historical questions. This difficulty is best settled by specific voluntary arrangements.

There is a not good deal about intellectual property in the CBD. Generally, the drafters seem to have assumed that IP was a problem rather than an opportunity. But the CBD clearly recognizes intellectual property rights. Article 16.2 requires transfers of technology under the Convention to take proper account of IP. I quote Article 16.5: "The Contracting Parties, recognizing that patents and other intellectual property rights may have an influence on the implementation of this Convention, shall cooperate in this regard subject to national legislation and international law in order to ensure that such rights are supportive of and do not run counter to its objectives."

While it is generally assumed that this is a warrant for limiting the application of IP to genetic resources, it can also be argued that IP can support the objectives of the Convention and therefore should be extended.

There is another very important international convention that relates to IP and is often seen as being directly opposed to the CBD. This is TRIPs (Trade-Related aspects of Intellectual Property), a creature of the World Trade Organization that lays down minimum IP standards for members. I quote and paraphrase parts of Article 27:

27.1 "Patents shall be available... *without discrimination as to...the field of technology.*"

27.2 "Inventions, the prevention within their territory of the commercial exploitation of which is necessary to protect public order or morality, including ...to avoid serious damage to the environment" *need not be patented.* [emphasis added]

27.3 Plants and animals need not be patented, but plant varieties must have some form of effective protection.

The general rule is that all types of invention must be allowed patents, regardless of the field of technology (27.1). However there are public policy exceptions (27.2). If commercial exploitation of an invention has to be prevented for various public policy reasons, including serious damage to the environment, no patent need be granted. It does not include ethical objections to patenting lifeforms, unless these are so serious that commercial exploitation of such lifeforms is also forbidden.

Article 27.3 provides further special exceptions. According to 27.3, not all lifeforms are required to be patented: it is not obligatory under TRIPs to offer patent protection for plants and animals. But plant varieties have to have some form of protection; for example, by plant variety rights, in accordance with the Union for the Protection of Varieties Convention.

The negotiation of Article 27.3 was extremely controversial, and the ultimate compromise suited few. In consequence it was agreed that it would be reviewed four years from the start of the Convention; that is, in 1999. There are widely differing views about what will happen. One view is that the only option will be to narrow the restriction on patenting, or even to abolish it. This is said to be supported by the history of the negotiations. Another view is that this will be a splendid opportunity to confirm and widen the existing exceptions, which many TRIPs participants want.

To conclude, I have two questions. First, is there a conflict between the CBD and TRIPs? Some people see these two conventions as being in partial or even direct opposition. If this were correct, it is not clear how the conflict would be settled. I suggest that there is no inevitable conflict. One would not expect one, since over 100 countries have subscribed to both conventions and they can readily be construed to be consistent with one another. Second, in the face of all these rights, of so many diverse kinds, how can anything new and useful ever be developed and exploited? It is not simple, and there are no easy answers— such as hoping that some of the rights will go away. We will have to work out practical accommodations. Above all we shall need moderation and patience.

Note

1. J. Laddie, "Copyright: Over-strength, Over-regulated, Over-rated?" Stephen Stewart Memorial Lecture, 1995.

Discussion
Moderator: Hamdallah Zedan

Sivramiah Shantharam: I would like to comment on the statement that the intellectual property rights (IPR) issue may not have much to do with biosafety, which should be the focus of discussion here. In every forum I have gone to in developing countries, these biosafety, IPR, and ethical issues in biotechnology get so intertwined that you can make very little progress towards facilitating safe deployment of genetically engineered organisms.

Biosafety should be delinked from discussions on ethics and IPR because at this stage, in most of the developing countries, what we are looking for is safe, effectively terminated field testing under closely monitored conditions using reasonable available physical, biological, and temporal biosafety safeguards.

We seem not to be making any progress towards that goal at all.

Audience comment: Desmond Mahon raised some very serious issues about the Convention on Biological Diversity and the biosafety protocol. One issue is that there is no socioeconomic factor in the risk management or risk assessment process. Should the protocol take into account the socioeconomic factor?

Second, he stated that the decisionmaking process is not scientific in nature and the sovereign state makes decisions based on political and other factors. Are there safeguards in the event that industry does not buy the decision? This is not done only in developing countries; it has hap-

pened in industrial countries. What if they let an unsafe product pass?

Finally, should the protocol have a clause to state liability of the producer if, down the road, the product shows safety hazards in developing countries, away from the countries that have really strong laws on that?

Desmond Mahon: I did not say there is no socioeconomic factor in the protocol. I said that what is happening is that socioeconomics is currently one of the major items to be discussed, and there are two views on it.

One is that it should be included in the risk assessment. Another is that it should not be in the risk assessment or potentially even in the protocol.

The question was, if you make a science-based risk assessment, whereas there is relative agreement on the Western sciences in molecular biology and many of the risk assessment components, there is not international agreement on the science of socioeconomics. So it is extremely difficult to put it into an instrument.

Should the protocol include it? That is for the Parties to the Convention to decide. It is not an issue that the secretariat can have a position on. It is something the Parties are going to discuss in great detail and potentially at great length.

Clearly the decisionmaking process is not science-based. If we use a science-based risk assessment, the determination of risk is science-based. The determination of acceptable risk is not. It is a political decision that stays with the sovereign states.

When risk is assessed for any given LMO, the importing country will make a decision. It may not be based upon the level of risk. It might be based upon a dozen different factors. That is true in every country in the world. But the determination of risk should be singular and unique. That is a different thing.

Mae-Wan Ho: Many countries have been arguing within the protocol process for a legally binding international biosafety protocol. Desmond Mahon seemed to say that that is not true and that it was up to the importing and exporting parties themselves to decide on the precise nature of what information is going to be given and accepted.

He did say that the importing country has the sovereign right to make a decision on whether to accept. I wonder whether that is part of the legally binding international biosafety protocol, because if it is not, then it is still up to individual countries to intimidate another country into accepting their products.

There is a natural link between intellectual property rights and biosafety, which is the issue of responsibility and liability. The biotechnology company, or whoever is benefiting commercially from the patent, should also have responsibility for liability. This brings up another very crucial biosafety issue—segregation and labeling, without which there is no way we can trace or prosecute the liable party.

Timothy Roberts: Regarding the point about responsibility of the patentee in cases where the invention proves dangerous, I can see that this is a very attractive proposition, but I really do not think it is accurate. The responsibility if anything goes wrong lies with the person who put it on the market.

An invention will be exploited in a particular form, and that particular form is the form that must be tested and regulated to make sure that it is safe. It is the responsibility of whoever puts that on the market to make sure that it is safe. It is not the responsibility of the patentee. The patentee is somebody who has had a broad idea, like somebody writing a book.

Desmond Mahon: With respect to the comment on the protocol, by definition the biotechnology protocol—any protocol under a convention—is a legally binding instrument for those who become parties to the protocol. It is a nested series. Currently 169 countries and organizations have ratified the Convention. That means the Convention is binding on those 169. Some countries have not, so it is not binding on them.

Under the Convention a protocol is developed. The process is the same. The 169 countries who ratified the Convention are asked to ratify the protocol. If 110 of them do, it is binding on those 110. It is not binding on the others. So it is a legally binding instrument for those who ratify it.

On the second question, you must remember that I am in the position of telling you what other people have done, not what they are going to agree to in the end. They are in the middle stage.

In that middle stage they are developing articles. Potentially the articles will include a description of the information that must be provided to an importing competent authority. There are a variety of options in that. There are options that say the company must provide the information, that the state must provide the information, that the state must do the risk assessment or the state must not do the risk assessment.

These decisions have not been made by the parties yet. There is now a series of options laid down upon which a consensus will eventually be reached as to which ones will be included in the Convention. But it is relatively clear that there will be an identification of the information that should be provided in the notification under the protocol, and that will be binding. That will be the minimum. Clearly an importing country will always have the option to state "we want more."

Safe handling and use is included in the context of the protocol. It is transboundary movement of living, modified organisms and it is a biosafety protocol on transport, handling, and use. But that will clearly be interpreted different ways by parties in the discussions, so I have no final say on what they will mean by "use."

Regarding labeling and segregation: segregation is not an issue that has been dealt with yet; labeling is an issue that has been dealt with in packaging, in terms of transboundary movement and transport, so that will be within a component of the protocol.

Finally, liability and responsibility: if as a sovereign state you have to make a decision as to whether or not to import, then with sovereign responsibility goes sovereign liability. It is something you choose or do not choose. The strength of liability or compensation will be determined by the Parties.

Jeremy Wright: I am from the Wellness Foundation, and I have a question on patents and intellectual property. The intent of the law, as I understand it, is to give a certain group of people the right to exploit something "for profit."

But when it comes to who assumes responsibility when something goes wrong, it is fine, in theory, when you say it is the sovereign nation or the corporation that introduces it. When you come to the actual case though, suddenly there is bankruptcy and nobody can get compensated, or the public health authorities take over or something like that. Arguments over who will pay the cost of the cleanup can go on for decades.

So the issue of accountability and responsibility is not nearly as clear-cut as you indicated that it might be, from a very practical point of view.

Timothy Roberts: Intellectual property is generally not the right to exploit something for profit. It is the right to stop other people from exploiting it. And it may well be that it cannot be safely exploited; if not, then there is a need for appropriate laws to stop people from exploiting it. That is quite separate from the intellectual property side.

But I maintain my view that those who actually do something are responsible for the consequences of their actions, not those who suggested that it might be done or even those who have acquired the legal right to prevent others from doing it. It is the form in which it is done that is crucial to whether it is safe or profitable or ethical or anything else. It is the specific form that is chosen that is crucial there.

Jeremy Wright: I agree with you totally on the principle that whoever introduces something should be held responsible. My question was to do with the fact that, in practice, there is no recourse and no enforceability of that theoretical responsibility.

Kheryn Klubnikin: When the Biodiversity Convention was being assembled, one of the problems was the disconnect between the traditional English notion of rights—in this case intellectual rights—and traditional rights.

The recent application for quinoa patents might be a good example of indigenous knowledge about the use of plants. The knowledge was developed under a different system of rights and a different understanding, which is about the rights of the community. It has nothing to do with rights of individuals.

Is it moral and appropriate to impose the Western world's notion of intellectual property rights on a traditional group, or is there a need to bring the two different concepts of rights and law together in a more equitable way?

Timothy Roberts: The point on traditional rights is a very serious question. The quinoa patents, on the face of it, look like a serious injustice to the people of South America, whose material has been appropriated without their permission, as well as a defect in a patent system.

As a patent attorney I would be inclined to come up with a technical solution for that, but the point is that these things happen. I do not know how traditional rights are to be reconciled with a Western system. This is not going to be a problem only in the intellectual property sphere. It may be a more general problem, but I am all in favor of keeping an open mind as to what the answer is.

Reviewing the Evidence

Are the Opportunities of Genetically Modified Organisms Being Fully Exploited?

Panel Presentation
George Tzotzos

In the late 1970s and early 1980s there was widespread belief that biotechnology could revolutionize agriculture by genetically engineering plants to fix nitrogen or resist biotic and abiotic stresses. Accomplishing research goals has been a more painstaking exercise than originally thought, and it is only now that we are observing the first commercial applications of biotechnology. Yet the pace of scientific advancement has been such that many breakthrough technological innovations are used routinely, and an increasing number of laboratories in the developing world make use of powerful and sophisticated technologies and equipment. As a consequence the scope of National Agricultural Research Systems (NARS) has been expanded tremendously.

Nonetheless, attempting to assess biotechnology's potential impact—or lack thereof—as a source of economic growth and social benefit in the developing world is a task confounded by the infancy of technological commercialization and the concomitant lack of paradigms.

The derivative question of whether the opportunities presented by transgenic crop plants are being fully exploited, with particular reference to poor farmers in rural areas, requires the following to be addressed:

- Is biotechnology responding to the needs of farmers?
- Are selected farming sectors benefiting from biotechnology at the expense of others?
- Are farmers playing a role in shaping the innovation strategies of agrobiotechnological research?

Indirect answers may be afforded by an assessment of the transgenic crops that are currently undergoing field trials or being commercialized. This reveals the dominant role of international agrobiotechnology enterprises in setting priority research and development (R&D) targets. Transformation of crops of importance for the developing world (such as sweet potato or cassava), perennials such as cocoa and coffee, and legumes are conspicuous for their absence from the list of priorities of the agrobiotechnology industry. However this situation is likely to change as several national and international research programs focus on the transformation of some of these crops (for example, cassava and sweet potato). Should this be the case, some of the potential socioeconomic benefits of biotechnology at the level of small-scale farming communities may materialize.

Although technological innovation in agriculture has been driven by the private sector, it cannot be taken for granted that efficiency and profit are the exclusive criteria for the development of new products. In industrialized countries research has often been guided toward products with greater public acceptance. The situation is different in the developing world, where consumers' purchasing power does not provide a significant incentive for private investment into research directed to local needs.

Nonetheless technological innovation and diffusion are not determined by commercial considerations alone. The role of mediators, such as

60

venture capital institutions and other financial brokers, also influences the capital flow to public and private institutions and firms, particularly the new technology-based firms. Government policies, likewise, have often been instrumental in guiding the pathways of innovation through funding of research, regulation, technology transfer legislation, and appropriate patenting policies.

In the nonindustrialized world, market failure, coupled with the absence of mediator mechanisms and inappropriate government policies on biosafety, intellectual property protection, and technology transfer constitute significant impediments to private investment and innovation in biotechnology. In this regard the effectiveness with which biotechnology can meet domestic needs is crucially dependent upon actions that strengthen the capacity of public and private research systems. Such actions include both the absorption of technological spin-offs that can be adapted to serve domestic needs, and the introduction of policy and institutional reforms conducive to investment in biotechnology.

It is therefore expedient that developing countries gear an important part of their biotechnology research capacity building toward the effective exploitation of existing knowledge, rather than the generation of new knowledge. The use, assimilation, and adaptation of new knowledge should be an integral part of the cumulative learning process that would increase a country's potential for upgrading its R&D capability. Clearly biotechnology alone is not the be-

all and end-all. It is, nonetheless, critical in overcoming some severe bottlenecks of conventional agricultural programs and enhancing their delivery prospects.

The role of the international research system in supporting national R&D programs cannot be overemphasized. However the situation to date is not promising. International donor and technical support agencies have been reluctant to redirect funds from conventional types of capacity building and R&D programs in favor of biotechnology. This is attested to by the fact that funding for biotechnology-related R&D pales in comparison with public-sector investment in agricultural research in industrialized countries—U.S. federal funding for agricultural research in 1996 was an order of magnitude higher—and is totally eclipsed by private investment.

Due to the shortcomings mentioned above, it is likely that the major impacts on the farming systems of the developing world will come from the importation of transgenic crop varieties. Although trade globalization makes this inevitable, the pace at which such varieties are introduced will depend on the price premium they carry, and consequently, on the purchasing power of farmers. The push of transgenic seed upon developing countries is seen at times to be part of a strategy of the agrobiotechnology industry to generate export markets rather than solve agricultural problems. Even if this were so, there are occasions where the two may coincide. Such coincidental convergence of interest should be exploited whenever possible.

Are the Opportunities of Genetically Modified Organisms Being Fully Exploited?

Panel Presentation
Gabrielle Persley

I would like to approach this discussion by looking at five different areas: perceptions, issues, objectives, activities, and outcomes. It has struck me over the past few days that when the international development community thinks about biotechnology, we tend to take a top-down approach, focusing on perceptions and, in decreasing order of priority, issues, objectives, activities, and outcomes.

It might enliven the debate if we focused more on what are the desirable outcomes to which biotechnology could contribute, and then work up the list discussing what activities and objectives would help us achieve those outcomes. What are the key issues that impact on achieving the outcomes? And finally, what are the perceptions from which we will derive the key issues?

In terms of outcomes I think we could all agree that increasing the wealth of people in developing countries, increasing people's health, reducing environmental damage, and conserving biodiversity would be desired outcomes. We could have a lively debate as to how biotechnology can contribute to these outcomes.

In terms of objectives and activities, obviously, it is very important to identify specific problems that could be tackled through biotechnology, particularly those which have proved to be intractable to more conventional approaches. The *Striga* in Africa comes to mind, as do a number of plant diseases and malaria.

A second key objective is to build national capability, not only in terms of scientific capability, but also legal capability and investment. Business communities must be able to look at adequately funding both the research and development aspects of biotechnology and at new paths toward public and private sector partnerships.

If we look, then, at the issues that might affect these programs, we must also consider the implications of international treaties and regulatory frameworks, management of intellectual property rights, public and private investment, and lest we forget, the need to attract the best and brightest science and the best and brightest young scientists to deal with global issues. This gives a key role to the universities in both developing and industrial countries.

Such an approach might help put in perspective the public perception of risk associated with new technologies, consumer acceptance of the new products, and the ethics associated with risk assessment and patenting.

Are the Opportunities of Genetically Modified Organisms Being Fully Exploited?

Panel Presentation
Carlienne Brenner

I propose to bring a somewhat different perspective to the discussion, based on the current status of agricultural biotechnology in a number of developing countries.

At the outset I would like make it clear that I firmly believe that most countries should have their own national science and agricultural research capacity and that there is a need for technological innovation *within* developing countries. There are clear limits to how much technology can be "imported" unless the know-how to make the best use of the technology is available. It is also important that there be a proper balance between the share of research and technology development conducted within developing countries and the share of imported technology, because the kinds of agricultural biotechnology being developed in industrialized countries may not be those most appropriate for production conditions in developing countries.

My presentation is based on the experiences of a number of countries I have studied in the course of my research at the Organisation for Economic Co-operation and Development (OECD) Development Centre. These countries include: in Africa, Kenya and Zimbabwe; in Asia, India, Indonesia, and Thailand; and in Latin America, Colombia and Mexico. I hope that the evidence drawn from these countries might present a middle-of-the-road approach between the diametrically opposed views that were expressed yesterday.

The presentation will cover three sets of issues. The first is agricultural biotechnology research and development (R&D) in developing countries; the second, changing public and private sector roles; and the third, the regulatory framework (including biosafety) and public policy.

With respect to the first set of issues I would like to place biotechnology R&D in the broader context of global trends in investment in agricultural research. One particularly significant statistic that should be kept in mind is that in OECD member countries agricultural research intensity ratios—that is, public agricultural R&D as a share of agricultural gross domestic product—averages about 2.39 percent. For developing countries this ratio is only 0.51 percent.

Against that background a growing number of developing countries are investing in agricultural biotechnology R&D. In some cases they are even setting up new biotechnology institutes. The fact that biotechnology is perceived as offering potential for more environmentally friendly technologies in agricultural production provides a strong incentive.

Pressure is also strong simply to "get into the act." Countries are very susceptible to the real or perceived fear that the technological gap may be widening. Thus in many situations biotechnology R&D has been very much science-driven. In other cases, as George Tzotzos has pointed out, it has been donor-driven.

Thus far biotechnology R&D in developing countries is largely uncoordinated. In most cases institutions conduct their research quite independently of any national coordination effort. Research is also undertaken without a sense of national priorities for biotechnology research and with very little awareness of what would be appropriate given the priorities that have been set for agriculture.

The research taking place is still very predominantly public-sector research carried out in national agriculture research institutes and, increasingly (depending on the country), in universities. Levels of investment are nevertheless still very low compared with those of industrialized countries.

If we think about innovation in agriculture we have to admit that research is only a small part—and perhaps the easiest and least costly part—of creating a new technology and having that technology transferred to the farmer's field. It is what happens beyond successful laboratory research, during the development phase and the distribution or marketing of a new agricultural biotechnology, when the difficulties occur for national agricultural research institutes and universities.

This brings me to the second set of issues: changing public and private sector roles. Following the advice of the World Bank and the International Monetary Fund, a growing number of countries have adopted structural adjustment and liberalization policies. This has meant strong pressure to privatize economic activities formerly undertaken by the public sector.

It has also resulted in problems of maintaining levels of investment for research and development in public research institutions. In addition the development aspect of R&D—usually more costly and time-consuming than the research phase—has often been neglected, with the result that no funds have been allocated.

A third problem facing national agricultural research systems at present is that traditional channels for technology transfer (public extension systems) are in many cases in the process of being either dismantled or privatized, without alternative mechanisms to replace them. In some instances nongovernmental organizations are stepping in to perform that role.

In most countries there is still very little private sector investment in agricultural biotechnology research. There are, however, a growing number of small biotechnology companies, particularly in tissue culture. A growing number of small tissue culture companies are providing improved, disease-free planting material for an increasing number of plants. It is unlikely, however, that in the short term the private sector is going to become involved in segments of the market where growth prospects are poor or in crops grown by smallholders.

There is therefore a need to foster public-private sector collaboration and to seek a better balance in the roles played by the two sectors. This is reflected in a diversity of new public-private sector initiatives for technology development and transfer occurring in developing countries, although there is no time to go into detail here. It is important that incentives be given to promote private sector activity in areas where there is strong potential demand for technology. Such incentives would enable the public sector to focus more sharply on those areas where there is a perceived social need, but where short-term market prospects are poor. An example of such an area is where poor farmers, rather than purchasing seed from the market, exchange it among themselves.

Finally, with respect to the third set of issues and, more specifically, intellectual property rights, most countries have signed the Trade-Related aspects of Intellectual Property Rights Agreement. Governments are therefore committed to the establishment of some kind of national system for intellectual property protection. While the agreement allows some scope with regard to the forms of protection allowed for plants and animals (patents, plant breeder's rights, or a sui generis system) the timeframe is limited. It is important, in deciding what system is most appropriate for a given country's needs, that governments help to create an environment that stimulates local innovation.

Although there is no time to go into it, I would be happy to answer questions on the impact of strengthening and extending intellectual property rights. Overall, impact is likely to be mixed, but it does pose important questions with respect to the future of "public-good technologies." This is something all of us need to be thinking about.

Finally, and of particular relevance to this meeting, if developing countries are to take advantage of what agricultural biotechnology has to offer, it is important that biosafety policy be addressed—whether as national legislation or simply as guidelines. Thus far very few countries have established national biosafety procedures and practices.

Are the Risks of Developing and Releasing Genetically Modified Organisms Being Adequately Evaluated and Assessed?

Panel Presentation
Rita R. Colwell

I plan to very briefly cover the changing perceptions from the first cloning of genes in the early 1970s to the present. The 15-plus years that have intervened have not resulted in any documentable adverse effect of the use of genetically engineered organisms, whether they be plants, microorganisms, insects, or any other forms. The record is fairly clear.

The only report that I know of with regard to use of genetically engineered microorganisms is a study done by a team at the U.S. Environmental Protection Agency, in which they showed some changes in the mixture of fungi after the introduction of an engineered organism into soil. This was reproducible, but subsequent studies did not confirm such a change.

I think that it is important to review the remarkable progress that has been made in the last 15 or so years, especially since the first structure analysis was done by Watson and Crick in the cracking of the code, cloning of genes in the 1970s, and formation of monoclonal antibodies. We now have a good portion of the human genome sequence, some half-dozen microorganisms are fully sequenced, and the plant genome sequencing initiative is well on its way.

One aspect of application is phytoremediation. I think this provides a very dramatic example of the potential application of biotechnology. In this case it is simply using plants, (phytoextraction, filtration of plant roots) to remove toxic metals from polluted waters and soils, and phytostabilization.

This process is being used in the Chernobyl area of Russia, where weedy plants are being put in place and the concentration of the radionucleides allows transformation of sites such as this in a reasonable period of time. It has been carried out in plots by several investigators at Rutgers University, at Savannah in Georgia, and current studies in the Chernobyl area of Russia, where phytoremediation allows reclamation and a translocation capture of radionucleides and heavy metals.

The phytoextraction allows recycling of materials, and by using engineered organisms for heavy metal uptake and concentration it is possible to restore to use farmland that would otherwise be unable to be utilized for decades.

It is important to look at the potential in terms of economic value, and I think the potential is being realized. In most cases the biotechnology promise has been exceeded by practice.

We have come quite a long way from the furor over the use of the bovine hormone. I have seen an advertisement from a farmer in Wisconsin who guaranteed synthetic-hormone free milk. That claim that might have been challenged, since there are many synthetic hormones other than bovine growth hormone.

We should also remember the planting of engineered strawberries in which moon-suited scientists were spraying the strawberries as reporters from several publications stood on the sideline in blue jeans and tennis shoes. So, as to perceptions we have come quite a long way.

The familiarity principle, as espoused and promulgated in a U.S. National Academy of Sciences report about a decade ago, is that when an organism about which relatively little genetic information is known is introduced to a new environment, it may pose an example in which regulation might be more acute.

Introducing a rhizobium into a field from which it had been isolated prior to being engineered for specific properties represents a familiar application of a familiar organism; the restrictions, if any, need not be severe.

Nevertheless the concerns are really for safe application of biotechnologies for agriculture and environmental applications. I think the example of the Swedish Institute of the Environment's Special Committee on Biotechnology is instructive. This mechanism provided developing countries lacking expertise with a committee to advise when a question or an opportunity to employ engineered crops or engineered organisms came up. The team from the Swedish Institute of the Environment was available, and it included experts from countries around the world.

The pattern of analysis outlined by that particular committee, I think, is useful and takes into account harmonizing biosafety guidelines. That is probably the most important message I would like to convey. It is time now for an organization, such as the International Council of Scientific Unions or an international body such as the U.N. Development Programme, to bring together scientists from all countries and develop harmonized, international regulations.

Release of engineered organisms has been extraordinary. By 1991 about 150 field tests had been carried out in the U.S.; by 1997 more than 1,000 field tests had been carried out. As I said in my introductory comment, there has been no adverse effect.

Neither those who hyperbolized biotechnology and said it was going to accomplish great things—such as the giant potato—nor those who were concerned about adverse effects at the other extreme have had their predictions realized. It is time to take a more balanced perspective, analyze the successes, and declare victory in that the regulations that are in place and the procedures that have been employed have allowed us to utilize biotechnology productively, if perhaps a bit more slowly than we would have preferred.

Are the Risks of Developing and Releasing Genetically Modified Organisms Being Adequately Evaluated and Assessed?

Panel Presentation
L. Val Giddings

First, I want to follow up on some of the material that was presented yesterday and give some updated numbers from the Animal and Plant Health Inspection Service (APHIS) of the U.S. Department of Agriculture. APHIS carries out regulatory oversight for genetically engineered organisms in the environment.

I do not see any of my colleagues from APHIS here today, so we are in the ironic position of having someone from the regulated community defending the regulators.

Based on field trials conducted in the United States through March of this year, 27 percent of research and development (R&D) activities subject to regulatory oversight by APHIS was related to herbicide-tolerant plants. Most of the numbers presented by critics of biotechnology in agriculture dramatically overstate the extent of work that is being done with herbicide-tolerant plants and misstate some of the implications of the extent of R&D in this area.

We are seeing substantial and dramatic declines in the amount of herbicides used as weed-control technologies. Furthermore some of the ancillary benefits lead to reductions in the amount of chemical pesticides for associated pests and insect pests.

Most of the research being done is aimed at solving problems of production resulting from constraints due to diseases or insect pests. Viral resistance constitutes about 10 percent, and fungal resistance and other applications about 12 percent, of the current activities subject to regulatory oversight. The most rapidly growing category is related to product quality, such as improved nutritional profiles of commodity crops and other areas that will lead to more direct benefits to the ultimate consumers. It currently constitutes 27 percent of the activities.

Not only is work being done on the majority of cash-producing commodity crops—an area where existing market incentives encourage private investment—but there is a great deal of work being done on smaller crops of interest to smallholders. This information represents only the work that is being done in the United States, as indicated by regulatory approvals carried out by APHIS over the past decade.

Now I would like to talk about the subject that I am supposed to talk about—whether or not the risks of developing and releasing genetically modified organisms (GMOs) are being adequately evaluated and assessed.

First, I would like to distill things and present some essential messages that I think all too often get lost. If we can introduce this perspective into our discussions of biosafety, it will help move organizations like the World Bank beyond the paralysis that was described yesterday, in which they are caught between conflicting viewpoints and cannot resolve the situation and move forward.

Although it is absolutely essential that regulation be firmly grounded in science, regulations themselves and the regulatory decisions made by regulators are not acts of science. They more closely approximate art. This means that much of the discussion about conflicting views over whether or not something is adequately regulated is more akin to a debate over taste in art than a scientific debate over a testable proposition.

Much of our discussion on risk has been framed in terms of inappropriate context; that is, in terms of trying to avoid risk altogether; trying to apply a standard of zero risk. This is the path to paralysis. You cannot achieve zero risk. It is unattainable.

I submit that it is far more useful to frame our discussion in terms of what *acceptable* risk might be—zero risk versus acceptable risk. This is where differences of viewpoint come into play. How much weight do you put upon this or that potential for harm? What kind of context do you put that in?

Talking about risk and trying to apply rigid, quantitative standards is extremely difficult because many of the questions do not have the kinds of ultimately perfect answers that we would like to see, that science strives for. So I think it is more appropriate to couch discussions in terms of absolute versus relative risk.

As we consider how to calibrate our decision-making on risk, there is a great temptation to approximate, to try to reach absolute certainty on questions where there is, in fact, insufficient research data or experience. The regulator is faced with making a decision on a particular proposition—for example: "Is this herbicide-tolerant plant safe enough to allow to go forward in a field trial?" The regulator must ask whether the weight of R&D experience available on this herbicide-tolerant plant is adequate to demonstrate that it generates no risk different from nontransgenic plants and, therefore, that the organism is more than sufficiently safe to be allowed to enter into commercialization.

As we weigh those sorts of questions, it is useful to keep one bellwether in mind. We must bear in mind the distinction between what is nice to know and what is needed to know to make a decision about the relative costs and benefits, or the relative risks; to make a wise decision about whether or not something should go forward.

Are the Risks of Developing and Releasing Genetically Modified Organisms Being Adequately Evaluated and Assessed?

Panel Presentation
Rebecca Goldburg

I am going to examine the question of whether the risks of biotechnology products are being adequately evaluated and assessed, based on my experience working in the United States. Experience in the U.S. is especially relevant because it is here that the majority of field testing and commercialization of genetically engineered crops has occurred to date.

I will argue that even in the "advanced" United States we have not done enough to address biosafety, in terms of both developing scientific information and regulatory capacity. I will use two examples, one in the area of science and one in the regulatory field.

To begin, I will discuss the development of resistance-management plans for so-called "Bt crops"—crops genetically engineered to contain insecticidal proteins from the bacterium *bacillus thurengiensis*. The development of these plants has generated considerable concern that pests will evolve resistance to Bt toxins, which have been widely used in the U.S. in nonengineered spray formulations for several decades. Bt sprays are used both by conventional and organic farmers and are some of our safest insecticides. As a result there is considerable interest in retaining the efficacy of Bt toxins, rather than squandering them on a few years of use in Bt crops.

Three such crops, cotton, corn, and potatoes are now sold commercially in the U.S. Several different varieties of Bt corn containing different genetic constructs of Bt toxins are on the market. The U.S. Environmental Protection Agency (EPA) has compelled companies to develop resistance-management plans for these crops to slow the evolution of Bt-resistant pests.

These plans are based on sound scientific theory, including mathematical models and some small-scale greenhouse and laboratory experiments, but there is no large-scale experimentation or field experience on which to base these resistance-management plans. In other words our current resistance-management plans for Bt crops have not been scientifically validated.

There are a number of other scientific issues regarding Bt resistance-management plans that remain unresolved. For example:

- Current resistance-management plans assume a very simple genetic model of pest resistance to Bt. What steps should be taken if data show that resistance traits involve more than one allele or do not follow patterns of Mendelian inheritance?

- Most of resistance-management theory is designed to prevent one target pest from evolving resistance. But Bt corn and cotton have multiple pests that are affected by their Bt toxins. How do resistance-management plans address the different susceptibilities and behaviors of different pests?

- What action should be taken if resistance is detected?

- How should integrated pest management (IPM) practices be integrated with resistance-management plans?

Given the rather primitive state of resistance management for Bt crops, it is no surprise that experience is revealing significant problems with current resistance-management plans. At least two examples of insect pests have been demonstrated to have substantial survival rates on Bt crops. The survival of these pests violates one of the two fundamental principles underlying resistance-management plans: Bt crops should express very high doses of toxins to kill virtually all the pests on the crop. In short, in some instances current resistance-management plans are being invalidated by experience.

Yet we in the United States seem to be merrily forging ahead without revising resistance-management plans. Bt crops are being planted on huge numbers of acres; enough area, for example, that the EPA is having to consider resistance-management measures for locales where 75 percent of cotton acreage is planted with Bt cotton.

It appears that we are being rather reckless with Bt. We are not taking adequate, scientifically cautious, iterative steps because we do not appear to have the societal restraint to go forward in a more cautious fashion.

Regarding biosafety regulation in the U.S., I will consider two examples: one concerning field releases of genetically engineered organisms and one concerning food safety. I argue that the U.S. regulatory system does not adequately protect public health and the environment from the risks of genetically engineered organisms.

Field releases of genetically engineered crops in the U.S. now receive minimal oversight. Virtually any genetically engineered crop can be field tested after simply notifying the U.S. Department of Agriculture, even if the crop can potentially transfer genetic material, via pollination, to wild relatives. In other words even if a crop exhibits the characteristic that most scientists agree is the foremost biosafety concern for genetically engineered crops, no formal public risk assessment is necessary before field testing.

A similar situation exists in regard to food safety regulation. The U.S. Food and Drug Administration requests that companies voluntarily consult with the agency before marketing genetically engineered crops.

For both field releases and food safety the relevant government agencies have admittedly established safety standards that companies are supposed to meet. But as I have indicated, the U.S. is virtually dependent on companies' good behavior in order to implement these standards. Although many corporations may comply with these standards and follow through on promises to the public of safe practices, there are at least two instances where they have not.

First, Northrup King Company produced and marketed Bt corn without having obtained the registration legally required by the EPA. The agency fined the company in 1996.

Second, Calgene, Inc. violated promises to label its FLAVR SAVR genetically engineered tomato. Calgene commercialized this tomato at a time when issues concerning labeling of genetically engineered foods were new and contentious in the U.S. The company promised the public that the company would label all of its genetically engineered tomatoes as such. However Calgene experienced quality problems with its genetically engineered tomatoes and decided not to sell many of them as branded products. The company then sold many of its genetically engineered tomatoes as ordinary, unlabeled fresh-market tomatoes, violating Calgene's promises to the public.

To sum up, the risks of genetically modified organisms are not being adequately evaluated and addressed in the United States. Since the U.S. is the world's largest producer of biotechnology products and a country with considerable resources, this conclusion is extremely troubling.

I would like to make one last point in response to Rita Colwell's remark that there have not been any adverse effects to date of genetically engineered organisms. She is correct that there have not been any biotechnology disasters. Biotechnology has not, to date, resulted in any Andromeda Strains—or more realistically, in any new pests.

But experience with biotechnology products has not been entirely smooth either. Unexpected events continue to raise a cautionary flag. As I mentioned, there are now a couple of examples of biotechnology crops that do not adequately control pests for purposes of resistance management.

Genetically engineered crops have also unexpectedly exhibited agronomic problems. For example, a recent headline from the *Clarion Ledger* in Jackson, Mississippi read: "Genetic Cotton Misfire." The story discusses recent problems of

Mississippi farmers with genetically engineered, herbicide-tolerant cotton plants in which the cotton bolls shed or are misshapen.

Shedding cotton bolls is not strictly a biosafety concern. Nevertheless, this problem raises a real red flag. Biotechnology companies focus on developing crops with particular agronomic traits and expend considerable effort testing for good agronomic performance. If companies cannot make a number of these crops perform as expected, what does that imply about the results of generally less rigorous, largely voluntary tests for biosafety, which is far less central to companies' mission?

Discussion
Moderator: Michel Petit

Donald Winkelmann: I am chair of the Technical Advisory Committee of the Consultative Group on International Agricultural Research, and I have a question for George Tzotzos.

Typically one would expect the output of biotechnology to lead to increased productivity, hence higher output, hence lower prices, so that consumers should be the ultimate beneficiary of the bulk of the effort in biotechnology. Would consumers be willing to pay the extra costs associated with the product? And can farmers pay the potential extra technology costs of transgenic seeds?

Judith Chambers: My question is directed to Rebecca Goldburg. I get concerned when the products of biotechnology, such as transgenic plants, are held up to a different standard of safety and environmental management than the traditional forms of biotechnology have been. The very first reported incident of biotechnology resistance took place approximately seven years ago, before any transgenic plants were on the market, and was written up in a reputable, peer-reviewed scientific journal. The incident took place in Thailand where biotechnology was being used to control insects, mostly on cruciferous plants, and being intensively used by people who are advocates of the traditional form of biotechnology.

There we had a form of resistance occurring, and I was wondering where the environmental community was in complaining about that particular incident, in which we had a nonengineered biotechnology showing resistance as a result of intensive use.

Desmond Mahon: Two concepts were brought up in the presentations of Rita Colwell and Val Giddings: the concept of familiarity and uncertainty in assessing risk from Rita Colwell, and then acceptable risk from Val Giddings. I do not think there is anybody in the room who can live with zero risk. This is nonsense scientifically and as a regulation.

What I would like you to comment on is coupling the two, specifically for the developing world and for agriculture. When you couple uncertainty with acceptable risk, who sets the level of acceptable risk? Has it got to be equivalent in every scenario, or should it be set for the situation in which the product is going to be developed, and by whom?

Audience comment: We have a situation in which both as a community of scientists and as part of the public, we have to think: do we want zero risk or do we want a low risk, or is it acceptable or not? But you cannot just say zero risk is intolerable. Therefore, I would like to have the panel address the question of whether there has been a good risk assessment.

Mae-Wan Ho: I am dismayed at the complacency shown by the first two speakers of the second panel. Such attitudes make me feel that the only alternative is to have a moratorium and an independent inquiry into all the risks, based on the most up-to-date scientific findings in peer-reviewed, well-referenced journals.

Let me comment on what I regard as fatal flaws in food safety assessment. The joint Food And Agriculture Organization/World Health Organization biotechnology and food safety report proposes a model of risk assessment based on the "no need, don't look, and don't see" triangle. Effectively, the biotechnology industry is given carte blanche to pass whatever they like.

If we are not careful, a list of gruesome products is going to appear on our dinner tables, including failed transgenic experiments and possibly also the residues of plants from which industrial chemicals have been extracted, after which they can be processed for food or animal feed.

The Kendall report has excluded that from its scope, so now I ask: Who or what is responsible for regulating all these things?

Rita Colwell: I apologize for my brevity, which may have been misinterpreted as complacency. I chaired the Environmental Protection Agency's Biotechnology Advisory Committee for about six years. I served on the National Institutes of Health Panel on Biotechnology and also on the Food and Drug Administration's Food Advisory Committee, where we spent at least three days hearing evidence and discussing risks with respect to the FLAVR SAVR® tomato. An enormous amount of work has been done over the last 10-to-15 years looking at risks and assessing benefits for the population.

In the case of some of the issues that are mentioned with respect to biotechnology products, such as allergenicity, I think this is, in general, something that has to be faced whether it is engineered or not. That is a function of proper labeling of food.

Val Giddings: The number of field trials that have been conducted in the United States to date exceeds 3,000 at over 12,000 field-trial test sites. Until five months ago I was with the division of APHIS that conducted the environmental assessments of these, and far from being complacent or from being guided by a "no need, don't look, don't see" criterion, we applied a rigorous criterion of "turn over every stone."

There is a level of scrutiny applied to these new products that exceeds any level that has been applied to other products in agriculture in the history of humanity. It may be argued that this is appropriate, but it certainly cannot be argued that we are underscrutinizing things.

Even under existing notification standards of the U.S. Department of Agriculture (USDA), field trials that are allowed to go forward must be conducted in accordance with performance criteria that essentially amount to biological isolation. Although the potential for gene flow may occur, the field trial is conducted under circumstances that prohibit or prevent such gene flow. So there are still rigorous criteria applied, even under the most streamlined avenue of regulation available under USDA.

Rebecca Goldburg: I was asked some questions about resistance management with Bt crops. First of all, are we applying a different standard to biotechnology crops than we have for other crop plants? The answer is most definitely yes. Is there a good reason for that? Yes, there are two good reasons.

One is that in many ways Bt (*Bacillus thuringiensis*) toxins are different than synthetic chemicals, which have historically been applied as commercial insecticides. Synthetic chemical pesticides are developed by particular companies and are proprietary. Bt has a long history of use. It is a natural chemical. Many people would argue that it is a public good; I would argue that as a public good, it is appropriate for us to have strong public stewardship of Bt.

Second, I would argue that even regarding synthetic chemicals, insecticides, or drugs the U.S.—and probably almost every other country in the world—is only now really beginning to face up to problems with the evolution of resistant diseases. We need to know more to do more. What we are doing with Bt is a step in the right direction, and we should start looking for other types of products as well for resistance management.

Finally, the example was brought up of the evolution of resistance to Bt products with naturally occurring Bt spore preparations, an example from Thailand. That is not the only example; there are several examples in which overuse of Bt spore products has led to the evolution of local resistant insects, and that concerns me greatly.

The difference between these incidents and those of transgenic Bt crops is that Bt microbial spore preparations are still used on very little acreage in most of the world. Transgenic crops are catching on at a tremendous rate; they are being used on millions and millions of acres and have the potential to exert a much stronger selection pressure on pests, in part because most of these crops express Bt toxins in virtually all of their tissues virtually all of the time.

Gabrielle Persley: Some have expressed surprise that some of the findings from experimentation were not as predicted. I would simply say that this is the nature of science. It would be very strange if experimentation did not yield new knowledge both in terms of ecology and genetics. Within the international development community we have two choices, to be either observers of the progress of science or participants.

George Tzotzos: With respect to the question about purchasing ability of farmers in the developing world to absorb transgenic seed, one finds that productivity will increase by bringing in trans-genic seed. Prices may even drop. But small-scale farmers simply do not have the purchasing capacity to buy transgenic seed, or even hybrid seed.

This discussion seems to have been polarized and has addressed only the transgenic applications of genetic engineering. There are other applications of genetic engineering, and they might have significantly higher impacts in increasing productivity in the developing world, for example, molecular-assisted breeding.

Michel Petit: There seems to be a consensus that what is at stake in risk assessment is the level of acceptable risk. But we do not agree on what level of risk is acceptable or even what scientific considerations need to be involved.

Role of International Agricultural Research

Biotechnology and Biosafety in the CGIAR System:
An Efficient, Equitable, and Ethical Path
Timothy G. Reeves

The issues of biotechnology and biosafety are often viewed only through the eyes of the developed world. When those of us in the development community think about these issues, however, the images that come to mind often differ greatly from stereotypical notions of biotechnology and biosafety in industrial countries. It is often forgotten that the biotechnological revolution occurring in the industrial world is gaining momentum in developing countries, and for this reason biosafety issues are assuming even greater importance worldwide. In this paper I would like to discuss these issues as they are perceived by the Consultative Group on International Agricultural Research (CGIAR), the family of international agricultural research centers whose mandate is to help the poor people of this world.

We believe that every man, woman, and child has the right to sufficient food to lead a healthy, productive life, and we are affronted by the fact that this right is not yet a reality. Every day 40,000 people still die from hunger-related diseases. Every day about 1 billion people have less than US$1 to meet their basic needs. This is the world that the CGIAR has resolved to change for the better through research; yet this goal becomes more elusive as our population continues to grow. During the next three decades the population of the developing world will grow by around 200 people per minute. Where will these people get the secure supply of food that should be their birthright? To feed us all, within the next 50 years we will have to produce as much food as the world has produced since 10,000 B.C., which is almost all the food that has been produced since people first began to practice agriculture.

We know that technology, including biotechnology, is one means of transforming food scarcity into food security; but technology alone is not the answer. The technologies that we develop to feed the world must meet four important criteria: they must be environmentally sound, economically viable, socially acceptable, and politically supportable—the four pillars of agriculture. In addition they should promote equity between people, regions, and generations. Agricultural systems that meet these criteria are critical for resource-poor farmers, and they are certainly critical for developing countries relying upon agriculture to power economic growth. Biosafety must be a key component of such systems to ensure that the well-being of future generations is not imperiled.

We also know that technological development has to occur within the right policy framework. Without political will the best agricultural technologies and systems may never benefit the world's poor.

It is within this framework of fostering sustainable, socially just agriculture that I wish to discuss the potential contributions of biotechnology research by the CGIAR centers. I will briefly describe the kinds of research in which the centers are engaged, with a view to highlighting the ways that this research differs from much biotechnology research pursued elsewhere. Next I will discuss how this different research orientation has implications for the way that we and our partners must approach the challenges that are emerging as we attempt to apply the newest agricultural research tools to solving some of the world's oldest problems: poverty and hunger.

Biotechnology Research and the CGIAR

The CGIAR has an investment in biotechnology of around US$30 million per year. This investment may seem small, but it differs greatly from most investments in biotechnology because it focuses on research that is appropriate to the needs of the poor. For example, the International Crops Research Institute for the Semi-Arid Tropics (ICRISAT) is using biotechnology to develop downy, mildew-resistant pearl millet, and the International Institute for Tropical Agriculture (IITA) is developing insect-resistant cowpeas. These areas of research are far from being high priorities for private-sector investment.

At the International Maize and Wheat Improvement Center (CIMMYT) we are using biotechnology to deliver research results to farmers more efficiently and effectively. To cite just one example, we are using molecular marker techniques to shorten the time needed to develop drought-tolerant maize. The approach currently under evaluation could cut the development time for drought-tolerant maize in half, as well as substitute selection in the laboratory for much work in the field. Given that the world is still too familiar with the macabre effects of drought, the merit of this research is obvious.

Another significant research effort at CIMMYT seeks to take advantage of a trait called "apomixis" (asexual reproduction through seed), which results in plants that are exact clones of the mother plant. For several years scientists from the French National Research Institute for Development Cooperation (ORSTOM), working at CIMMYT, have sought to transfer apomixis to maize from Tripsacum, a relative of maize. If farmers had apomictic versions of improved maize varieties and hybrids, they could replant seed from their own harvests each year and still maintain high yields, instead of having to purchase fresh seed. Numerous studies in the developing world have emphasized that the real barriers to farmers' adoption of improved maize

varieties and hybrids are inadequate infrastructure and policies for effective maize-seed industries. In many areas the private sector is not yet delivering improved seed to small-scale farmers, and the private sector may never have sufficient incentives to meet the needs of the most marginal farmers. For farmers who cannot obtain or afford commercial seed, apomictic maize would be nothing short of revolutionary. We regard this research as true biotechnology for poor people.

The work on apomixis, like many other efforts in biotechnology, has considerably widened the scope for genetic resources to contribute to plant-improvement research. Biotechnology research is also changing our view of how research can ultimately enhance agrobiodiversity. We believe that agrobiodiversity can be enhanced directly through greater diversity in the pedigrees of the varieties that we develop with our partners and through prebreeding research, and indirectly by allowing a greater diversity of plant and animal species to flourish in agricultural systems.

Pedigree Diversity

Recent evidence from CIMMYT suggests that the bread wheats that have been most widely adopted in the fields of developing country farmers also possess some of the most complex pedigrees. The top ten crosses grown in the developing world in 1990 are genetic powerhouses. They contain an average of 44 landraces, 19 generations, and 1,192 parental combinations in their pedigrees, of which about 20 percent were used only once. (For comparison, note that for all of the different crosses grown in the developing world in 1990, the average number of distinct landraces per pedigree is 36.) This gives some idea of the considerable, and continuing, investment made by farmers (landraces) and by scientific plant breeders (generations and parental combinations) in the diversity of the world's bread wheat crop.

Prebreeding Research

The plant improvement centers of the CGIAR, including CIMMYT, also concentrate on prebreeding. Through innovative breeding techniques, desirable genetic traits from landraces and wild relatives of crop species are continually built into breeding lines that our partners in developing countries can use to develop varieties of interest to local farmers. Biotechnology is a significant contributor to prebreeding research.

Indirect Effects on Species Diversity

Finally, in developing new varieties that enable farmers to obtain higher yields from the same amount of land, biotechnology and conventional breeding can contribute to greater biodiversity in the cropping system. Varietal diversity is critical. CIMMYT, for example, is not working to cover the Earth with maize and wheat varieties. We do not want one variety of any crop dominating the landscape. We want diverse cropping systems and agricultural enterprises, because we think that is the way to achieve sustainability. We want a patchwork of modern varieties, good varieties, different varieties, because we believe that this is important for agrobiodiversity. By developing a continuous stream of new varieties and working with our colleagues in national agricultural research systems and public and private organizations, we can facilitate that diversity.

A poor farmer in Africa, for example, needs her whole farm to produce the 1,000 kilograms of maize that will keep her family alive. If in some way we can help to produce that 1,000 kilograms of maize on half of the farm area, the other half is freed for other crops, exotic or indigenous, or for wood lots or agroforestry. If that farmer can get a more diverse, sustainable, and profitable rotation going thanks to the results of sensible and safe biotechnology research, that would be an achievement to celebrate.

All of these examples of biotechnology research and its potential benefits highlight our concern that the technologies we develop with our research partners should be environmentally and economically sound and easily available to poor people. However other important and often controversial issues may strongly influence the potential effectiveness of biotechnology research, and the CGIAR centers are extremely concerned about them. These issues include biosafety and related issues of ethics and equity.

Efficient, Equitable, and Ethical Research: Challenges Ahead

In partnership with our colleagues throughout the world, the CGIAR has developed working guidelines in relation to intellectual property rights. A key feature of these guidelines is that CGIAR centers will not work with biotechnology processes, particularly with transgenic material, in any country that lacks biosafety legislation and regulations. We believe that this is a good practice. But we also know that many of our partners lack biosafety legislation or a regulatory framework to support such legislation, though they urgently wish to conduct biotechnology research. One of our sister centers, the International Service for National Agricultural Research (ISNAR), is helping national programs to develop appropriate technology and establish legislative guidelines that will enable new technologies to be tested safely. We think that this sort of hands-on approach helps governments and public sector research institutions consider complex biosafety issues in a careful, timely fashion, with respect for the interests of less powerful members of society.

In Mexico, where very good biosafety legislation is in place, CIMMYT is helping the government examine particular dilemmas arising from biotechnology research, such as sound biosafety procedures for working with transgenic maize in a center of genetic diversity still populated by wild relatives of maize. The procedures developed in Mexico are designed to deal with real issues, and they are expected to be extremely useful for the rest of the world.

The CGIAR is also concerned about drafting ethical guidelines that will enable us to do all in our power to ensure that we and our partners can engage in biotechnology research in a way that is efficient, equitable, and ethical. One of the most pressing issues is to determine what approach the CGIAR should take with respect to biosafety in relation to biotechnology. If we were to take a hands-off approach, we would have nothing to do with biotechnology, because there is a debate over biosafety in the public arena at the moment and we do not want to get criticized. Is that the right way to go? Or should we adopt a hands-on approach and try to help solve some of the problems related to biosafety and find a way forward? Under that scenario we would work with our partners in the South, jointly resolving such issues as licensing agreements, helping to define appropriate financial involvement and assess ways of meeting costs. These are all very real issues that research systems and governments must confront sooner or later.

Although the world remains divided over which approach might be better—a hands-on or a hands-off approach—it is our belief that we cannot abandon our research partners to the vagaries of an increasingly competitive, profit-oriented environment for research and development. For example, we have colleagues in Africa who wish to study the potential of using transgenic maize as part of an integrated pest management (IPM) strategy to combat *Striga*, a parasitic weed species. Do we leave our colleagues to deal directly with companies that want to work in this area? Or do we help them investi-

gate how transgenic maize fits into IPM programs; help them conduct the research necessary to ensure that the resistance in transgenic maize is useful over the long run?

We believe that partnerships can offer a way forward through the welter of complex issues transforming agricultural research. Our range of partners is much greater than it used to be, including national research systems, CGIAR centers, advanced research institutions, nongovernmental organizations, and increasingly, the private sector. The CGIAR is listening to and attempting to understand the needs of these partners, because only successful partnerships can foster efficient, equitable, and ethical research arrangements. Together we must devise solutions to the many challenges for agricultural research, including the new challenges posed by biotechnology and biosafety. Together we must work towards a sustainable and socially just agriculture.

Research Partnerships in Biotechnology:
Role of the Global Forum on Agricultural Research

Fernando Osorio Chaparro

This conference provides us with an excellent opportunity to exchange ideas on the role biotechnology plays in agricultural research for development, on the forces that are shaping this process, and on the role different actors play in this area of research. I will approach these issues from the perspective of the National Agricultural Research Systems (NARS) of developing countries; thus one of the issues I will address is the participation of developing countries in global biotechnology research. In this paper I will address three main issues:

1. A brief analysis of some of the important trends shaping the present context in which research and technological development for sustainable agriculture is taking place

2. New opportunities and challenges that are being generated by the development of biotechnology and other strategic research areas, in the present context of more science-intensive agricultural production systems

3. The role of research partnerships and transnational research networks in seeking more cost-effective approaches to agricultural research; integrating research groups in developing countries (NARS) into these efforts; and mobilizing the research capacity of different actors in the global scientific community and applying it to development research. In this third point I will analyze the role the Global Forum on Agricultural Research can play in this process, as an initiative aimed at facilitating and promoting such research partnerships.

Changing Context of Agricultural Research

There are four dimensions in the present context of agricultural research that are having a deep influence on the present and future directions of agricultural research. These are: (1) the socioeconomic context, (2) the knowledge, or science, context, (3) the institutional context, and (4) the process of globalization.

Socioeconomic Context

Despite the very important technological advances of this century, including those of the Green Revolution, the world is still faced with increasing poverty in both urban and rural areas. The figures are staggering:

- More than 800 million people remain undernourished.
- One third of pre-school-age children are in this situation, which has a severe impact on school performance and future productivity.
- In some countries more than 65 percent of the population live below the poverty line.

Recent studies carried out by the International Food Policy Research Institute and other organizations have clearly pointed out a set of contradictory trends that are presently taking place and will tend to dominate the coming decades. The aggregate supply and demand picture for food, as compared to population, presents a relatively balanced picture— if present investment levels in agricultural research are maintained or increased. But despite this positive picture at the global level, the world will continue to face a dual and contradictory situation, based on two different realities. Wealthy countries, together with a small number of developing countries (mainly from Asia), will enjoy low food prices and food surpluses, or affordable imports. But less developed, slowly growing countries will face a growing problem of food security that will have to be solved through food imports.

Food surpluses will be generated in industrial countries, especially the United States, and a growing food deficit requiring growing food imports will predominate in developing countries. The proportion of the malnourished population, especially in the case of vulnerable populations, will continue to increase. If instead of maintaining present rates of investment in agricultural research, national and international institutions further cut back their investments the relatively favorable aggregate food situation could worsen, generating a global food security crisis and worsening environmental problems and sustainability.

Desertification, deforestation, and environmental deterioration are growing problems, even in countries well endowed with natural resources. With the population likely to increase by another four billion by the year 2020 and the problems of growing natural resource degradation, agricultural research is faced with a series of daunting challenges: to improve farm family income to alleviate poverty, increase food production, provide employment opportunities for the resource poor and landless farmers to ensure household food security, while at the same time conserving natural resources in a sustainable fashion.

The Knowledge, or Science, Context

Agricultural production is becoming increasingly knowledge-based and science-intensive. New strategic research areas have emerged and developed, with profound effects on our capacity to produce food and manage natural resources and the environment. There are three new key areas of knowledge that could play a critical role in strengthening our capacity to respond to these growing challenges:

1. Biotechnology and its various applications
2. Research areas related to sustainable agriculture
3. Information and communications technology (ICT).

These new research areas do not replace plant breeding and production systems research (including on-farm research). On the contrary the new research areas are generating *enabling technologies* that complement and deepen previous approaches. They provide new tools for addressing these issues, which can be combined with other, very important research tools related to crop improvement and crop management. The latter will continue to be the mainstream of agricultural research.

These new areas of science and the enabling technologies they generate represent a great potential for increasing our capacity to respond to the social and economic challenges we face: poverty, resource degradation, and food security. If well utilized, they can significantly increase our capacity to cope with these problems and promote development. At the same time we also face the clear possibility of widening technology gaps between industrial and developing countries, due to differentials in research capacities and the increasing limitations of accessing these technologies, given their nature as proprietary technologies. This is what a recent report of the Consultative Group on International Agricultural Research (CGIAR) Private Sector Committee calls "barriers to the freedom to operate" that research institutions and developing countries will face, due to the increasing number of proprietary technologies.

This trend reflects an important change taking place in the nature of biological technologies. In evolving from technologies that manipulate plants (species, varieties) to technologies that manipulate cells and molecules, we have witnessed the emergence of technologies that are much more easily appropriated. It is not easy to reproduce or duplicate either the biotechnological process that has led to the final product or the final product itself, given the complexity of the knowledge involved and the investment requirements. The fact that an increasing proportion of the relevant knowledge and techniques are of a proprietary nature has two important implications. First, the flow of knowledge is increasingly constrained by this new reality. Second, in order to participate in the technology development process it is important for any research institute (such as NARS) to develop a research capacity as well as generate research results (a knowledge asset), that enables it to participate in active knowledge exchanges, through joint ventures or other relevant research partnerships. As a recent report points out: "If a global 'trait market' evolves, developing countries and [research] centers will be able to participate in this market more effectively if they have a cache of 'trading chips' in the form of traits generated through their own research." The knowledge-exchange capacity and bargaining power of research institutions becomes an important element in the new context.

The challenge here is to develop a framework or environment that may facilitate strategic alliances and joint ventures between the various actors involved in these research efforts, bringing closer together the normative framework and incentive structure related to the development of technologies of a public good nature, with the framework and incentives that prevail in the biotechnology industry and the development of proprietary technologies.

Institutional Context

A more diversified institutional structure of stakeholders has developed in recent years in the area of agricultural research and natural resource management, at both the national and global levels. Traditionally, given the nature of the knowledge and technology related to these fields, most research has been carried out by national public research institutes or by international research centers concerned with the generation of knowledge that could be characterized as "international public goods." Given the fact that the technology was not easily appropriated, the private sector played a relatively marginal role, especially in the area of development research. The other two important actors were universities (especially in industrial countries) and advanced research institutes or centers of excellence, quite often with close links to universities.

In more recent years three other actors have started to play a central role in this process: farmers' organizations, nongovernmental organizations (NGOs), and the private sector. Farmers have become more organized, and have been able to build on the learning experience generated by a variety of participatory research schemes and rural development projects. This has allowed for the emergence of approaches to research and extension that places the farmer at the center of the process, as a key actor, and not just as a user of technology. Similarly, in many countries NGOs have either complemented the role of the State or filled in the gap generated by the weakness of public research institutions, especially in terms of reaching and working with farmers (inefficient technology transfer mechanisms). In Latin America and the Caribbean, in Africa and in Asia there is an increasingly rich experience with NGOs, community organizations, and participatory research approaches that could provide the basis for more efficient research and technology transfer systems.

The role of the private sector has become increasingly important, reflecting the fact that biological research and the technology generated by it has become more privatized, as a result of investment incentives. Presently it is estimated that the private sector is responsible for approximately 80 percent of the research in plant biotechnology worldwide. By 1992 the U.S. private sector alone was spending $US559 million in agricultural biotechnology research, reflecting a 50 percent increase over 1985. One reason for this surge is that the market for agricultural inputs is large. Farmers in the U.S. purchase US$3.5 billion of planting seed per year. It is estimated that total global sales of agricultural biotechnology products will reach US$3 to 5 billion by the year 2000.

The private sector has thus become an important player in the basic research end of the range of activities that constitute the basic-strategic-applied-adaptive research continuum. This is a fundamental change with respect to the traditional role this sector traditionally played, which was basically being an user of knowledge and research findings generated by the public sector (as public goods). These changes also raise the related issue of property rights and plant breeder's rights and the role they play in the knowledge generation and dissemination process.

This evolving institutional environment has to be taken into consideration in the process of strengthening science and technology for sustainable agriculture, and in developing new approaches to cooperation in this area through strategic alliances and research partnerships. These partnerships, built on *collaboration* and *mutual benefit*, are becoming much more effective than traditional "aid programs." This is an important dimension of the new joint ventures among interested stakeholders, especially in the present context of diminishing funds for traditional overseas development assistance.

Process of Globalization

The fourth dimension of the present context in which we operate is the process of globalization, the symptoms of which are all around us. Globalization has clearly changed the way financial markets and the economy operate, where the transnational dimension, a global view of markets, and a capacity to operate in them, has become an essential part of being competitive in the present world. This is true even for the smallholder, given the increasing importance of the global context for everyday life and well-being. The global dimension is no longer of interest only to large and export-oriented producers. It is part of the context in which everyone operates, with a direct impact on farmers' viability as producers and the well-being of their families.

But globalization is also reflected in changes that are taking place in the scientific community and the organization of research. Technological innovations are seldom generated by individual research institutions or firms. They are increasingly the product of transnational research networks, or "networks of learning" that are playing a central role in the process of knowledge generation, dissemination, and application. In some areas of research, such as sugar cane, these transnational networks are responsible for having generated most of the varieties with present commercial utilization. We will return to this point in a subsequent analysis of the role of research partnerships and strategic alliances.

Given the increasing importance of proprietary technology, the process of globalization is characterized by two contrasting trends. On the one hand globalization is taking place in terms of markets and final products. But on the other, we are witnessing increasing constraints in terms of knowledge flows and technology transfer because of the increasing importance of proprietary technology.

There is another important aspect of the impact of globalization as it affects agriculture, research, and development. This is the fact that the challenges represented by poverty, food security, and environmental deterioration in developing countries are no longer an issue of concern only to those countries. Given the increasing interdependence of the world, they are rapidly becoming global issues. Much in the same way that the global context has an impact on smallholders and peasants and their viability as producers, these development issues have an impact on the well-being of urban dwellers in New York or in any large metropolitan center, and on the global capacity to assure sustainable development. Globalization requires us to take a fresh look at institutional arrangements and collaborative mechanisms, based on common interests and mutual benefits to those involved.

Biotechnology Research in Developing Countries: Role of NARS

In biotechnology we are witnessing the very rapid development of the application of molecular biology to a range of agricultural production problems and issues of sustainability. The best known application is that of genetic engineering that is leading to an increasing availability of transgenic plants with the specific characteristics that one wants to maximize. This is quite a recent development, since the first transgenic plants were sold in the United States in 1996. But their commercial success is clearly encouraging an increasing effort of the private sector in that direction.

But the role of biotechnology goes beyond genetic engineering in addressing the problems of development. In this section I will analyze three related aspects: (a) the development of a relevant biotechnology research agenda in the context of developing countries, (b) the development of a research capacity in this area, and (c) the development of an appropriate environment for the establishment of research partnerships between the public and private sectors, as well as participation in transnational research networks. The first two points will be analyzed in the first subsection.

The use of biotechnology in developing countries goes far beyond genetic engineering, covering a broad range of research techniques and their applications. As an example of the biotechnology research agenda that is presently being discussed in developing countries, I would like to summarize the results of a recent strategic planning exercise carried out by the Colombian National Research Organization, known as "CORPOICA," on this topic. The objective of this exercise was to identify the main research issues that should orient local research efforts, in many cases through strategic alliances with international agricultural research centers (IARCs), such as the International Center on Agricultural Research (CIAT) in Colombia, or with agricultural research institutions in Europe or North America.

The research strategy that CORPOICA is developing involves two dimensions. For some topics research programs are being put in place, in most cases on the basis of strategic alliances with other partners in the region or in industrial countries. In other cases, where it is considered that the required investments are too high to tackle or the critical mass of researchers is not yet available, a clear strategy is being put in place to follow the cutting edge of research very closely simply to understand what is going on and be able to have easier access to, and stronger absorptive capacity of, the technologies and the know-how that is being generated in these research areas. The training of researchers, through graduate training and joint ventures with advanced research institutions, is an important component of this strategy.

Five research areas of biotechnology were identified in this strategic planning exercise as having a particularly important role in development oriented research.

1. *Tissue culture*, through which we can make massive multiplication of genetic material, as well as carry out genetic improvement and germplasm conservation. The main applications are in cleaning of plant material and protoplast fusion. This is the most established research area in developing countries, but it still faces many problems of quality control and dominating the relevant research techniques.

2. *Molecular markers* play a key role in characterization of genetic variability and in genetic improvement. Coupled with the use of computers and the development of relevant research software, this research technique can speed up genetic improvement research of value to developing countries. An example of this can be found in the development of maize and soya varieties resistant to acid soils that may be integrated into sustainable production systems of the savanna regions found in different parts of Latin America, Africa, and Asia (such as the *llanos* in Colombia and Venezuela or the *cerrados* of Brazil). The maize research program carried out in Colombia, Venezuela, and Brazil in collaboration with CIMMYT and CIAT, took many years to develop the first varieties resistant to acid soils. After that first effort, the introduction of molecular marker techniques and computers has significantly accelerated the research process.

3. *Genetic engineering* is leading to increasing availability of transgenic plants with the specific characteristics that one wants to maximize. The new products being developed are having profound effects on production costs and environmental impact as well as sustainability, markets, and competitiveness. These technological changes may totally change the comparative advantages among countries in the production of basic foodstuffs (and thus world trade). These technological breakthroughs can increase our global capacity to cope with food security, but they can also deepen inequalities among industrial and developing countries, if not well managed. Until now most of the work related to transgenic plants has been related to temperate crops, such as soybeans; 60 percent of the production in North America already comes from these varieties. This concentration generates "orphan market-segments," where the private sector has not had any incentive to invest. When these coincide with national priorities, they represent potential areas of concentration for NARS.

4. *Bolstering of immune systems* through biotechnological applications in vaccines and in diagnostic kits.

5. *Applications of biotechnology in developing sustainable agriculture*, where some of the most rapid developments are taking place in terms of biopesticide research and new products being introduced on the market as part of efforts to use biological control or integrated pest management (IPM) techniques. Research on management of genetic resources, through which the gene pools

of commercial agricultural products have been enriched with those of wild varieties, also plays an important role.

Within each of these five research areas, the strategic planning exercise identified the principal research techniques and main applications relevant for the effective use of biotechnology in tackling the development problems of the country. This information is presented in a series of tables in an annex to this paper. It should be pointed out that this effort of identifying key research areas and research techniques that are relevant for the country is presently being complemented with an analysis of the development needs of the country and opportunities for new production efforts, in order to relate the research techniques to priority crops and the sustainable production problems of Colombia. The technology supply approach that was used in identifying the "research map" presented in the annex is being complemented with a more in-depth analysis of development needs and opportunities in this field.

Although this part of the exercise is still under way, five criteria have been defined to identify priorities among the different research lines and applications that could be pursued.

1. Since most of the private sector's involvement with agricultural biotechnology in industrial countries is related to temperate crops, priority will be given to tropical or Andean crops of importance to Colombia in genetic engineering research (orphan market-segments argument).

2. The development of strategic alliances with firms or research centers that could provide genes or "traits" that could facilitate the development of the desired characteristics in these crops. This requires developing a capacity to use the techniques related to inserting and manipulating the genes in cells, through plant transformation systems and selectable markers.

3. Priority is being given to IPM, and thus to the applications of biotechnology in the area of biopesticides.

4. Biotechnology research related to biodiversity management, especially germplasm conservation, is of high priority.

5. Biotechnology research related to the characterization of ecosystems, management of natural resources, and farm practices (agroecology).

A specific effort is being made to identify the applications of biotechnology that are relevant to the small producer and to peasant economies. Biotechnology is not only related to the development of transgenic plants. Many of the research areas and techniques mentioned above have applications that are of clear interest to the production problems of smallholders and peasant economies. In the case of Colombia's CORPOICA an emerging biotechnology research program aimed at addressing the needs of small-scale producers is starting to produce its first results. They include the development of high-quality seed for peasant communities obtained through tissue culture (plantain, cassava) and participatory technology-transfer schemes for the dissemination of different biotechnological applications relevant to small-scale producers.

Developing an Appropriate Environment: Policy Issues

Besides developing an appropriate research agenda and building up the research capacity to carry it out, it is of great importance to promote the development of an environment with incentives to facilitate the establishment of strategic research partnerships, within the country and with firms and research institutions abroad. Four policy issues have to be addressed in doing so:

1. Establishing intellectual property rights (IPR)

2. Establishing biosafety regulations

3. Developing information and communication technology capacity as a means of facilitating research partnerships and alliances

4. Funding mechanisms and direct State support.

The growing importance of proprietary technology and of the private sector in agricultural research and development (R&D), is leading to the need to develop IPR regulations in each country. It is equally important to be able to influence the establishment of the main principles and criteria that will shape the IPR frameworks of the future, since once established, they will determine very basic questions of accessibility to technology. This is particularly important in light of the emergence of a "trait market" for technologies at the molecular level, which provides critical inputs to the process of bundling several traits into germplasm, or enriching existing germplasm to solve food security problems of developing countries.

In order to promote the involvement of the private sector and facilitate the establishment of strategic alliances between the public and the private sector in pursuing common objectives, it is important to develop a regulatory environment that, while protecting the public good, also provides the proper incentives for the private sector to invest.

The IPR issue in biotechnology is not limited to the establishment of appropriate regulations. It is also related to the development of research capacities in the CGIAR and in NARS, in partnership with the private sector, to be able to effectively participate in the biotechnology market of the future. Given the number of new, proprietary technologies that are being generated and the critical role certain "traits" or genes can play in controlling the development of valuable germplasm, smaller players will be facing increasing barriers to the "freedom to operate" and have access to the enabling technologies that the biotechnology revolution is generating.

The development of biosafety regulations is equally important, given the potential impact of new varieties with regard to people and the environment. Existing regulatory schemes pay attention to both the impact of the new variety on human health and on the immediate ecosystem, as well as to the process used in the production of a transgenic plant, because of environmental concerns.

Third, the development of an ICT capacity in developing countries and in NARS is of great importance to enable research institutes in these countries to interact with their peers through transnational research networks and different types of research partnerships. The latter play a particularly important role in the area of biotechnology research. The different forms they take is analyzed in the next section.

A fourth important aspect of the process of establishing an appropriate environment for the development of biotechnology has to do with funding mechanisms, incentives, and the role of the state in developing countries. In addition to IPR, it is important to establish fiscal incentives and risk capital facilities to promote private sector investment from both multinational and na-

tional firms. This is a particularly important element in developing countries given the weakness of their financial systems. A variety of interesting experiences in terms of funding mechanisms and schemes have emerged in various industrial and developing countries.

A very important factor in developing countries is the role of the state in producing, through research, public goods related to important biotechnological inputs. Due to limited private-sector capacity to respond to the above-mentioned incentives, the role of the state is particularly important in these countries. Public research institutions, either through their own programs or in partnership with other research institutions, have tended to move to upstream technologies that provide basic inputs to other institutional actors. Examples of this are: identification of genes with potential to be transformed through biotechnological processes; development of gene maps for the main crops of the country; and research on critical metabolism processes that could lead to the identification of potential new products.

Research Partnerships, Strategic Alliances, and the Global Forum on Agricultural Research

It is now clear that the recent advances in science and technology achieved in new strategic research areas—mainly biotechnology and ICT—can play a key role in overcoming the global problems of poverty, food security, and environmental degradation in developing countries. Biotechnology alone cannot solve these problems. But if used in conjunction with other research tools related to plant breeding and crop management, biotechnology can contribute to a quantum leap in agricultural production, reducing production costs, and increasing sustainability.

If we are to take advantage of the opportunities generated by this knowledge revolution, however, a strategy of facilitating and developing research partnerships and strategic alliances among the different stakeholders should be followed, on the basis of the following considerations:

- Increasing research needs and requirements, and thus expanding research agendas

- Decreasing availability of public resources devoted to research, as reflected in both real expenditure per researcher and the annual growth rate in research expenditure
- The impact of globalization on promoting cooperation in tackling global issues
- Innovation and technical change is increasingly the product of transnational research networks facilitated by advances in ICT, making communication among researchers across the globe faster and less costly.

This last point is particularly important. Research carried out on innovative processes and systems has clearly emphasized the role of "innovation networks" as the main agent of knowledge generation and technical change in different industrial and agroindustrial sectors. The same is true of biotechnology, in which corporations form partnerships as part of a strategy to increase their competitive advantage. A recent CGIAR report points out that: "Having an internal research capacity is necessary but not sufficient for innovation. The complexity of the problems faced and the rapidity of the advances in knowledge compel companies and their researchers to reach out widely for partners." Another study points out that "when the knowledge base of an industry is both complex and expanding and the sources of expertise are widely dispersed, the locus of innovation will be found in *networks of learning*, rather than in individual firms."

These partnerships may involve universities, research institutes, international research centers, and private firms, and thus they involve *strategic alliances between the public and the private sectors*. For this to be feasible, it is important to develop a regulatory framework that, while protecting the public good, also provides adequate incentives for the private sector to invest. This environment requires a change in organizational culture in many research institutions, since it requires new attitudes and forms of interaction between public research centers oriented towards the development of public goods, and firms which are profit-oriented and interested in proprietary technologies. It also involves transnational research networks from both North and South, especially if we want to integrate NARS and avoid the dangers of increasing technology gaps.

In order to participate actively in such networks, NARS and their institutions have to develop a collaborative advantage or capability permitting them to do so. This involves having sufficient research capacity to contribute to and profit from such exchanges, as well as needed skills and organizational flexibility for entering into such agreements.

These research partnerships take various forms, but the most common modalities are: (a) loose or open research networks, (b) research consortia (when the networks become more formalized), (c) joint ventures (in specific projects), and (d) licensing arrangements The relevance and advantage of each modality varies from case to case.

These four types of research partnerships define a range of options that go from the open research networks constituted by peers in the scientific community working in a specific area or topic, to other forms of collaborative R&D characterized by increasing levels of formality, often based on contractual relationships between partners that agree to collaborate in the development of a proprietary technology. Thus there is a strong commercial relationship in these cases. It is important to point out that in the case of the development of proprietary technologies, joint ventures and licensing agreements play a much more important role.

Open research networks are usually based on the flow of public information between researchers or research groups that share a common area of interest. These networks are better suited for the development of nonproprietary technologies (this is the case of some biotechnological applications in developing countries) or for the exchange of general information that does not lead to biotechnological access. Here they can play a very important role.

The commercial dimension becomes much more important in the case of the research partnerships located at the other end of this range of options: joint ventures and licensing arrangements. The latter also require partners with a clear possibility of exchanging research results and technologies, and thus having the basis for interacting in such types of strategic alliances. Thus this typology of research partnerships identifies different organizational modalities that play different roles, and that are better suited for different objectives and circumstances.

Global Forum on Agricultural Research

It is within this context that the question of new approaches to global cooperation in this area, through strategic alliances and research partnerships, becomes of paramount importance. Four key questions emerge in this regard:

1. How can we mobilize the global scientific community in a concerted effort to address these issues, facilitating the harnessing of knowledge to the solution of development and global problems, complementing and strengthening the work already being done by the CGIAR?

2. How can we develop a capacity in the developing world (in the NARS), to avoid the dangers of growing technology gaps that could emerge in the new strategic research areas (such as biotechnology), with the concomitant impact on equity, sustainability, and development possibilities?

3. How can we develop strategic alliances and research partnerships among the various stakeholders related to biotechnology and development-oriented agricultural and natural resources research, building on the strengths and comparative advantages of each one?

4. How can we take advantage of the new opportunities the development of science offers, as well as the ICT revolution, to develop a knowledge-brokerage capacity that could mobilize expertise and knowledge, wherever it may be, and apply it to the solution of specific problems of a policy, institutional or technological nature? This entails involving the high-technology groups into the agricultural research effort, addressing both the global and development problems we face.

These are the questions that led, at the end of last year, to the initiation of a process aimed at building up a Global Forum on Agricultural Research, as a collective endeavor to facilitates exchange of information and research partnerships among the various stakeholders involved in this area of research. The Global Forum emerged from the conviction that, in order to respond to the increasing challenges and research needs we presently face, as well as take advantage of the

new opportunities that are emerging, it is necessary to promote the development of a global system for agricultural research, based on cost-effective partnerships and strategic alliances among the various institutional actors related to agricultural research, aimed at three major objectives:

1. Reducing poverty
2. Ensuring food security
3. Ensuring the conservation and management of biodiversity and the natural resource base.

This involves the active participation of NARS, IARCS, advanced research institutes in universities or centers of excellence around the world, the private sector, NGOs and farmers' organizations. The IARCs are particularly well placed to play an important role in this process, given the high-quality research infrastructure they have, their knowledge of tropical agriculture, the network of contacts in developing countries, their germplasm collections, and the highly trained research staff that constitute one of their main assets. Many of the transnational research networks that can be generated through the Global Forum can be coordinated by specific IARCs, working in close collaboration with other stakeholders.

The origins of the Global Forum lie in the recent efforts of the CGIAR to broaden its partnerships with the above-mentioned institutions. This process involved consultation with groups of NARS at the regional level on the substance of research collaboration, leading to the emergence of representative regional groupings, and, finally, to the Global Forum.

In the last two years Regional Forums have been established by the NARS of developing countries in Africa, East Asia and Pacific, Eastern Europe, Central Asia, and Latin America and the Caribbean. These are the main components of the Global Forum. These Regional Forums are aimed at facilitating collaboration among NARS, at the regional and subregional levels, and at facilitating their insertion into the global research arena. In certain regions these collaborative efforts have crystallized into new and innovative cooperative mechanisms, such as the Regional Agricultural Technology Fund established in Latin America and the Caribbean, to promote and facilitate cooperation in this area, both within the region as well as with advanced research institutes around the world.

At the national level similar considerations have led to major institutional reforms in the NARS of developing countries, where new policy approaches and institutional frameworks are being tried out in seeking to develop new partnerships in a multi-stakeholder environment, and to increase the effectiveness of agricultural research systems. The evolution of national agricultural research institutes to NARS, and the integration of the latter, is generating major institutional and organizational reforms in many developing countries, leading to new organizational structures based on public-private sector cooperation and joint ventures. This is changing the structure of the traditional technology research institutes in both the agricultural and industrial sectors.

In developing the Global Forum on Agricultural Research, the new information and telecommunication technologies will be used, relying heavily on electronic networks organized around specific topics and on Internet linkages, and using the new institutional models of virtual organizations and dynamic learning processes. The different organizational modalities of research partnerships mentioned above will be explored and facilitated. However, a clear strategy for addressing the various issues raised in this paper will also have to be developed. A strategy is necessary to ensure the participation of NARS in this process and to make use of the full potential of biotechnology and the other strategic research areas in coping with the challenges of alleviating poverty, ensuring food security, and achieving sustainable development.

Annex. Research Techniques and Research Applications in Biotechnology Identified in the Strategic Planning Exercise of CORPOICA (Colombia)

Technique	*Application*
Plant tissue culture	
Conventional micropropagation methods	Cleaning and multiplication
Micropropagation in bioreactors	
• Artificial seed production	
Conventional methods of *in vitro* conservation	Germplasm banks
• Cryo-preservation	
• Haploid production	Plant breeding
• Protoplast fusion	
• Cell culture	Production of secondary metabolites
• Organ culture	
Genetic engineering	
Recombinant DNA	Use of transgenic plants in plant breeding
Ti plasmid-mediated genetic transformation	Broadening of crops genetic base to improve their characteristics
Biolistics	
Viral vectors	Conservation, characterization, and improvement of crop and microorganisms germplasm
Direct genetic transformation of plant proteins	Development of desired characteristics
Microinjection	• Tolerance to:
Electroporation	Herbicides (glyphosate)
Liposome fusion	Insects *(Bacillus thuringiensis)*
	Fungi (chitinase)
	Bacteria (lysozymes)
	Virus (protein envelope)
	• Protein quality (seeds, tubers)
	• Starch metabolism
	• Physiological characteristics
	Synthesis of ethylene
	Cold tolerance
	Lignin content
	Soluble sugars
	Delayed fruit ripening
	• Flower pigments
	• Male sterility
	Nuclear
	Cytoplasmic
Modification of structure or composition of plant lipids	Improvement of vegetable oil quality
• Production of monoclonal and polyclonal antibodies	Diagnosis
• DNA probes	
• DNA fingerprinting	
• PCR (polymerase chain reaction)	
• Vaccine production in fruits	Vaccines
Molecular markers	
• RFLPs	Evaluation of genetic variability
• RAPDs	Molecular animal and plant mapping
• DNA fingerprinting	Plant breeding
• PCR	Germplasm characterization
• Microsatellites (SSP)	Selection of desirable genotypes
• SCARs	Pedigree and population analysis
• AFLP	

Annex (continued)

Technique	Application
Bioprocessing enzymes	
Carbohydratases	Brewing, baking, sweets, sweeteners, textile fibers, fruit juices, drugs, foods, dairy products, sugar beet
Proteases	Brewing, meats, drugs, baking, cheese, detergents
Hydrolases	Drugs, foods, dairy products, baking, detergents, leather tanning
Oxidoreductases	

Perspectives from National Agricultural Research Systems
Maria José A. Sampaio

One of the main challenges to expanding agricultural production in the decades ahead is to develop new crops with increased yield, pest resistance, and drought tolerance. To drive agriculture towards sustainability is to add to those characteristics reduced dependency on pesticides and herbicides. These are some of the tasks that can be addressed by modern biotechnology.

However, as with all new tools, biotechnology must be assessed in terms of benefits and costs. Experience shows that some problems, such as gene flow from modified plants to wild relatives, potential development of new viruses, pathogen-derived resistance, or ecosystem damage are the same as those faced 30 years ago during the Green Revolution, and they need be addressed again to safeguard the environment and human health.

Not all development-oriented basic or applied research need be conducted in the country where engineered crops are to be grown. However selection of traits of interest, confirmation in the field of the agronomic value of the new crop, and the study of its interaction with a given ecosystem need to be done on site, thus creating an opportunity for the transfer of biotechnology to developing countries.

To evaluate potential risks and establish regulations to discipline the use of biotechnology, a new "scientific area" has been created, which is commonly known as biosafety. Discussions of biosafety began to receive more attention after the Earth Summit in Rio de Janeiro in 1992, when the Convention on Biological Diversity (CBD) was opened for signature.

In Latin America the first workshops for regional discussions of biosafety issues took place in 1990, sponsored by the Inter-American Institute for Cooperation on Agriculture. Harmonized proposals came out of meetings held in Argentina (1992), Colombia (1994), and Costa Rica (1994). These workshops were very valuable in the sense that participants, most of them working for National Agricultural Research Systems (NARS), had the chance to discuss scientific and policy issues. The United Nations Development Programme has played a major role by providing some countries with the possibility of developing joint biotechnology projects and raising awareness of biosafety and the need for risk assessment. Also, the U. S. Department of Agriculture, the Stockholm Environment Institute, and the United Nations Industrial Development Organization have been giving strong support to newly formed national committees for the organization of workshops and seminars in Latin America. Other developing countries, such as China and India, are receiving similar attention.

Under the CBD parties have decided to prepare a binding protocol that will establish rules for the transboundary movement of living modified organisms. A first draft is being prepared during a series of meetings of member-country representatives, and will be submitted to the Committee of the Whole during the fourth meeting of Conference of the Parties, scheduled for

May 1998. A final document should emerge before year 2000.

Since 1992 countries have been discussing the types of national legal infrastructure necessary for the implementation of biosafety. When discussing options such as guidelines, protocols, and directives for the management of genetically modified organisms (GMOs), decisions have to be made regarding binding instruments, such as a special law or ministerial decree, or nonbinding instruments, such as guidelines and directives.

Different countries in Latin America have decided to take different approaches. So far Brazil is the only country in the region to adopt a biosafety law. Other countries, while discussing the possibility of having a law in the future, are using ministerial decrees under existing quarantine laws or regulations; some have decided to start using guidelines, mostly based on the United Nations Environment Programme model. But almost all countries have already formed a national biosafety committee to deliberate about field tests and other issues related to GMOs. The committees are usually linked to ministries of agriculture, environment, or science and technology.

Biosafety in Latin America: Supervisory Authorities

Argentina	National Biotechnology Commission (CONABIA)
Bolivia	National Biosafety Committee
Brazil	National Technical Biosafety Committee (CTNBio)
Chile	National Biosafety Committee
Colombia	National Biosafety Committee
Costa Rica	National Biosafety Committee
Cuba	National Biosafety Committee
Ecuador	Under discussion
Mexico	National Biosafety Committee
Paraguay	National Biosafety Committee
Peru	National Biosafety Committee (under discussion)
Venezuela	National Biosafety Committee

Brazil is a good example of the early involvement of NARS in national-level decisionmaking about the management of biotechnology and related biosafety issues. In the early 1990s it could already be foreseen that genetically engineered crops would play an important role in Brazilian

agriculture by the turn of the century. Therefore regulations and regulating authorities would be needed to allow for the development of the technology and its further use in the country. In 1993 leading scientists from the Brazilian Agricultural Research Corporation (EMBRAPA), the major component of the NARS, with support from colleagues at the Oswaldo Cruz Foundation, a research institute linked to the Ministry of Health, prepared a proposal that was submitted to the Brazilian Congress for discussion. In January 1995 the Biosafety Law was enacted by Congress. In December of the same year, a complementary statute regulating the law was published.

The Biosafety Law establishes safety procedures and mechanisms for supervision of the use of genetic engineering techniques in the construction, cultivation, manipulation, transportation, commercialization, consumption, release, and disposal of GMOs, aiming to protect the health and lives of human beings, animals, plants, and the environment.

The mechanism proposed for implementation of activities comprises:

1. A National Technical Biosafety Committee, formed by representatives of the following ministries: science and technology, agriculture, health, environment, education, and foreign affairs. Other members are nominated by associations representing consumers' rights, corporations working with biotechnology, and workers' health. Finally, eight scientists nominated by the scientific community complement the group.

2. The formation of an Internal Biosafety Commission by every public or private institute or organization that deals with biotechnology and the manipulation of DNA. This Commission is ultimately responsible for all activities relating to GMOs under their supervision.

3. The need for every public or private laboratory working with biotechnology research to apply and obtain a Certificate of Quality in Biosafety, after having its infrastructure reviewed by the National Committee.

Under the law public or private institutions are considered technically and scientifically responsible for activities and projects in which they become involved, regardless of whether or not they are carried out on their own premises.

Supervisory responsibilities pertain to agencies of the Ministry of Agriculture, Ministry of

Environment, and Ministry of Health within their areas of jurisdiction, observing the conclusive technical analysis of the National Committee. The law establishes punishments for different violations and crimes, which range from the payment of fines to imprisonment for 20 years.

During 1997 the National Committee issued eight rulings covering: requirements for the issuance of the Certificate of Quality in Biosafety, importation for research of genetically modified plants and seeds, field release of GMOs, transportation of GMOs, classification of organisms according to risk and levels of containment, experimental and industrial management of GMOs under containment, genetic manipulation, and human cloning. The National Committee has received many petitions for field releases of GMOs. Small-scale releases started during the 1997 crop season. National Committee members, industry and governmental research institutes, and society are learning together the best way to design risk assessment and apply risk management. The important fact to be observed is that all of this, which seems to be taken for granted now, would not have been possible if the NARS had not reacted and acted in time.

The involvement of NARS, through their scientific leadership, has also been decisive in the design of biosafety measures adopted in Argentina, Chile, Costa Rica, Mexico, and Uruguay. The experience in the Latin American region has shown that the existence of a strong NARS facilitates the design and implementation of biosafety measures, because the system usually provides scientists from different fields of expertise with the necessary background knowledge to face the challenge and take on the coordination of the process. The latter is a strongly needed capacity due to the numerous lobbies that try to influence decisions in the biosafety arena. Countries lacking this capacity are systematically lagging behind, both in the acquisition, adaptation, and development of biotechnology for in-house use and the formulation of biosafety regulations. This in turn, and given present trends, will represent a tremendous bottleneck for the agricultural development of these nations.

As the use of GMOs in agriculture spreads worldwide, the coordination capacity of NARS in both industrial and developing countries will be critical for the design of national and regional monitoring programs, which will have to involve both private and public research initiatives. Potential problems could get out of control if these programs are not put in place in a very timely fashion. For these programs nothing will be more important than the gathering by NARS of basic ecological, botanical, and agronomic data on the undisturbed environment and its changes after the introduction of genetically modified crops.

References

Kendall, H.W., Beachy, R., Eisner,T., Gould, F., Herdt, R., Raven, P.H., Shell, J.S., and Swaminathan, M.S. 1997. *Bioengineering of Crops: Report of the World Bank Panel on Transgenic Crops.* Washington, D.C.: World Bank. Reprinted in this volume as appendix C.

Sampaio, M.J.A. 1995. "Biosafety Regulations in Brazil." *African Crop Journal* 3: 315-17.

———. 1998 (forthcoming). "Biosafety in Latin America: Building up Experience and a Framework for Genetically Modified Organisms Management since 1990." *Biosafety Workshop on the Environmental Impact Analysis of Transgenic Plants in the Asia Pacific Region.* London: Oxford Press.

Genetic Engineering: Addressing Agricultural Development in Egypt
Magdy Madkour

The challenge facing the world today is to provide food, fiber, and industrial raw materials for an ever-growing world population without harming the environment or affecting the future productivity of natural resources. Meeting this challenge will require the continued support of science, research, and education. A high demand for attention to these problems lies in developing countries, where 90 percent of the world's population growth will take place within the next two decades.

In Egypt agriculture represents the spearhead of socioeconomic development, accounting for almost 28 percent of national income and employing almost 50 percent of the workforce. Agricultural commodities generate more than 20 percent of the country's total export earnings. A limited arable land base, coupled with an ever-growing population (annual birth rate 2.7 percent), are the main reasons for the increasing food production/consumption gap. Egypt's population will grow to about 70 million by the year 2000 and swell to 110 million by 2025. In recent years only 15 percent of production for total agricultural commodity exports in Egypt has been exported, which is indicative of increased domestic demand due to increased population growth. Increasing the agricultural land base from a 7.4– to a 14–million feddans cropping area would satisfy only 50 percent of the requirement of the current population of 59 million. To bridge the food gap and fulfill the goal of self reliance, an expansion of the land base and optimization of agricultural outputs are urgently needed.

National Perceptions

The Government of Egypt is increasingly aware that it must use its own limited resources in a cost-effective way. Failure to develop its own appropriate biotechnology applications and inability to acquire technology developed worldwide could deny Egypt timely access to important new advances capable of overcoming significant constraints to increased agricultural productivity.

A very significant contribution to increased food production could be made by protecting more crops from losses to pests, pathogens, and weeds. The total loss of worldwide agricultural production ranges from 20 to 40 percent, including both pre– and post–harvest losses, which occur despite the widespread use of synthetic pesticides.

It is in areas such as crop protection that biotechnology, especially genetic engineering, could offer great benefits to the environment by replacing the present policy of blanket sprayings of crops with herbicides, fungicides, and pesticides, with a combination of inherent engineered resistance to pests and diseases. Thus genetic engineering is very suitable to agriculture in the developing world, since it is "user-friendly." If it is applied in a sensible manner, there can be no doubt that this technology is "green."

One of the major targets of the application of genetic engineering is the production of transgenic plants conferring resistance to both biotic stress resulting from pathogenic viruses, fungi, and insect pests and abiotic stress, including such unfavorable environmental conditions as salinity in the soil and irrigation water, drought, and high temperatures.

The production of transgenic plants tolerant to environmental stress could significantly help Egypt's efforts toward horizontal expansion of agricultural lands toward the desert. This would increase the agricultural land base by about 1 million acres.

The Agricultural Genetic Engineering Research Institute (AGERI) represents a vehicle within the agricultural arena for the transfer and application of this new technology. The original establishment of AGERI in 1990 was the result of a commitment of expertise in agricultural biotechnology. At the time of it's genesis, AGERI was named the National Agricultural Genetic Engineering Laboratory (NAGEL). The rapid progress of its activities during the first three years encouraged the Ministry of Agriculture and Land Reclamation to authorize the foundation of AGERI, which represents phase two of the national goal for excellence in genetic engineering and biotechnology. AGERI is now aiming to adopt the most advanced technologies available worldwide and apply them to contemporary problems facing agriculture in Egypt.

AGERI is housed within the Agricultural Research Center (ARC), which not only facilitates an interface with ARC's ongoing research programs, but also provides a focal point for biotechnology and genetic engineering for crop applications in Egypt.

AGERI runs its present activities from a building with a net space of 1,500 square meters, which houses 13 modern, well-equipped laboratories, a central facility containing major equipment used commonly, and a controlled environment chambers facility (11 units) to host transgenic plant material for acclimatization.

A state-of-the-art Biocontainment Greenhouse Facility is now in full function. This facility complies with the most advanced regulations of the U.S. Environmental Protection Agency and Animal and Plant Health Inspection Service, as well as United Nations Environment Programme guidelines for containment and isolation. The facility is dedicated to confined testing of genetically modified plants prior to their release to the field.

Moreover AGERI has dedicated 1.5 acres of land to serve as an open-field experimental station for field testing of genetically engineered plant material.

The staff of AGERI is composed of 17 highly accomplished senior scientists. Each is a vital link in the program's goals for crop improvement. The senior scientists have institutional affiliation in six Egyptian universities, in addition to their scientific responsibilities within AGERI. They work at AGERI on a joint-appointment basis, which maximizes their interaction between the academic and research domains.

AGERI continues to play a role as the interface between the international scientific community and Egypt. Various seminars and conferences have been held at AGERI with the participation of highly qualified international consultants. Some 40 study tours have taken both senior scientists and junior assistants from AGERI to various international biotechnology centers in Asia, Europe, and North America to attend conferences or training courses.

Condensed short courses and seminars concentrating on vital basics of biotechnology have been conducted by AGERI. Educational activities have been promoted as a result of this linkage and cooperation with international researchers and laboratories, and opportunities have arisen for the exchange of genes, genetic probes, DNA libraries, and vectors. Such contacts with centers worldwide have been initiated and encouraged to facilitate meaningful interactions.

Research and Scientific Collaboration

AGERI has been successful in attracting funds to sponsor its research from the following international organizations:

- United Nations Development Programme, as a cofunding agency supporting the initial research at NAGEL (currently AGERI).
- A cooperative research agreement between AGERI and the Agricultural Biotechnology for Sustainable Productivity Project based at Michigan State University, which is funded by the U.S. Agency for International Development/Cairo under the National Agricultural

Research Project. This activity allowed inter-action between AGERI's scientists and re-searchers from a number of eminent American universities, including Michigan State University, Cornell University, University of California, the Scripps Research Institute, University of Maryland, University of Wyoming, University of Arizona, and the Agricultural Research Service of the U.S. Department of Agriculture.

• Recently, the International Center for Agricultural Research in Dry Areas, located in Aleppo, Syria, contracted AGERI to conduct research on some of their mandated crops.

The projects carried out at AGERI are based on the concept of maintaining a program focused on the problems of Egypt. The immediate objectives are to develop and deliver transgenic cultivars of major economically important crops in Egypt. Thus the most recent and successful genetic engineering techniques are being employed to address this need. These projects also represent a spectrum of increasingly complex scientific challenges requiring state-of-the-art genetic engineering and gene transfer technologies. Gene manipulation techniques such as cloning, sequencing, modifications, construction of genomic and cDNA libraries, plant transformation, and regeneration in tissue culture are just few examples of the cellular and molecular biology methodologies that are utilized for production of transgenic plants.

The successful implementation of these projects would build a national capacity within Egypt for the sustainable production of crops crucial to the economy and to a safer, cleaner environment.

Examples of Projects Carried Out at AGERI

1. Genetic engineering of virus-resistant potato to the most important viruses in Egypt (PVX, PVY, PLRV); production of transgenic tomatoes resistant to geminiviruses such as Tomato Yellow Leaf Curl Virus (TYLCV); introduction of virus resistance in squash and melon against Zuccini Yellow Mosaic Virus (ZYMV); and finally, the production of transgenic faba bean conferring resistance to Bean Yellow Mosaic Virus (BYMV) and Faba Bean Necrotic Yellow Virus (FBNYV).

2. Engineering of insect-resistant plants with Bacillus thuringiensis crystal protein genes. Bt genes are used for the transformation of cotton, maize, potato, and tomato plants to resist their major insect pests.

3. Genetic engineering for fungal resistance using the chitinase gene concept for the development of transgenic maize, tomato, and faba bean expressing resistance to fungal diseases caused by *Fusarium sp.*, *Alternaria sp.*, and *Botrytis fabae*.

4. Enhancing the nutritional quality of faba bean seed protein by the successful transfer of the sulphur-rich genes to faba bean plants.

5. Cloning the genes' encoding for important economic traits in tomatoes, faba beans, and cotton, especially those related to stress tolerance (that is, heat shock proteins and osmoregulation genes).

6. Mapping the rapeseed genome in order to develop cultivars adapted to the constraints of the Egyptian environment, thus securing a good source of edible oil.

7. Developing efficient diagnostic tools for the identification and characterization of major viruses in Egypt.

These projects are relevant to Egyptian agriculture, since they reflect a significant positive impact on agricultural productivity and foreign exchange. For example, Egyptian Bt transgenic cotton, resistant to major insect pests, would result in substantial savings of the US$50 million spent annually on the purchase of imported pesticides. Mapping of rapeseed oil has a potential to substantially reduce the 400,000 tons of edible oil imported into Egypt annually. Similarly, transgenic potato varieties resistant to selected viruses and insect pests would prevent the expenditure of approximately US$33 million per year in the import of seed potatoes.

The goals of AGERI in the agricultural community are summarized below:

• Advance Egyptian agriculture using biotechnology and genetic engineering capabilities available worldwide to meet contemporary problems of Egyptian agriculture

• Broaden the research and development capabilities and scope of the Agricultural Research Center in the public and private sectors (for example, initiation of new program areas and application to a wider array of crop species)

- Expand and diversify the pool of highly qualified, trained professionals in the area of biotechnology and genetic engineering
- Provide opportunities for university-trained professionals (faculty, researchers, and teachers), the Ministry of Agriculture (professional researchers), and private venture companies to cooperate in agricultural genetic engineering research
- Promote opportunities for private sector development
- Achieve the desired level of self-reliance and self-financing within AGERI to mobilize the funds necessary for maintaining laboratories.

AGERI is seeking to fulfill a role in Africa and the Middle East as an emerging center of excellence for plant genetic engineering and biotechnology. AGERI will act as an interface between elite centers and laboratories from the international scientific community and research centers, universities, and the private sector in Egypt, Africa, and the Middle East. The major goal is to assist and provide the mechanism for proper technology transfer to benefit their respective agriculture mandates.

Overview of Biosafety Status in Egypt

In Egypt, as in other developing countries, a national biosafety system will ensure the safe development of biotechnology products and facilitate collaborative research activities with other countries. Until 1995 Egypt's regulations did not include guidelines for handling transgenic materials under contained conditions, nor did they cover the release of genetically modified organisms into the environment.

AGERI is the primary institute dealing with biotechnology in Egypt. As AGERI's research projects have now reached the stage of field evaluation of genetically modified organisms, the Egyptian government has moved forward to build a national biosafety policy to regulate such activities.

The Egyptian National Biosafety Committee (NBC) was established by Ministerial Decree 85 in January 1995. This committee is responsible for putting together policies and procedures to govern the use of biotechnology in the country.

To formulate a biosafety system for Egypt, information was gathered from different counties regarding their regulations, guidelines, and systems design. A draft document entitled "The Establishment of a National Biosafety System in Egypt: Regulations and Guidelines," was prepared by AGERI, with regulations and guidelines adapted to Egyptian conditions. This document was revised by the NBC and approved by government authorities as a binding law for biosafety in Egypt (Ministerial Decree 136, February 1995).

The NBC includes representatives from the ministries of agriculture, health, industry, environment, education, and scientific research. Representatives from the private sector, policymakers, and consultants knowledgeable in policies and applicable law, as well as nontechnical members representing community interests (nongovernmental organizaions) are also active members of the NBC.

NBC Activities

- Formulation, implementation, and updating of safety codes
- Risk assessment and license issuance
- Training and technical advice
- Annual reporting to government authorities
- Coordination with national and international organizations

Principal Investigator

The principal investigator is an NBC member with the following scope of duties:
- Receive permit requests for the release of GMOs
- Visit locations for inspection of facilities
- Submit a report to the NBC upon which a permit will be issued or denied
- Instruct and advise staff in practices and techniques to assure level of safety concern.

Institutional Biosafety Committees

Each institute or organization actively involved in genetic engineering research is mandated to establish its own biosafety committee. Institutional Biosafety Committees (IBCs) should include:

- Experts in r-DNA technology
- Experts in biological safety and physical containment
- Consultants knowledgeable in institutional committees, policies, and applicable law
- A biological safety officer.

IBC Activities

- Establish an inspection program
- Assemble a set of oriented guidelines that comply with NBC guidelines
- Assess facilities, practices, and procedures
- Periodically review r-DNA research conducted in the institute
- Adopt emergency plans covering accidental spills and personal contamination
- Periodically review containment measures
- Monitor changes in intellectual property rights
- Report annually to the NBC.

Biological Safety Officer

The Biological Safety Officer (BSO) is an active member of the IBC responsible for:

- Enforcing policies and regulations approved in the institute
- Ensuring that all facility standards are rigorously followed
- Ensuring safety of all facility work and preventing the accidental escape of GMOs
- Maintaining a database on all aspects of biosafety related to mandated crops
- Checking and giving advice on biosafety issues on a day-to-day basis
- Monitoring worldwide biosafety requirements for the r-DNA technology.

Overview of Intellectual Property Rights Status in Egypt

Intellectual property rights (IPR) are important for biotechnology; they can provide incentives to local researchers and firms, they have come to be required by international law, and they can assist in the international transfer of technology.

As Egypt moves toward genetic engineering, it needs to ensure that the developer of a novel gene can obtain appropriate protection. Egypt is already moving to strengthen its law. The old 1949 patent law had no food or pharmaceutical product protection, only a possibility of a 10-year process protection. According to the law's explanatory memorandum, food products are excluded on the grounds that they do not constitute an invention and that a monopoly over producing such products is harmful to the public's health.

As Egypt undergoes a major agricultural reform, in which the private sector will play an essential role, the government is modifying the existing patent law. Under a new law agriculture, foodstuffs, medical drugs, pharmaceutical compounds, plant and animal species, and microbiological organisms and products are included as patentable subject matter. This is a significant strengthening of the previous law and brings Egypt in line with international standards.

New laws such as this, along with an expanded understanding of IPR, should assist Egypt to acquire technology earlier and enter into more effective scientific strategic alliances that will help in developing new technologies and strengthening local research capabilities.

Discussion
Moderator: Louise O. Fresco

Wanda Collins: I would like for Magdy Madkour and Maria José Sampaio to tell us what the public perception is in their countries of existing biosafety provisions. Has there been a change in public perception, or at what level is it?

Also, I got a fair idea of how Brazil approaches the magnitude of risk that they are willing to accept. Could Magdy Madkour give us more information on how Egypt will approach that issue.

Maria José Sampaio: Public perception has been changing slowly. Remember that Brazil is field testing for the first time this year, and even though every proposal for the committee has been published in the press, there has not been much of a reaction from the public so far. Let us see when the field crops start to be planted in October, November.

Magdy Madkour: Regarding the public perception in Egypt, so far we have been doing small-scale field trials, which are confined to a certain stand. We have not yet gone for a large-scale field trial. The first large-scale field trial that will take place in Egypt will be on potatoes.

We have not yet encountered any public resistance in terms of accepting the concept of biotechnology in Egypt. In Egypt we cannot produce any more from the existing crop and crop packages that we have and the technology package we have. We have another tool to use, which is biotechnology.

We see that biotechnology can address expansion into the desert. We know that we can grow wheat in the desert now using such genes, and yesterday there was some discussion that stress and salinity are multigenic traits. Well, we are talking now about a single-gene trait. In the Ministry of Agriculture we do not have alternatives. We have the desert, and we have to increase our vertical production. We have no other new technology that would allow us to do this.

Public perception in terms of biosafety has not yet been tested, but there was one incident in which the Egyptian Ministry of Health released a decree to ban imports of genetically engineered food. This was done after a recommendation by the committee on food safety within the Ministry of Health in response to some wrong information.

This is where coordination and collaboration should take place. The national biosafety committee existed in Egypt, but it was not consulted on this issue. We brought members of the food safety committee and Ministry of Health together with the national biosafety committee. As a result we amended the earlier Health Ministry decree to allow for the importation of genetically engineered material as long as it has been approved in the country of origin and we have enough evidence of the kind of technology used to develop this kind of transgenic material.

This was tested for two months in Egypt, and I think the public has responded very favorably. Both the opposition and the government party have been involved, and we have come to this resolution. I think the public perception is in favor of providing safe technology that will allow Egypt to meet its demand for food production.

Peter Matlon: Maria José Sampaio concluded her statement by underlining the need for regional harmonization in biosafety regulations, and I would like to explore with the panel what might be a more proactive and ambitious approach, depending upon subregional organizations. When we look at Africa right now, as far as I know we have biosafety regulations in place only in Egypt, South Africa, and Zimbabwe. The capacities of national programs are extremely weak. They will require outside assistance to develop regulations. To do this on a country-by-country basis, I think most optimistically, would take 15 to 20 years before regulations are in place. The risks posed by different transgenic crops that might be introduced are identical across neighboring countries in similar agricultural systems.

Would it be feasible politically to consider using subregional organizations as a base to develop intergovernmental agreements whereby a single set of biosafety legislation, perhaps model legislation, could be developed? A single set of regulations would be applied uniformly, through government agreement, through subregional organizations, to identify points of entry—countries with the strongest infrastructural and human resource capacities—so that containment facilities would be concentrated in one or two countries in the subregion.

Once the materials have passed through and been verified as being of acceptable risk, they could then be circulated to other countries that have agreed to this approach without requiring additional containment and field testing.

Is this politically feasible? Is it technically acceptable?

Maria José Sampaio: In relation to South America, when you ask whether it would be possible to have intergovernmental agreements, the answer is yes. But the problem is that you have to analyze every case and every trait. For instance if I had something to analyze between Argentina and southern Brazil, it would be very easy to have one field test organized between both countries. But if a crop is going to be planted near the Amazon, for instance, there is no reason why data acquired in the south would be the same.

Harmonization has to happen, at least for the minimum requirements. But you do have to decide case by case, because of the ecological variation, which brings new challenges every time.

Louise Fresco: Maybe one idea that could be explored further in this context is to see how we can use the approach developed in the Consultative Group on International Agricultural Research (CGIAR) on agroecological zoning. This would identify areas of broad ecological homogeneity as a basis for extrapolation of field testing and regulations.

Fernando Osorio Chaparro: The issue that Peter Matlon has brought up is one that has been discussed mainly at the subregional level, where you can get easier consensus on action and on common legal frameworks.

For example, the Andean countries already have approved a broad common framework within which the national regulatory mechanisms are being approved.

The Latin American and Caribbean region is probably the only subregion that has been able to move in that direction. I am aware of the fact that in the Southern Cone, within Mercosur, there are also discussions along those lines.

But that is a broad framework for national legislation to be formulated and enforced. A second common element that is being carried out at the subregional level is capacity building. There you do have collective efforts to develop economies of scale and a larger impact, because if we go on a country-by-country basis, as Peter Matlon was pointing out, probably time will run out on us.

Third, campaigns of public awareness. In Prociandino there is an effort to move in that direction. The issue of having joint mechanisms for screening has been discussed, but without much agreement. It is much more complicated to have formal collective action at the transnational level.

Samuel Dryden: I would like to address the partnership question that Louise Fresco posed. I think that introducing a private sector perspective might be important to this discussion, because it helps to think in terms of the collaborative advantages and respective roles that a partnership might have and that each party brings to it.

There are two private sector perspectives that I would like to identify, and then ask for comments. One has to do with a market perspective.

The private sector views many of the developing countries in a more refined way, as emerging markets and then within a given country, there are relevant market segments.

That leaves by subtraction those countries that are noncommercial and not really within the view of the private sector. Even within countries where there is a commercial market, there are noncommercial market segments. I think that public sector participants would do well to dialogue with the private sector enough to understand what are the emerging commercial countries and what are the market segments within those, as well.

A second perspective has to do with developing countries as technology collaborators. From a private sector perspective, the comparative and collaborative advantage that any particular country has as a developer of germplasm is important; in the end, while the technology that is being developed is important, the ability to integrate that into the relevant germplasm is going to be the most important.

Beyond that, in terms of the more advanced technologies, I think the private sector is viewing countries in two ways. First, as a group of countries that are technology innovators (here I think of countries that have large, integrated programs, such as Brazil, China, Egypt, India, and Mexico, and a critical mass to develop technologies; over the next 10 years such countries will actually be innovators of these technologies); and second, countries that are technology integrators—those that have the ability to take technology that has been innovated elsewhere and integrate it into the germplasm.

If the public sector and the private sector can dialogue on market issues as well as technology issues, it will provide the opportunity for better partnerships and collaboration.

Charles Jumbe: In reference to Timothy Reeves' presentation, we are faced now with a problem where technology was introduced to the farmers, but the farmers have gone back to their local varieties. These technologies came with some additional inputs that the farmers could not accept.

What would be the potential of the technologies that are being developed amid this environment? Another issue that I would like to ask about is how do you incorporate the ideas and

thoughts of different groups of local farmers? Often we have incorporated farmers only at later stages or using them as a testing ground.

Timothy Reeves: The way that CIMMYT approaches its priorities is very much to try to get all of the partners around the table. A good example is that we are thinking of starting some work on risk management in southern Africa. The approach has been to have a number of round-table meetings, national programs, involving farmers and the local community, to identify the risks that farmers face each day. How do they categorize the risks? What are their current levels of managing those risks? And what ways do they see to better manage risk, both climatic and the associated economic risk, and, of course, environmental risk?

The sort of approach that we believe that we need to adhere to is to have a win-win situation. A major emphasis, for example, of our current work in Africa is to develop maize varieties that are more drought resistant and more tolerant of low-nitrogen conditions. This material does not depend on inputs; it performs better at the low-nitrogen, low-water end of the scale. But when you are able to provide inputs to it, it is also better at the top end of the scale. This is the win-win sort of technology that we look for.

Robert Blake: I am chair of a committee on agricultural sustainability, and I have some conceptual problems regarding how to bring the private sector together with the CGIAR centers and national systems.

You need some leadership to find ways to bring incentives to bear, to bring more research possibilities to the fore at a time when the needs are enormous and we have to move very fast.

How do we do that? Could the World Bank, for example, be designated to, and provide some monies to, begin to find ways to tap the vast resources of the private sector for many things that do not have any immediate profit, to bring those resources to "poor person's agriculture?"

Somehow we have got to get over that gap between the huge potential of the work being done by the private sector and the access of developing country scientists to it, as well as the finances to work. We do not have any time. We need some kind of leadership. Where will we get it?

Derek Byerlee: I am from the World Bank Group, and I want to make one small comment on a particular question that we struggled with during a recent agricultural research project in India; that is, the relationship between national programs and the private sector, particularly the multinational private sector.

We had earmarked funds to try to develop that collaboration, particularly interchanges between multinational companies that may have technology and Indian agricultural research institutions. It is a small step in trying to develop the linkages to be able to access the technology. It is an experimental step, because we do not know really how it is going to work out.

Mahendra Shah: I am with the CGIAR systems review. I would like to ask about what opportunities we can create for the private sector in this area? What strategies are we going to have to obtain private sector involvement?

Maria José Sampaio: Private sector involvement in Brazil is coming. We do not need to force it, because the market is so huge. The private sector is interested, however, only in a commodity that can produce profit. We want to involve the private sector in also working in crops that have a social value, and this is the major opportunity and task for a national system, to try to promote that link.

Louise Fresco: I think we ought to focus this discussion a little bit back to the issue of biosafety. One of the inferences from what both Maria Sampaio and Fernando Chaparro have said is that the private sector is, or should be, very interested in developing biosafety regulations in close conjunction with the government. In the long term it is also to their benefit, not just for the local situation but certainly for the international situation. This is something to be capitalized upon in possibly varying partnerships depending on who and what commodity will be involved.

Mae-Wan Ho: Just a short comment to bring us back to biosafety. I think the previous speaker

contrasting incentive with regulation does bring up the main issue, which is how can we have public accountability from the private sector? For consumers this is the most worrying aspect, because it is not just a matter of regulation or incentives.

Louise Fresco: I think one of the things coming forward from this discussion is that the more open the partnership, the earlier you sit around a table to discuss this, the greater the chances are that public accountability will be part of the operations.

Michel Petit: The issue raised by Robert Blake, as I understand it, is what can the World Bank Group do—and is it the proper role of the World Bank Group—to provide incentives to foster collaboration? I will try to answer, because I think it is important for all the partners around this room to understand what the Bank can do; it can be influential, undoubtedly, but there are limitations under which we work.

The Bank is an important financial institution, but bear in mind that most of its resources are in loans to government. So we are not going to come up with subsidies to promote partnership. It is not an instrument that we are able to utilize.

What do we do? We make loans to governments and we, in turn, dialogue with governments. So clearly, in helping governments create an environment favorable to partnerships with the private sector, we can play a useful role.

Another instrument is that we provide financial resources to the CGIAR. I believe that what the Bank says in the CGIAR is listened to and heard. They do not necessarily do what we say, but they do not ignore what we say. So our role, together with others, in the governance of the CGIAR has an impact.

Finally, a small but effective role that we can play has to do with our ability to conduct pilot operations. We get involved in some activities. Some of you are familiar with the fact that, for instance, we administered and are still administering a banana improvement project for which we receive funding from the Common Fund for Commodities; we are the implementing agency for that project.

We are in the process of exploring with the private sector, which plays a very important role in the export banana business, whether they would be willing to fund at least part of that research. Of course, the World Bank Group is interested in the research because it would be of potential benefit also to the growers of plantain and cooking bananas and to the workers on plantations of export bananas, who suffer from pesticide use.

The point is that we are engaged in a pilot operation to see if we can develop a partnership with the private sector. One major limitation facing the World Bank Group is that it has never done this before. It has to deal with intellectual property rights. We would have to devise a policy, and we are on very tentative grounds. It seems like a very simple idea, but it is complicated to put it in place. I hope this has given you an idea of what the World Bank Group can do on those matters.

Val Giddings: I am with the Biotechnology Industry Organization, and I would like briefly to address the issue of accountability.

I think there is a great temptation in discussions in this arena, when our minds turn to the issue of accountability, to assume that the only means of effecting accountability—particularly of large transnational corporations—is through government mandates and formal regulations and laws.

I would point out that the most effective, immediate, and sometimes brutal mechanism for making accountability a reality lies in the decisions made by the individual consumer at the point of purchase. If the products we are talking about do not pass that muster, in the face of a relentlessly skeptical and conservative consuming public, these products will not survive. Preliminary indications to date are that these products have a bright but still somewhat rocky future.

Louise Fresco: The devil's advocate would say that the public needs to be informed before it can make a choice, and I think accountability also is about information.

Maria José Sampaio: I agree with Val Giddings. Accountability will be done by the final consumer, but the consumer will need to be very well informed in all senses of the word. If we were

the government, we should be very worried about that and make it happen.

Audience comment: I will address my comments to Robert Blake's important point, which is that there is no time to hang around, no time to waste when talking about fruitful and positive partnerships.

One of the big opportunities of marshaling a public-private partnership relates to genome mapping. This is going on already to a certain extent, but if we understood a lot more about the genomes of all of these crops that we want to work with, both the big ones and the small ones, this would be a real win-win situation.

It would help the companies, of course, and it would also help the public sector tremendously. It would also help in the characterizing of genetic diversity. It would help, I believe, in understanding a little better some of the issues of biosafety. So that is the one area where we could get together and make things move ahead. The reality is that the competitive advantage for any company in making a little more progress in the short term will be short-lived, because in the end we will have this information. The sooner we get there and everyone has it, the better it will be.

Louise Fresco: Let me highlight what I think are the major issues that came across in this meeting, which I found very stimulating and very important.

First, there are obviously major differences between national systems in developing countries. Sam Dryden used the typology of technology innovators and technology integrators. Their needs are different, but some of the needs are similar. Some of those have to do with the need for information, for a monitoring system, for skills development, and for national capacity building. There is also a need to learn from the example of others in terms of regulatory measures, and legislation.

The differences between national programs, as well as the experiences within the CGIAR and advanced research institutions in Western countries, can help provide a basis for what is proposed as a proactive regional partnership, where some regional problems, rather than being solved on a country-by-country basis, could be tackled on a regional basis. Possibly the CGIAR could play an important role through its bases of networks of research stations according to certain ecological zones, which would help harmonize some of the field testing.

The other issue that came forward very strongly is accountability. While we did not speak very much about it, another area for possible collaboration is the review of participatory approaches to get consumers and society at large much more involved early in the process of priority setting and understanding some of the regulation measures.

Last but not least, the plea for more massive efforts to get biotechnology going in developing countries, not just for commercially inter-esting crops but also for crops that are essential to livelihoods. The focus needs to be on those crops or varieties that may be in the process of disappearing. I wonder whether we should somehow visit the idea of a more massive effort in terms of mobilizing the world community in the same way that our fellow scientists from the climate community have done through, for example, the Intergovernmental Panel on Climate Change.

The time may have come, in a period where agriculture has fallen from grace in so many urban communities, for urban-based decision-makers to think about a global coalition for biotechnology to solve the food problem.

Role of Public Policy

Panel Presentation
Vernon W. Ruttan

As we look at the role of public policy, including support for research; the evolution of intellectual property rights; and environmental, health, and market regulation it is useful to remind ourselves of its importance in the development of the biotechnology industry.

Research Support

More than any other industry, the biotechnology industry in the United States owes its origin to public support. Prior to the mid-1970s almost all research in molecular biology and biotechnology had been conducted by universities (with foundation and federal funding) and by federal government (primarily the National Institutes of Health) laboratories. The initial motivation was the potential contribution to the solution of human health problems. The flow of federal funding into biomedical research associated with President Nixon's "war on cancer" focused much of the early research in the biomedical area.

Plant molecular biology and agricultural biotechnology developed later and more slowly. Progress was inhibited by: (a) the dramatic success of plant breeders, drawing on the techniques of "classical" Mendelian genetics; (b) initial skepticism by plant breeders about the claims being made by molecular biologists; and (c) funding constraints in the field of plant molecular biology.

Safety

The initiative taken by leading researchers in molecular biology and biotechnology in calling attention to potential health and environmental dangers was unprecedented in any field of science. The 1975 Asilomar Conference, organized by Paul Berg and Maxine Singer, was the landmark event. The conference concluded that "there are certain experiments in which the potential risks are of such a serious nature that they ought not to be taken given presently available containment facilities" and recommended a moratorium on such experiments until more secure facilities could be built and appropriate protocols developed.

By the mid-1980s the legacy of the Asilomar Conference had largely been reversed. In the biomedical area almost the entire spectrum of living things had been opened to genetic manipulation, with controls remaining only for limited classes of experiments. One observer noted: "It is quite remarkable how quickly doubts about safety receded once it appeared that profits could be made in this new technology."

As this conference indicates, however, safety concerns have remained stronger in the area of agricultural than pharmaceutical biotechnology. These concerns include the effects of introducing transgenic crops on the genetic integrity of wild species and the emergence of new and more troublesome weeds and other pests and pathogens.

Intellectual Property Rights

Plant patent and patent-like (plant variety registration) property rights have evolved slowly in the U.S. and other industrial countries since 1930. The landmark in intellectual property rights for biotechnology was the 1980 decision by the U.S. Supreme Court (Diamond vs. Chakrabasty) that extended patent protection to new microorganisms.

A major issue that remains unresolved is how broadly life forms can be patented. Recent decisions by the U.S. patent and trademark office seem to favor broad interpretations. For example:

1. The decision to grant a patent for gene therapy that encompasses virtually all gene therapy involving in vivo technique (to Kelly, Palella, and Levine)

2. The Abbott-Geneit application to patent genetic markers (of the single nucleotide polymorphism-SWPS type).

Students of patent policy have generally concluded that broad grants of property rights are more likely to inhibit competition than more narrow rights. Researchers are concerned that the broader grants could inhibit research.

Commercial Development

Commercial development of biotechnology has been slower than was anticipated two decades ago. By the mid-1990s there were still fewer than 30 biotechnology therapeutics and vaccines on the market. During the last several years, however, new product approvals by the U.S. Food and Drug Administration have increased rapidly. Profitability and sustainability of specialized biotechnology firms have remained problematic. It seems clear, in retrospect, that in addition to a potentially promising commercial product, a few "delusion genes" have also been important in starting up a new biotechnology company.

In the case of agriculture it is only in the last two years that biotechnology products have become commercially important (bovine somatotropin, herbicide resistant soybeans, Bt corn and cotton). Agricultural biotechnology is, at present, a very small industry. Pharmaceuticals account for 90 percent of total sales. However agrochemical and agrobiological biotechnology, which accounted for only about 2 percent of sales in 1995, are now the most rapidly growing segment of the industry.

The field of nonmedical diagnostics (to detect chemicals, pathogens, and other contaminants in the food supply and environment) is also growing rapidly.

Industrial Organization

During the 1990s the market structure of the pharmaceutical industry underwent a major transformation. For much of the postwar period the industry had been composed of large, research-intensive, vertically integrated (from laboratory to distribution) firms. The rise of specialized computational biology centers is dramatically altering the structure of the industry. It is now composed of a few marketing firms; many small, knowledge-intensive biotechnology firms; associated university research laboratories; and the foundations and government agencies that support biological, biochemical, and biotechnology research. We are now, however, seeing a wave of consolidation among the major pharmaceutical companies.

The structure of the agricultural biotechnology industry is becoming consolidated even more rapidly than that of the pharmaceutical industry. Four (possibly five) corporate groupings, including Monsanto, Novartis (formed by Ciba-Geigy and Sandoz) and Dow-Elanco, AgrEvo (Hoechst and Sheriny), and Pioneer-DuPont are evolving.

Developing Countries

The experience of Japan, which tried to develop a biotechnology industry based on its dominance in fermentation products, seems to indicate that sufficient depth in both basic science and bioengineering are difficult to acquire for those who lag behind, such as developing countries.

A country may not need to be at the leading edge in the development of either biomedical or agricultural biotechnology to make effective use of the technology. China may be the leading country in the development, testing, and utilization of transgenic plants. Brazil, Egypt, India, and Mexico are also making rapid progress.

Another culture and genetic marker techniques are being used by plant breeders in many developing countries. Biopesticides based on biotechnology are being used in a number of developing countries.

Substantial scientific and technical capacity will be required in developing countries if they are to introduce and manage the diffusion of these technologies safely and productively.

There will be winners and losers in both industrial and developing countries. The health concerns of the rich, the old, and the fat will continue to be served, while the institutional reforms necessary to enable the poor to lead a healthier life will be neglected. Producers of agricultural products that continue to be sold as "commodities" (undifferentiated maize, oil seeds, and cotton) will lose while those who produce the higher value-added fibers, grains, and oilseeds will gain.

Capacity to Respond to Surprise

No one in the 1950s, and few in the 1960s or 1970s, would have anticipated that agricultural commodity prices would continue their long-term decline into the 1990s. Wheat prices have declined since the middle of 19th century; rice prices have declined since the middle of the 20th century.

Almost no one, particularly the World Bank Group, anticipated that in the mid-1990s petroleum prices would be below the levels of the early 1970s.

It is not possible to anticipate surprises. The future will be different than the past because it has not yet occurred! It is not unreasonable to expect "surprises" in population, health, agricultural production, and the environment. The capacity to advance knowledge and technology is the only "reserve army" available to deal with surprise. Most of the time our research is focused on normal science and incremental technical change. When confronted by surprise, the trajectory of technical change can be redirected—but only if the "reserve army" is in place.

My sense is that the biotechnology industry stands, in its development, at about the same stage as computers in the late 1950s, before vacuum tubes were replaced by transistors. No one committed to 1950s mainframe computer development anticipated the personal computer.

We are just emerging from the first-generation stage: doing what we can do by working with single genes. The second generation will involve multiple genes and the modification of plants, animals, and human components. The third generation will involve the modification of whole organisms. An excessive commitment to avoiding surprise will also mean that we avoid the benefits of biotechnology.

Panel Presentation
Michel Dron

The question of public policy for the safe management of biotechnology products and processes in developing countries cannot be fully covered within the framework of a short presentation. Therefore this overview will leave aside many important considerations and focus instead on a small number of features stemming from the direct experience of scientists active in this field. It will selectively highlight a few questions or personal feelings on current debates, rather than advance many certainties. When speaking of biotechnology in general, this overview will mostly refer implicitly to genetic engineering for agricultural purposes, or even more specifically to the release of genetically modified organisms.

Biotechnology for the South

Biotechnology is obviously not the only solution to the development problems of agriculture in developing countries, and such basics as sound agricultural practices, conventional breeding, or integrated pest management will remain predominant concerns.

Unique Opportunities of Biotechnology

Nevertheless, it is widely recognized that biotechnology holds exceptional promise for improving agricultural production and ensuring that such improvements are environmentally sound.

Biotechnology may provide original and easy-to-use solutions to general problems that will prove more appropriate in some local contexts than those adopted in the North, such as human or animal vaccination through plants or mosquito bites or high-yield plant varieties needing only limited agrochemical inputs.

Biotechnology may also partially help to overcome problems more specific to the South: development of hardier plant varieties tolerant to different stresses, maize apomixy avoiding the annual purchase of higher-yielding hybrid seeds, and clonal propagation of rubber trees resistant to South American leaf blight.

Expansion of Biotechnology in the South

With the world population forecast to double over the next 50 years, there is no way that the required increase in productivity can be reached without a technological breakthrough, which can hardly be envisioned without the intensive use of biotechnology. The same reasoning may be applied to sustainability, since the doubling of present food-production levels with current techniques would undoubtedly prove disastrous for the environment.

Biotechnology must also be considered from a defensive point of view. Developing countries must anticipate the development of new techniques in the North that may displace some of their commercial markets: the production of lauric oil from rapeseed will reduce the demand for copra; aroma culture in bioreactors is a threat to vanilla, coffee, cocoa, and orange production.

Less than 5 percent of all transgenic plant field trials in the world take place in the South at the present time.

Characteristics of Biotechnology Development in the South

Not all development-oriented research, whether basic or applied, need necessarily be conducted in developing countries. Conversely, there is no reason not to perform such research in the South whenever the prerequisites for efficiency prevail, let alone whenever it is imperative. Gene transfer may be carried out anywhere, but the same is not true for selection of traits of interest, confirmation in the field of the agronomic value of the plants, or the study of tropical ecosystems.

Safety issues should not be treated more superficially in the South than in the North. This is both a moral imperative (let us not repeat with biotechnology the counterexample of the use of pesticides) and a global necessity stemming from the fact that environmental hazards cannot be contained within national borders.

Safety issues are matters of national sovereignty. However the implementation of this principle is dependent on the capacity of each country to exercise its prerogatives, the responsibility of the technique or product provider, and transborder cooperation needs.

Not all countries can develop high-performance research in the different fields of biotechnology, but all countries should aim at building up the minimum level of expertise needed to define their own policies (including regulation and monitoring) and carry out a fruitful exchange with foreign specialists. The first step toward a safety policy is the creation of an endogenous technical capacity.

Role of Science in Defining Public Policy

Science currently plays a key role in establishing the founding principles of public policies: defining their content, implementing them, and creating the conditions for their social acceptance. It is now mainly at the implementation stage that doubts and uncertainties, or even paradoxes, arise.

Policy Issues

Public policy is directly responsible for many factors affecting the development of biotechnology. To name but a few: training; defining a regulatory framework that will take into account the advantages and constraints of genetically modified organisms (GMOs) and respect the interests of every partner (seed grower, farmer, agribusiness, consumer); specifying the respective roles of the public and private sectors; creating appropriate incentives; ensuring public acceptance; and orienting public research.

Governments must direct resources toward research topics that will enable a better assessment of the ecological, toxicological, or economic risks associated with GMOs, such as the consequences of induced changes in plant metabolism, gene flows, or the prevention of insect resistance.

Concerning plants, priority should probably be given:

- In the short term to the application of well-mastered biotechnology techniques; to the species of major importance in the South, which are of little concern to the private sector; and to a better knowledge of these species
- In the medium term to physiological mechanisms, resistance to pests or diseases, or environmental impacts
- In the long term to resistance to salt or drought stress and nitrogen fixation.

The growing appropriation of public-interest transformation techniques and genes is of prime concern for public research and developing countries. Excesses are becoming apparent. While recognizing the necessity for maintaining financial inducements that enable strong private investment in these areas, new balances will have to be found. This will not be an easy task since opposing needs must be reconciled not only between economic interests, but also between national and international legislation, cultures, and values.

Overview of National Regulatory Approaches

An overview of national regulatory approaches and sensibilities leads to contrasting pictures.
- In North America, which relies on a product-based approach, several million hectares of genetically engineered cotton, corn, soybean,

rapeseed, or tomatoes were sown this year with overall acceptance from a public that rejected GMOs until fairly recently. Risk assessment and regulation controls are carried out by the same authority. The bulk of legal liability is borne by the companies marketing the products. When hazards are still conjectural, guidelines are usually considered more appropriate than laws.

- Europe has also built up extensive experience in laboratory research and field trials under stringent regulations and monitoring. Recent major problems in areas that are related in people's minds (blood contamination, bovine spongiform encephalopathy—BSE) or ethical considerations (the first cloning of mammals) have kept alive significant public distrust, which has prevented the cultivation of any transgenic crop on an industrial scale. Consumer groups are very sensitive to the issues of traceability and product labeling, which have not yet been fully settled. Aware of these trends, governments have occasionally dissociated themselves from the advice of their own expert commissions, as was demonstrated recently in France in the case of an herbicide-resistant maize. Risk assessment and regulation controls are usually carried out by different bodies, and governments are more directly involved in legal responsibilities.

- China is engaged in the large-scale growing of transgenic rice, tobacco, and tomatoes, with apparent priority given to quantitative results, little heed to public opinion, and a general lack of sensitivity among farmers to environmental issues.

- Emerging countries such as Brazil, India, and Mexico have developed a substantial domestic research base, which provides them with a large absorption capacity. The regulatory systems that are progressively being set up in these countries usually follow closely those of other countries or regions, mainly the U.S. and Europe.

- Many developing countries have a simultaneous fear of being left behind by progress—which will further increase the inequalities between nations—and becoming risk experimentation grounds for industrialized countries. Nongovernmental organizations have substantial influence on some governments and opinion leaders. A large number of countries have expressed a will to take common stands in international negotiations, most African countries having at one point endorsed a proposal calling for a moratorium on all GMO releases. These countries are pressing for compulsory international biosafety regulations within the framework of the Rio Earth Summit Convention on Biological Diversity. On the entire African continent only Egypt and South Africa have set up effective biosafety regulatory procedures so far. Kenya, Zimbabwe, and a few other countries have made headway in that direction.

The representative of the Group of 77 demands a protocol that would cover research and development (R&D), transfer, use, and disposal involving any biotechnologically altered organism that may adversely affect the conservation and sustainable use of biological diversity. These countries wish to be protected by an international instrument from any harm resulting from imported modified organisms. They emphasize the need to consider liability and compensation issues.

However most industrialized countries prefer restricting the protocol to transboundary movements. They consider R&D, domestic handling, use, and disposal to be matters of national sovereignty not subject to regulation by international protocol.

Root Safety Policies in Local Societies and Cultures

Science alone cannot define good practice rules capable of universal application. Regarding GMOs, for example, and stemming from the same range of proven knowledge, the United States has adopted a more clearly "product-based" approach than the European Union (EU). Before the EU harmonized its national regulations, Denmark and Spain had developed radically opposing philosophies from the same data, the former practically banning GMOs on the grounds that they involved new types of risks, and the latter considering that none of their characteristics called for new rules.

Administrative cultures also differ from country to country; while some may enact laws providing for preliminary authorizations, others may exert a posteriori controls and rely on individual and business liabilities.

More importantly, problems are necessarily weighed differently in different countries. International conferences on such global issues as deforestation or emissions of polluting gases are proof enough that, to some extent, environment and development issues may be in conflict and priorities cannot be the same in different contexts.

Role and Duties of Scientists

To be better prepared to answer the questions of tomorrow, scientists must be able to anticipate emerging problems or potential crises and translate them into scientific approaches

Helping Define and Implement Public Choices

The experience and evolution of the French Biomolecular Engineering Commission (FBEC) may be of interest in this regard. Created to prepare administrative approval for GMO field trials, the commission has expanded its role to include early interaction with applicants, with a view to improving the quality of the projects submitted. Capitalizing on a growing body of experience, it has also engaged in in-depth analyses of the philosophy of dissemination, exploring some of the possible consequences of a generalization of genetically engineered specific products in agriculture. The FBEC then characterized different scenarios that could enable decisionmakers to better assess situations with which they might be confronted and help them react more appropriately. The goal would then be to offer a decisionmaking tree for biomonitoring purposes.

Acting as Experts

Increasingly, scientists are requested to give expert advice to decisionmakers. The questions are most frequently asked in a form, and with time constraints, that require experts to express clear answers that go well beyond their own competence and what they consider to have been scientifically proven. Their opinions necessarily stem from both the state of current knowledge and their convictions as individuals, which are natu-

rally subjective and vulnerable to outside influences. It is reasonable to assume that an expert's advice may be formulated differently according to the perceived stakes. For example, will the certainties and doubts of a person questioned about "mad cow" disease be expressed in the same way if he or she feels the objective is to protect Europeans from a potentially dramatic epidemic, manage cattle health, or straighten out the beef market?

Scientists acting as experts are too often asked to make decisions when their role should be limited to providing knowledge. But they cannot refuse to answer, for where else can politicians and civil servants go for enlightened advice?

On major issues expertise should be organized in a collective form with debates that feature both sides of the issue, do not hide minority opinions, and clearly distinguish between conclusions drawn from scientific certainties and those related to economic or political choices. In areas such as biosafety, where the need is greatest, permanent networks or committees might be set up to discuss potential problems before action is needed. Many disciplines, including the social sciences, should be represented in these fora, as should nonspecialists. The conclusions should be worth publishing as actual contributions to knowledge, even when still not final. It is more important to create a procedure capable of expanding the scope for scientific critiques of possible options than to reach premature consensus.

Increasing Public Awareness

Public anxiety about biotechnology is fed as much by the progress of science, which simultaneously produces and warns about new dangers, as by the feeling that experts are unable to reach certainties and provide solutions.

Scientists have a duty to bring references to the public, so that the latter becomes less sensitive to campaigns organized by particular lobbies or irrational and demagogic postures. If the permanent expert networks or committees alluded to previously were to be set up, one of their main tasks would be to provide credible benchmarks for public opinion and the media, so that subsequent decisions might be taken in the most transparent way.

But popularizing knowledge is not enough. Individually, or as a group, scientists are also responsible for the image of science in society. They must take part directly in debates with non-specialists—either decisionmakers (what proportion of a country's representatives who will vote on bioethics or biosafety laws really grasp their significance?) or the general public, which can demand or prevent technically justified measures according to its feelings about their legitimacy.

Acting Ethically

A number of the points raised above deal with the ethics of science itself: making scientific controversies explicit, clearly indicating the nature of "personal convictions" when providing expert advice, calling for real debate, and maintaining a responsible relationship with the media (announcement of unproved results, formulation of unlikely hypotheses).

Safety Issues

There is no need to elaborate upon why safety issues must be addressed with extreme caution. The main reasons are: the number of unsolved questions, the extent and dimension of potential damage, the irreversibility of some environmental consequences, our responsibility toward future generations, and the fact that GMOs ignore national borders.

Precautionary Principle

Everybody will agree on the necessity to take preventive measures, even before the reality of the risks involved is fully demonstrated. However, implementation of the "precautionary principle" raises many conceptual and practical difficulties.

The first major debate focuses on the intrinsic danger of biotechnology processes. There seems to be a fairly broad consensus within the scientific community that biotechnology bears no particular danger in and of itself, and that risk assessments must be carried out exclusively on the products resulting from its use. "Traditional" techniques may present the same kind of risks, associated, for example, with the toxicity or allergenicity of a new plant variety obtained

through classical breeding (the border between "classical breeding" and "biotechnology-assisted breeding" itself being somewhat fuzzy), or with the disruption of an ecological balance through the introduction of an exogenous organism into a given environment. Some go as far as to estimate that the potentially undesirable consequences of biotechnology products are indeed fewer, due to greater concern for their safety and better control of that which is being inserted into the organisms.

Most existing authorization committees have developed a common "philosophy" that can be summarized as follows:

- Assessment of the potential risks associated with a transgenic plant requires a precise characterization of the plant, the transgene actually integrated, and the transgenic plant's behavior in its natural ecosystem.
- The ideal transgenic fragment inserted into a plant should be short, fully characterized, stable, and restricted to whatever is strictly necessary to obtain the desired effect.
- The goal of genetic engineering in agriculture is not only to produce more, but also to produce with increased safety standards.
- Some phenomena undetectable in small-scale tests could be observed under conditions of large-scale cultivation of transgenic plants.

Science frequently proves unable to provide in due time the required certainties for a fully enlightened decision. Conversely, just as too much information may result in confusion, too great a perception of potential risks may paralyze decisionmaking capacities, since researchers will find it increasingly difficult to certify the total harmlessness for human health or the environment of a given substance or technique.

Nevertheless the precautionary approach means seriously taking into account marginal or dissident opinions within the scientific community (for example, the initial appraisal of the Acquired Immunodeficiency Syndrome, or AIDS, epidemic)—even the most dubious ones—despite the risk of creating unjustified anxiety or economic disruption (such as the drop in consumption of red meat in Europe following the BSE crisis).

It must be borne in mind that most modern or traditional human activities or techniques that might have an impact on the environment would be banned if the precautionary principle were to be strictly applied, demanding that proof be given of the nonexistence of any kind of risk in the long run, or focusing exclusively on disaster scenarios. The very high resulting costs would be considered unbearable. The same excesses threaten biotechnology. One must therefore revert to the notion of "tolerable risk," which raises new questions:

- How can we define "tolerable risk" from the social or legal point of view? Jurisprudence is far from being settled in any country. It has evolved considerably in recent years in a context of sanitary and political disaster and emergency (AIDS virus-contaminated blood, the BSE epidemic), which may not be the most appropriate framework for due consideration of environmental issues.

- How can we foresee totally unknown dangers? Chlorinated fluorocarbons (CFCs) were widely used for decades before the hole in the ozone layer was discovered and attributed partially to the very chemical inertia that led them previously to be considered the safest of all gases.

- In our societies who will bear the costs of public interest? Total herbicides are very limited in number and bound to disappear with the development of resistant varieties through genetic engineering. Will the risk of escape of herbicide-resistant genes lead to the preservation of a few total herbicides? Who will make the decision? How will the proprietary firms be compensated for their loss of income?

Internationalization

GMO release agreements will increasingly tend to be granted by groups of countries, if only because international scientific cooperation will make risk assessment procedures more similar to one another. Some people even predict that some biotechnology products may be declared intrinsically safe by internationally recognized institutions and therefore receive simultaneous worldwide clearance. But paradoxically, environmental dangers should, in many instances, be appreciated for each specific ecosystem on a much smaller scale than that of most countries.

Most attention has focused thus far on the individual risk presented by new products. But other types of risks could be attached to the widespread use of more efficient techniques; for example, loss of more traditional agricultural know-how, reduction of biodiversity, disruption of ecological balance, or the emergence of new resistance in pests. These problems call for collective management of risks over long periods of time on a supranational level.

Specific Safety Issues in the South

The nature of the problem is not different in North and South, but coping with it may prove more difficult in the latter, due to less development in some key areas.

- Scientific knowledge is often more limited with regard to tropical plants, microorganisms, and ecosystems. Plant species such as cotton, rice, soybean, maize, or vegetables, which are of common interest to North and South, are already being genetically engineered and cultivated in large quantities in industrialized countries. Pressure will be strong to have similar seeds adapted everywhere, even though much less will be known about dissemination risks in other environments.

- Many countries will lag behind for some time in their domestic capacity to define their own regulatory systems—even when inspired by foreign experiences—and monitor their implementation. We have drawn up a proposal to alleviate this constraint as an appendix to this contribution.

- The large-scale use of new techniques will raise questions of compatibility between individual and collective interests, which may prove more difficult to reconcile in places where the average technical level is lower. This may be the case for good agricultural practices aimed at preventing the appearance of new resistance among insects.

- Generally speaking, it is likely that regional cooperation should be promoted to make up for the lack of domestic expertise.

- Last, without neglecting either the absolute necessity of acting with extreme care or legitimate national sovereignty concerns, there is a fear that biosafety matters may, in some instances, serve as excuses for two harmful, opposing attitudes: the refusal of high-performance products or processes for want of complete safety assurances, on the one hand, and the acceptance of dangerous practices by incompetent authorities on the other.

Conclusion

Risk

There is no such thing as "zero risk." Therefore, a "tolerable level of risk" has to be assessed. The acceptance by a community of a given level of risk will depend on the perceived potential benefits, the risk of nonintervention, and the local situation. The "precautionary principle" bears no meaning if its most rigorous application is not restricted to relatively exceptional circumstances.

Evolution of Scientists' Responsibilities and Role

Science is bound to create anxiety through the very questions and doubts it raises, but the rate of increase of proven knowledge is not sufficiently rapid to provide decisionmakers with the desired answers in due time.

Collective decisionmaking is becoming increasingly dependent upon scientific activity, and scientists now have to act more and more as go-betweens between knowledge and decision-making. This situation grants them considerable influence, if only through the public expression of mere speculation capable of upsetting entire industries.

Governments, which are called upon to enact regulations, solve environmental crises, and cope with all kinds of risks, are steadily becoming scientists' main "customers." Many social protagonists, including the numerous lobbies that try to influence policies or public opinion, have a similar need for scientific expertise. This leads to the increasing meddling of society as a whole into scientific affairs. Scientists are being submitted to pressures and may become instruments in power games. Both the quality of scientists' answers and their freedom to research could be protected through a collective organization of appraisal functions.

The role of economics and social sciences to help make and legitimize decisions in uncertain environments must not be underestimated.

Reasonable Management of Precautions

Science will be unable to provide clear answers to some essential problems for a considerable time. This uncertainty must not be used, deliberately or not, to prevent decsionmaking. We must accept a continuous evolution of risk assessments and a gradual approach to regulatory requirements that will improve the basis of further decisions.

Primacy of Politics

Biology is obviously not the only discipline concerned about biosafety matters. Industrial engineers, economists, lawyers, political scientists, and many others have to cooperate with biologists, since risk management clearly has ecological, economic, and social dimensions. But even all these experts together (fortunately) cannot dictate the choices of executive authorities or society in general.

In a democracy the final choices on matters affecting society are political. It is therefore the duty of society, or its representatives, to ensure that they are made in the public interest and to offer solutions that most people will consider reasonable.

We conclude by paraphrasing a famous statement: "Biosafety is too serious a matter to be left to biologists."

Annex. Proposal for the Establishment of an International Biomolecular Engineering Commission for Tropical Agriculture

The countries of the South cannot refrain from the use in agriculture of genetically modified organisms (GMOs), which may bring original, appropriate, and powerful solutions to some of their needs to increase productivity, limit inputs, and achieve sustainable development.

However many of them will not have access in the near future to the domestic expertise that would enable them to define their own policies regarding biosafety matters with full knowledge of the case or to implement their own regulatory mechanisms without outside help.

Countries of the North have begun to accumulate significant expertise, part—but not all—of which might be transferred, since their specialized commissions know little about tropical cultures or ecosystems.

Therefore it is suggested that a study be carried out to determine under what conditions an international biomolecular engineering commission for tropical agriculture might be established, the advice of which might be requested by governments on a case-by-case basis on the following topics:

- General policies regarding GMOs and regulations regarding releases; the mandate of the commission might be extended, if so desired, to encompass the release of all exogenous organisms.
- Definition of technical references regarding the assessment of different types of risks in specific tropical environments. The documents might result from syntheses made by the members of the commission themselves, from studies on the state of current knowledge commissioned from outside experts, or from the results of specific research, which could be initiated on issues insufficiently addressed. In all cases the resulting conclusions would be subject to rigorous debate within the international scientific community before their formal adoption. The commission could also act as a permanent forum in which similar national bodies might publicly discuss their experiences.
- The authorization of GMO releases for research or business purposes. Projects might be referred to the commission by governments, research institutes, or companies. Beyond formal approval, their study would provide the opportunity for in-depth dialogue between the project initiators and the commission, in order that safety requirements might be better accounted for in trial design or full-scale operations.

One of the ways to reach these goals might be to establish a small, permanent secretariat close to an existing institution. Its task would consist of mobilizing an international network of experts, both scientific and nonscientific, who would commit themselves to a minimum annual availability.

Panel Presentation
George A. Lloyd

First and foremost, I must acknowledge the contributions of technology in answering the vexing problems of uncontrolled population growth, nonavailability of sustainable land, and growing food demand. At the same time one cannot overlook the environmental concerns and fears of unknown safety implications when introducing new technology.

History has shown that it is very difficult to implement scientifically proven remedies if they come up against financial considerations. A good example of this is something that affects people from my region very directly; that is, the failure to implement the many resolutions of international agreements on anthropogenic gas emissions.

As a result one approaches new technology with a certain amount of trepidation. The main fear is that if technology is not well managed, the solution provided may become the root cause of other, often more serious, problems. Examination of this phenomenon leads to the belief that we appear to be treating the symptoms and not the root cause of many problems confronting mankind. Inaction is having a devastating impact on the environment. The political will to act appears to be lacking.

With the advent of information technology, decisionmakers are more apt to respond to public opinion polls than to correct, scientifically based studies. If any policy is to have a meaningful impact, we must take into consideration the fact that politicians will not take a stand on the side of unpopular decisions, irrespective of how correct they may be. Our major concern, therefore, is to ensure that sufficient safeguards are put in place when introducing new technology.

We have to accept that biotechnology is already having an impact on the marketplace and will play an ever-increasing role in the economics of the world. Our focus must now move to addressing the major concerns of health, environmental issues, ecological concerns, ethical considerations, and biosafety. While the risk remains, the role of public policy should be to ensure that sufficient safeguards are put into place. These safeguards must contain regulatory mechanisms that include enforcement through legislation on an internationally accepted basis.

It is imperative that the regulatory framework ensures safe, expeditious, and economic development and use of such products and processes to be developed. This will enable a country to capture the present and future benefits of biotechnology's introduction of new products.

To achieve this, there is a need to ensure that national regulatory frameworks and international frameworks are similar. We have been told that 169 countries have already signed the Convention on Biological Diversity. The negotiation of protocols, therefore, provides us with the last forum in which to address the fears expressed by the different lobbies.

There is undoubtedly a need for an international watchdog to ensure compliance. Some of the functions of such a watchdog should include control of introductions, field testing, import, and export. This point I particularly address to some of the smaller countries that would find it very difficult to finance some of these controls.

The developing countries have a need for new technologies, particularly those which are scale-neutral, to combat hunger. Unfortunately, biotechnology is only one of the tools in this fight. The developed world's governments must be made to realize that the real enemy is not in the trenches of some foreign country where they spend nearly one trillion U.S. dollars on military activity. The new war is being fought in laboratories that are trying to find solutions to the growing problems of poverty and hunger. Technologies such as biotechnology will help in this battle. However we must convince the world that we are losing the war against poverty and that the casualties are much higher than in all other human conflicts.

I must also address the imbalances between the haves and the have-nots, which is growing and will continue to grow until an equitable form of trade is established. The most well-intentioned policy is doomed to failure as long as these imbalances exist. There is a need for the world to change the way in which policies are made, because the whole world is influenced by the decisions and actions of each of its parts.

Technological solutions can be found in the developed world for many of the developed world's problems. However, these lead to a false sense of security. The climatic changes that are occurring may not have an immediate negative impact on the industrialized countries, and may even appear to have some beneficial effect. The problems also often appear remote. Most of the negative effects are taking place in the less-developed tropics, where climate change is compounding existing problems.

Poverty and ignorance often mean that mortality rates are high. Therefore, large families appear to be the answer for survival, labor, and security in old age. This further compounds the problem. The developing world must also take stock, and unpopular decisions will have to be made. Here, also, a new approach is necessary.

Interregional trade must be encouraged. The developing world must make itself attractive to entice investment. Reliance on aid cannot and should not be taken for granted. Instead, inter-national partnerships and commercial credits through governments to the private sector should be encouraged.

Markets and economies must be opened up. Impediments restricting trade, such as border tariffs and levies, should be gradually done away with. Intellectual property rights and patents must be recognized and enforced. Planning should be on a regional basis. The principle of comparative advantage should be exploited to the fullest if we are to avoid the white elephant projects of the past. This includes any biotechnology projects that might be undertaken.

The world has an uphill battle if it is to harness the full promise of biotechnology for the benefit of the world's poor, the environment, and the safe management of products and processes. No doubt this is another weapon against hunger, and its use should go a long way in combating this scourge.

Public policy should have at its core the concept of environmentally sustainable development, based on the idea that it is possible to improve the basic living of the world's growing population without necessarily depleting the world's finite natural resources. At the center of this policy should be the belief that emerging biotechnologies offer novel approaches for striking a balance between development needs and environmental conservation.

At the same time a wider diffusion of biotechnology is essential to giving the world access to its positive attributes. Since most of the world's poor come from countries whose economies are not in a position to finance much of the research required, innovative finance mechanisms should be explored and built into policy. Without such mechanisms most developing countries will not be able to build the infrastructure to acquire, absorb, and develop the technology, nor will they be able to build up local scientific and technological competence. There is a need to put in place mechanisms for technological transfer, training of scientists, creation of international partnerships, and transfer of spillover technology.

The approach in the developing world may have to include use of existing national scientific research centers. However, to achieve self-sustainability over the long term, it may be necessary to rethink the modes of financing, as most will not be high on the list of government spending.

It may be possible to innovate and develop ownership and responsibility-sharing between governments and organizations representing stakeholders at both the national and regional levels. I am convinced that, given the right environment, African private business will rise to the challenge.

Discussion
Moderator: Per Pinstrup-Andersen

Per Pinstrup-Andersen: I would like to hear comments by some of the panelists regarding the potential tradeoff between biosafety and poverty and hunger. In other words, whose biosafety are we looking after? Whose standards are we using, and do poor and rich have the same acceptable risk levels?

It seems to me that this is one of the issues that this session should address. If we set standards for "the rich, the fat, and the old," then it is possible that we are really not looking after the biosafety of the many millions of people who are trying to feed their children, but are unable to do so, by setting standards that are so high that we are plucking out of the market opportunities for using modern science to benefit poor people.

Would any of you like to comment on these tradeoffs, what kind of policies we need, and how we avoid the prediction made by Vernon Ruttan that we are going to run this show the way we run many other shows, namely that the rich are going to benefit and the poor are going to lose?

Panelist comment: I think the biosafety level in relation to the need of different populations, the poor compared to the rich, is an area where we must ask: Who will decide?

That is why countries have national sovereignty to decide what biosafety rules they need. They need to have information and, of course, we have to put together all the information. When they get the information, they will decide what they need in relation to their specific issues. For example, if there is a need for food, the biosafety level needed in that country will be a little different from the ones that we might have in Europe, where we have the luxury of imposing much more stringent regulations.

If you look at the world level, you might say that in China there is far less stringent regulation. It is probably important for them to have a more flexible regulatory system, but danger has no frontier and everybody is concerned. So it is really difficult to know how much international society has to be involved in this issue of regulatory issues in one country and who has to decide on that.

I think this is the reason why you are proposing an international panel that will involve all the different people who are concerned in it, but respect national sovereignty, because they are deciding what they need.

Vernon Ruttan: If we are interested in the health of the poor, then we do not need to wait for biotechnology. When you look at new pharmaceutical products coming out of the biotechnology industry, they are not the kinds that are going to reduce infant mortality or raise life expectancy. They are valuable to the limited numbers of people who are able to pay for the products. If directed to areas largely unattractive to the proprietary products and whose use would have to be substantially subsidized, one could visualize advances in biotechnology making important impacts, but not being profitable.

The problem in the U.S. is that we find it much easier to look for silver bullets than to make the institutional reforms that would go a long way toward improving the health of the poor.

Per Pinstrup-Andersen: Let me turn back to the specific proposal that is before us, Michel Dron's proposal for a committee. Does anybody have comments on that proposal? Is that what we need at this point?

Audience comment: I think this committee would only be useful if it were truly independent, interdisciplinary, and comprehensive, so that there would be an inquiry into the risk as well as assessment of the benefits; that is, how the technology can be used safely and to the benefit of all, not only the fat and the rich. But other than that, I think it will be yet another window dressing exercise.

Val Giddings: I do not like to be argumentative, but I have to take at least partial exception to the suggestion from Vernon Ruttan that we do not need to wait for biotechnology to help the poor. This is certainly true. There are many things that could be done—but have not been done—that do not rely upon biotechnology. But it is a mistake to lead others to infer that important health improvements cannot be accomplished with the use of biotechnology.

I mention a couple of examples that should be well known. There have been a number of recombinant hepatitis vaccines produced in the recent years. Hepatitis has been a scourge, especially in developing countries. This is an unprecedentedly effective way of solving a serious problem.

There are vast possibilities for improvements of human nutrition via the improvements in various commodity crops, or what is coming to be known as "nutraceuticals." There are all sorts of possibilities for meeting presently unmet nutritional or health needs of people in the developing world to benefit from biotechnology innovations.

There may be some merit in the committee idea, but there is also a problem. The Stockholm Environment Institute has had over the past decade a Biotechnology Advisory Commission to perform many of the same sorts of functions now being suggested for the committee we are talking about. The Commission was largely independent and multidisciplinary, with the possibility of enhancing specific efficiencies in its standing membership with ad hoc members as necessary.

However it was very difficult for them to get people to come to them with requests for assistance for a whole variety of reasons related to governance, responsibility, and to the sovereignty attached to decisions about safety for products in individual countries.

These sorts of problems need to be overcome in order to make this kind of committee work effectively. Perhaps the World Bank Group could make some progress in this direction by providing such a committee-based service to its members or to states that take out loans for biotechnology products. But there are a whole host of practical problems of that sort that will have to be overcome before such a committee could have the confidence necessary to elicit requests for help that result in the kinds of decision-facilitating exercises we hope for.

Vince Morton: I am a private agricultural consultant, and I would like to address not so much policy but implementation.

At the present time biotechnology is being introduced via the seed. I would suggest that one of the things we have to address is how to get the most out of seed and emergence—one seed in the ground, one plant emerging—and that includes getting it into the ground, getting it to the farmer, and maybe, as UNIDO has done, offering seed treatment. But this certainly will have to be addressed if biotechnology is introduced into developing countries, because it will be through the seed.

Vernon Ruttan: Many of the things that we are discussing now were discussed 20 years ago in connection with the Green Revolution. Issues of equity, of whether poor farmers could afford it, whether short, stiff-strawed varieties would keep farmers from feeding straw to their buffalo, a whole set of issues. Most of them were wrong.

Farmers in a municipality in Central Luzon, in the Philippines, where the IR6 was first introduced, adopted it faster than Iowa farmers adopted hybrid corn, even though they had to pay for seed, because the cost of the seed was so small relative to increment and use.

If we introduce biotechnology in that form, I think it will be adopted very rapidly. If it is introduced in forms that involve a technology fee, diffusion will occur more slowly. I always remember the farmer in the Philippines with a sixth-grade education who, when asked whether he would adopt something, said: "I am going to push my pencil first." Farmers are pretty good at pushing their pencils, even small-scale farmers.

Peasant farmers all over the world are tied into the market already. Only in extremely remote areas do you find farmers not tied into the market. When technology is made available, it is incredible. If you find a new technology being introduced but not being adopted, ask what is wrong with the technology.

George Lloyd: I wanted to respond to the question about introduction of biotechnology through seed. Even in the least developed countries mechanisms for supplying seed to the most remote areas actually exist.

In Zambia we have what is called an outgrower scheme. Normally this entails commercial farmers actually having on their periphery smaller-scale farmers whom they look after and supply inputs to. And vice-versa, the small-scale farmers market their produce back through the commercial system. We have found that even the smallest of farmers actually buys hybrid seed if it is available and is given to them on time, and that they can actually see the benefits derived from using hybrids.

Recommendations for Action

Synopsis
Wanda Collins

This Associated Event was held in conjunction with the Fifth Annual World Bank Conference on Environmentally and Socially Sustainable Development. The focal point for the event was the recently released *Bioengineering of Crops: Report of the World Bank Panel on Transgenic Crops*, prepared under the leadership of Dr. Henry Kendall. This particular event was organized to focus on the question of biosafety. We were exhorted by World Bank Group Vice President Ismail Serageldin in his opening speech to disentangle ourselves from the other controversial issues surrounding the application of biotechnology and focus on the issue at hand.

We have had wide-ranging, provocative discussions over the past two days. During these discussions we demonstrated again and again how difficult it is to look at a single issue in a dispassionate, unbiased way and to disentangle it from other issues. But it was equally obvious that there is broad agreement on many points, and I hope I can summarize them without bias. There are areas where consensus or agreement was not possible, but I believe we have given a clearer focus to those areas where our opinions continue to diverge. I will try to summarize these as well.

Biotechnology: Areas of Agreement and Lack of Agreement

1. Related issues such as ethics, morals, and worldviews are entangled with the science of biotechnology and biosafety and make it very difficult for us to address those issues dispassionately.

2. Biotechnology is here, will continue to be here, and is proceeding slowly but surely forward.

3. Biotechnology-derived solutions are *part* of a strategy to solve problems. They may or may not become the *major part* of a particular solution to a particular problem; agricultural biotechnology products must be adjusted for regions and for crops.

4. Many biotechnology tools of use in agriculture are uniformly seen as helpful (for example, marker-aided selection and diagnostic tools).

5. There are risks in biotechnological solutions, as is the case with any other solutions (including plant-breeding methodologies that do not use molecular techniques). There are no zero-risk solutions, but we do not agree on the level of acceptable risk or who should make this determination.

6. There are also benefits; and there are potentially undesirable outcomes in food issues, health, and public safety if available technology is *not* used to solve intractable problems.

7. There are dangers in unduly lax or unduly stringent regulation. In the U.S., regulations governing biotechnology products have been much more rigorous than those governing equivalent products developed using nonmolecular techniques.

8. There is genuine lack of agreement over the potential benefits of biotechnology. Neither the eternal optimists nor the eternal pessimists have

had their dreams realized! In the long term, however, benefits will emerge through market forces. The resulting level of benefits will be an aggregate of failures and successes, which may or may not allow an evaluation of the value of the technology itself.

What Must We Do?

- We must, insofar as possible, separate the issues and view biosafety dispassionately.
- We must be unbiased in attributing the effects of biotechnological solutions. For example: monoculture exists; added biotechnological solutions may exacerbate the problems of mono-culture, or they may be totally neutral, or they may contribute added stability and diversity. Only when we can attain that unbiased view can we ask if our scientific information is such that we have a sufficient database to say that a biotechnology-derived risk is no larger than a nonbiotechnology-derived risk.
- We must clearly and scientifically define the risks in categories such as:
  1. Gene flows to wild plants (ecological risks)
  2. Development of new and more virulent pathogens (viruses)
  3. Effects of plant-produced insecticides (Bt)
  4. Ecosystem damage (transfer of DNA to other organisms).
- We must clearly and cautiously define the relative magnitude of the risks within categories; not generally, but crop-by-crop and region-by-region, and based on available, sound scientific data, not speculation.
- Choices will be made about relative risks. We must leave choices about acceptance of those risks where those choices will be made (for example: at the national government level, will we or won't we *allow* the technology; at the individual client level, will we or won't we *use* the embodied technology; and at the individual consumer level, will we or won't we *use* this product of the technology). These are political or personal choices and are seldom based on scientific evidence alone.
- We must, however, provide science-based mechanisms by which choices of acceptance can be made in an informed way. For example: What magnitude of risk is acceptable by a government in accepting the technology? What are

the likely outcomes in high-risk situations? What additional risks do individual users face at the farm level (opportunity costs and direct costs; probably mainly an economic issue)? What risks do consumers face in choosing the product and how do they recognize those individual risks? Two issues are involved:

1. *Food safety* is not, for the most part, an individual choice. There are national guidelines, rules, and regulations (such as those of the Food and Drug Administration in the U.S.) that determine the safety of foods; unsafe foods are not allowed on the market. In countries where the opposite extreme is the case (there is no legal framework for food safety) then it is impossible to address relative food safety questions without the appropriate reference points from which to make comparisons.

2. *Food choice* is a matter of choosing among safe foods, or foods that are allowed by a ountry to be marketed. The consumer can and should be informed through labeling the contents of a food choice. Labeling has little to do with safety and everything to do with informed choice).

- We must also provide science-based mechanisms to monitor relative risks; for example, how does a country follow the changes as technologies are implemented and continue to make informed decisions as information accumulates?
- As possible risks are being monitored, we must provide as much scientific underpinning as possible to the understanding of how to manage the risks. Risk management is not a science-based activity; it is pragmatic and resource dependent. But we can provide scientific information that allows the best decisions to be made.
- We must understand the complexity of biotechnology and biosafety within a development and international context; that is, economically, distributionally, and scientifically.

It appears that throughout the two days of the Conference on Biotechnology and Biosafety, these positions were agreed upon by participants from all perspectives.

The most basic point of disagreement concerned the relative magnitude of the risks posed by the use of the tools of biotechnology and the resulting products. To a lesser extent, there was divergence of opinion on the subsequent management of risk. Reconciliation regarding the magnitude of the risks will only occur through sound science directed towards specific solutions to specific questions. It will most likely be based on a matrix of crop-x-region solutions rather than generalized, speculative, all-encompassing statements. There was agreement that an element of caution must be included.

Scientific data are already being collected; in some cases years of data have been collected. Some of these data point to very safe solutions to very difficult problems, such as transferring plant genes for resistance to devastating diseases. Some data point to potential magnitudes of risk, such as biotechnology resistance in insects. As was stated during the conference, there is not yet sufficient, large-scale experience with management of resistance. However at the present time no data point to obvious adverse results to human health or to the environment from any of the biotechnology products on the market.

Are these data derived through reductionist approaches? Yes, and they are appropriate approaches. However the value of more holistic agroecological approaches must be incorporated in the translation of these data to effective criteria for decisionmaking. They must be utilized in a similarly appropriate, broader context that takes into account the complexities of farming systems and farmers' choices, needs, and preferences.

The overriding factor is that the scientific data must be very carefully scrutinized and considered in order to make science-based, informed decisions and provide sound advice.

However, in trying to resolve this divergence of opinion on relative magnitude of risks, we must not forget that risk has to be weighed against potential benefit; for example, the case of black *Sigatoga* in bananas—where no other solution has yet emerged and both smallholders and the environment are suffering—and late blight of potato, the most economically devastating disease in the world. The issue comes down to information and the proper use of information, both for better management practices and to avoid the paralysis associated with unwillingness or inability to make decisions.

Opportunities and Needs Are Evident

There is much potential for biotechnology; the vastness of its potential is unknown to us, and we have barely scratched the surface of its capabilities. The question posed was: "Is that potential being fully exploited for small farmers?" These sessions of the conference reinforced the critical nature of effective partnerships. Discussion focused on the roles and complementarities of the public and private sectors and the necessity of finding a balance that will allow the private sector to reach its financial objectives, while also providing opportunities to contribute to the public good. What are their incentives?

There are major differences between national systems to address the issues associated with biosafety. They have some similar needs (for example, information, monitoring, skills, good practice examples), but they also have differing needs (for example, for internal processes and experiences in each country and site-specific determinations of biosafety risks). Capacity building within national systems of developing countries was seen as a particularly critical necessity.

The value of proactive regional partnerships for efficiency was recognized during the conference, as was the potential value of the international agricultural research centers of the Consultative Group on International Agricultural Research. Regional cooperation was seen as being of overriding importance in assisting in the development of competence in developing countries, particularly in conducting biosafety reviews.

Moving Forward Is Necessary

Positions and points were identified upon which all agreed, at least implicitly. On other issues, which are now more narrowly focused, disagreement remains. How do we address those issues?

Continuing dialogue is needed to arrive at consensus opinions on the magnitude of the risks associated with the use of biotechnology. This should involve very careful scrutiny of scientific evidence, identification of gaps in the research that are critical for immediate decisions, and interpretations that are unbiased and realistic. Eventually viewpoints will begin to converge, whether based on scientific data or on simple experience.

We must move forward, in the words of Miguel Altieri, to allow the partnerships to develop, get into the field, work together, and provide solutions to maximize the potential of biotechnology in complex systems.

These steps are necessary to build on those areas where agreement was identified and build effective partnerships to address those areas where disagreement still abounds. It is essential, in the words of two participants, to move from a "dialogue of the deaf" to a dialogue of "mutual learning."

Suggestions by Participants

As a result of the two days of discussions, several participants offered suggestions for future actions. No mechanism was in place by which these suggestions could be agreed upon by the entire group, so they are presented here as individual suggestions.

1. To promote mutual understanding and make progress, concrete projects and concrete actions must be a result of this event.

2. A comprehensive inquiry is needed, including socioeconomic impacts of biotechnology-derived products.

3. Research should be supported in specific areas.

4. Safe and legitimate uses of biotechnology should be recognized (for example, in marker-aided genetic selection), and its power as a tool of research should not be undervalued.

5. Information exchanges should be supported so that both successes and failures can be made known.

6. Post-market monitoring of products is desirable.

7. Support should also be given to alternative approaches to biotechnology-derived solutions; that is, those which emphasize peoples' livelihoods and the conservation of biodiversity, agroecological approaches.

8. Another independent study should be conducted to further explore the issues raised during this event and on which opinions continue to diverge.

Discussion
Moderator: Alexander F. McCalla

Miguel Altieri: I think we all agree from the synopsis that we are calling for a more informed approach to risk. We want to avoid any approaches in biotechnology that are going to undermine the objectives of the agenda—reducing poverty and increasing food security and environmental protection—by emphasizing genetic uniformity or reducing the possibility of developing more sustainable systems. So if biotechnology can be geared in that direction, I think that mutual understanding is already happening.

Since this session is a call for action, I think we need to stress that the only way we are going to be able to come up with answers and an integration of approaches is by getting into concrete projects. I would like to see three or four pilot projects in which we integrate the different approaches of biotechnology that are offered by industry, the Consultative Group on International Agricultural Research (CGIAR), nongovernmental organizations (NGOs) and universities, obviously with the participation of farmers.

In that regard we could take a small farming system in which one portion is put into production with transgenic crops or biotechnologically appropriate crops, and the rest maintained in a diversified mode. That way we can start integrating the two approaches, avoiding the possibility of erosion of genetic diversity and maybe providing refuge and examples for delaying resistance development.

Timothy Roberts: One conclusion of the synopsis was that we had a basic disagreement on estimating the magnitude of risk. I am sure that is right. It was also pointed out that this had to be balanced against the potential benefits, but I would like to highlight that we have an equally basic disagreement about the value of the potential benefits. On one side, we perhaps overstate them wildly. On the other side, we perhaps minimize or say they are not really benefits at all. The variation is at least as great as with the disagreement about risk.

Mae-Wan Ho: I have a list of five recommendations for action that might be constructive. The first is to have a broad, comprehensive inquiry into the risks involved, including socioeconomic impacts. We really need to support targeted research into some of the risks that I and others have highlighted—such as horizontal gene transfer—in order to develop rational safety assessments and regulations, because in the opinion of some of us, these do not exist yet.

Second, this is an opportunity to consider the safe and legitimate uses of genetically engineered biotechnology; for example, using markers to aid in plant breeding. I do not undervalue the power of the technique as a research tool. It is potentially very valuable.

Third, there should be support for information exchange and total transparency, so that failures as well as successes will be completely transparent and available to the public, in order to encourage public participation.

Fourth, we should support post-market monitoring. This is very important; in order to do so, we really must have segregation and labeling. If we do not do that, it means we are not taking risks seriously at all.

My last point is a plea for support of alternative approaches, such as those discussed by Miguel Altieri, with emphasis on livelihoods and conservation of biodiversity as an ecological approach, which is in contrast to the reductionist approach.

Val Giddings: Like one of the earlier commentators, I had singled out one area of the synopsis where I was not sure I agreed, which was in the invocation of significant disagreement over the magnitude of risk involved. Let me illustrate with one example.

My eight years with the U.S. Department of Agriculture doing environmental assessments for these types of modified crops was marked by repeated disagreements with one of my closest colleagues. We would try to define the nature of our disagreement. Ultimately, we would reach the same conclusion: we agreed on the quantitative value of the risk, but differed in the way we judged whether or not it was acceptable.

I think that illustrates the need for making risk decisions based on analysis of relative risk. This point could be stressed more in the synopsis and serve as guidance to future consideration of these issues.

I also agree with Miguel Altieri that the real test will come as we move into the consideration of concrete proposals. This means that more donors will have to be galvanized to come up with more money to support worthwhile projects.

Desmond Mahon: What I got out of the discussions of the last two days was the overriding importance of the regional perspective in both biosafety and risk assessment and risk management in the application of biotechnology and its acceptability—the critical nature of the regional, as opposed to the global.

The second point is that if one were to make a recommendation on biosafety, purely in the regional context, it would be the need to assist in the development of competence based upon two components, training and information availability.

Donald Winkelmann: As I understood the observations about food safety, it was describing the circumstances in the U.S., where we know that if food is in the stores, it is safe. It seems to me that there was some discussion about food safety in countries that do not have these kinds of regulations, and I wonder if the synopsis should say something to that effect.

Second, to the extent that we encourage individual nations or regions to make judgments about acceptable levels of risk, implicit in that is the assumption that there will be no spillover from that region into other parts of the world. So what might be perfectly safe and perfectly tolerable in one place, were a spillover to occur, might be discovered to be unacceptable—in the sense that we have been using that word—in other parts of the world. This occurred to me because of the strength of that particular recommendation.

Alexander McCalla: The point you are making is that with each individual country making its own set of rules, there can be an influence on the freedom with which goods and products move in international trade and whether or not these kinds of activities can become technical barriers to trade. That is an issue that I did not hear in this discussion, but is worth raising.

I got the sense from the synopsis and the discussion that there is a general recognition that the challenge ahead of us is very large, very complicated, and will have no single solution. The solution will call for the best of our capacities, no matter where they come from, no matter what paradigm they use, no matter what way they go at this, to address the overall issue.

I sense an agreement, or some willingness to say let us get together, recognizing that there are differences in the way that we measure risk and the weights we attach to risk. But there is also a willingness to say, let us move ahead and see where we can cooperate, collaborate, to address what I think is an enormous challenge ahead: feeding the world over the next 25 to 30 years.

Wrap-up and Next Steps
Ismail Serageldin

First, I would like to say a profound thank you to the people who organized this event, specifically Wanda Collins and Sarwat Hussain, and more generally Joan Martin-Brown, who has been the impresario of the multiplicity of events this week, as well as Lisa Carlson and many other staff members from the CGIAR Secretariat, the World Bank Group, the International Food Policy Research Institute, and others who have worked so patiently, along with our cosponsors, to made this event possible.

It has, indeed, been a compelling two days and, if nothing else, serves as an interesting starting point. There are actually some 16 different organizations, including conservation groups, scientific groups, international agencies, and bilateral agencies that agreed to cosponsor this event, which speaks to the importance that we all attach to this issue.

I think that we have done reasonably well in trying to disentangle a number of the issues, including an effort to start with the more general ethical issues and then deal separately with legal regimes. But the comment that Alexander McCalla made at the end about World Trade Organization (WTO) and nontariff barriers brings back the whole issue of links between the WTO, other conventions, legal arrangements, and intellectual property rights, which is a topic that deserves a separate, in-depth discussion in its own right.

The decision was to confine this particular discussion to the safety issues related to biotechnology, and I feel that we have made considerable advances.

Sometimes there is a fear of setting reductionism up too much as a straw man, because many of the top scientists in the world would not adhere to the view of reductionist science. Roger Penrose, for example, who is a mathematician, wrote a beautiful essay in a book called *Nature's Imaginings* in which he shows why even the structure of mathematics, which due to its inherent structure is assumed to be the most reductionist, recognizes that there are things that remain outside of the reductionist approach.

In many instances we use the concept of reductionism as an artifact; the problems are too complex, and we try to bring them down to a more comprehensible level. I am fond of pointing out that on one level human beings are nothing more than three buckets of water and a handful of minerals held together by chemical reactions. That extreme reductionist view has served us extremely well in medicine, bringing about enormous advances in treatment and longevity of human beings.

Yet it is a view that misses the difference between a Mother Teresa and a Hitler, or between a Mozart and a Stalin. It fails to take into account everything that we refer to as a human being. In the same way no doctors or medical practitioners would assume that this reductionist view is the entire totality of human beings, even though they find it convenient to do so.

In some ways there has also been a tendency—perhaps less so in this group than in others—to hold up economics as a discipline as being reductionist in an unacceptable way, by reducing a society to the sum of its economic and financial transactions, which is equivalent to reducing a human being to three buckets of water and a handful of minerals.

I think there is something there of value. But I sense that the other side of that equation is really concern for the complexity of the interactions and synergistic effects present in the idea of understanding an ecosystem in its entirety, not just its individual organisms, and that takes a more holistic approach to sort out.

This is a debate that has also permeated the Convention on Biological Diversity, as one of protecting species or entire habitats in ecosystems, and that is where I think we need to have a larger discussion. I have spent much time debating with colleagues on how to bridge the differences between microbiologists and ecologists in their general perception of life.

I think we need to engage others in discussing this. Miguel Altieri said earlier that science is too serious to leave to the scientists, paraphrasing a famous leader talking about war being too serious to be left to the generals. Nevertheless there is a scientific basis and a scientific viewpoint for dealing with ecological interactions as well.

But we are not just about settling perceptions in science; we are also about trying to move forward with realities. With every passing minute we have 200 additional people on the planet, three per second. They will be demanding food, nutrition, shelter, housing, and habitats, and enormous pressure is going to be coming upon us. It is important that actions are being taken. Delaying action is an action. It is a choice. It is not postponing a choice; it *is* a choice.

The balance is between perception and reality. The tradeoffs are there and they are inescapable. They will require that we try to find ways of dealing with the disagreements that we have. Val Giddings, I think, rightly pointed out the disagreements about what is acceptable risk. Even if you have defined the level of risk, what is acceptable?

Acceptable risk is not really a scientific issue, but rather a social and political issue. We accept airlines as being safe, yet planes do crash. So there is a level of risk. We can build in a redundancy system and a second. There is no end to how far we can go, but it is implicit that at certain points

choices are being made about levels of acceptable risk, and they vary.

Defining the level of acceptable risk is not an issue that can be determined by science. Science may be able to help determine the magnitude of the risk or the probability of its occurrence, but ultimately the choices have got to be there. It is in that context that I think Wanda Collins' comment reminding us about the question of choice between things that have already passed acceptable risk is especially pertinent.

I would like to add two other dimensions to our concern, since much of what drives me and my colleagues is concern with the poor and the impoverished in the developing world. The first is that discussions of standards must always be weighed with the interests of those who do not have voice in many of these debates in mind. We need to remember that. We should not allow the noxious practices of dumping toxic materials on them. We should not allow the sale of expired medicines to developing countries or other practices of which we are fully aware.

At the same time we also must be concerned about the pressures of the counter-factual. For example, in another domain I have worked for many years on issues of accessibility to water and sanitation. When governments insisted that they would have a certain level of service—now, mind you, this is not risk, this is service, levels of service—the net result was that they rationed out a lot of people. They ended up having subsidized water running from the taps of the middle class, while very large numbers of poor people had no access to water. Women had to travel for five hours a day to get water; children were playing in the filth, causing all sorts of diseases. Meanwhile the claim was that: "We cannot reach those people because we are trying to provide water at a certain standard." That is counter-factual: we are trying to reach everyone, but our self-imposed standards do not actually allow us to reach the people who need it most.

In the same way I think that we have to look at a range of approaches capable of improving the productivity and income of the poor, including and only in part—and here I concur with Wanda Collins—the issue of biotechnology, which is being seen only as a subsidiary to that larger problem.

On the ecological side is the issue of pressure on habitats, which is important because debates around the Green Revolution still continue today. But at the same time it is important to know that if we had not had significant yield increases, we would have had 300 million more hectares under cultivation, and the net result of that in terms of additional forests destroyed and additional species lost would have been very severe—plus the fact that there would have been colonization of the hillsides, erosion of the soil, and a lot of other negative consequences.

So we need to balance these issues—the needs and demands versus the risks. None of these choices are easy. Many of them are not going to be scientific choices, but rather societal choices. On this point I join our colleagues from the Third World Network who spoke about the need for greater information sharing and transparency in public debate, and I hope that this event has contributed to that.

Disagreement about benefits is easier. To the extent that we can prevent fraudulent claims and safeguard with scientific scrutiny against fraudulence and incorrect claims, then the question as to who is making the claims of benefits (of course, mostly these are people on the industry side) is whether they are willing to bet their money that this will prove economically viable. If the benefits are there, farmers will use the technology and it will be economically viable. If not, the technology will disappear.

Our job as decisionmakers and informed people is to ensure that the prices are real and that they incorporate the full environmental and social costs. Because to the extent that you have distorted prices or hidden subsidies, decisionmaking about whether or not the alternative choices are more beneficial and more economical would be unsound and distorted. Therefore incorporation and internalization of the externalities becomes essential.

It seems to me, finally, that there are two points that can pull us together in terms of movement. If we look at everything that is being done and discussed in biotechnology, we can go from a level of comfort to less and less comfort. The highest level of comfort would be the use of genetic markers, tissue culture. It is mainstream. Nobody worries about it. It is being done very well.

Second is movement within the same species, wheat and wheat. We take genetic material from one wheat and put it into another wheat. We could probably produce the same result by conventional breeding over a longer period of time and, therefore, there is not much of a problem there in terms of acceptance.

Third would be closely related species. It happens in nature and it happens to conventional breeding programs. Triticale is the result of a cross between wheat and rye, so we are still fairly close to conventional techniques, even if we used a transfer technique that enabled us to do it more quickly and the gene to express itself. But, fundamentally, we are not breaching much of what could be achieved at a slower pace in a conventional manner.

Then we get into more complex areas of moving from organisms where the transfers would not likely occur, including, for example, the biotechnology gene coming from a bacterium into a plant. Then you enter into suggestions of entire restructuring of the genome and changing the architecture of plants by putting traits together.

I think we can start by building partnerships where people feel a common comfort level and then work outwards from that. To the extent that additional evidence comes in, additional safeguards are employed, and the comfort levels of people are satisfied, then we can move with all deliberate caution on all of these problems.

That requires us, finally, to add two more things to make it feasible to have an effective follow-up. One is to work on clusters of specific problems, and I think Wanda Collins' comment about black Sigatoga in bananas is a very pertinent one. Next week I will be meeting with a group of people from industry, developing countries, and research institutions to discuss whether such a partnership is feasible around the issue of black Sigatoga in bananas, and whether such a partnership could also benefit plantains, which would benefit some very poor people in another commercial crop, even if it also benefits the dessert banana, which is a commercial export crop.

To determine whether or not this is feasible, we will have to bring in the lawyers. It seems that nothing can be done without lawyers nowadays, but that is part of the bane of proprietary science and many other things. But lawyers also have fashioned wise constraints that keep us free, so I hope that the lawyers will live up to that lofty and noble description of their profession.

And that, of course, is where we need to move towards a partnership. Partnership, we said, moves beyond the dialogue of the deaf toward a learning relationship. Yes, but it also has to be a definition and understanding of what it is that each one of us brings to the table. What we bring to the table is different knowledge, different perspectives, different abilities, so this is where we will have to work together.

In that working together around specific clusters of problems in specific projects, I take up Miguel Altieri's appeal to the noble forum: when you have the ability to say let us fuse our efforts around a specific problem, and in so doing you go on a journey, not just for the discovery of the other but also for discovery of the self. That is our goal in partnerships, and that is what will allow us to finally reach mutual agreement on more issues.

I have always been an optimist, and I am convinced that we will be able to forge the partnerships that we have been talking about in a manner that will benefit the poor generations to come and the environment as a whole.

I am also optimistic that we will be able to raise additional funds if they are required, but to do so will require that we define more accurately the scope of the interventions for which these funds need to be raised. I hope it will not be at the expense of some of the other activities that we want to undertake.

It is with these notes that I would like to leave you, with a deep vote of thanks to each and every one of you that have taken time from your busy schedules to share with us your concerns, your visions, your knowledge, your experience, your expertise, your fears, and your hopes. For in the end there is nothing that exists today that was not once before imagined, and there is nothing that will exist in the future that we will not ourselves imagine.

The future is very much what we will make of it, and I believe that by our thoughts and our actions we are creating the future right now, this instant, in this room, in the very crucible of our minds, by defining the limits of the possible.

PART II. ETHICS AND BIOTECHNOLOGY: REALITIES AND UNCERTAINTIES

(excerpted from *Ethics and Values: A Global Perspective*)

Introduction

Kamla Chowdhry

In this session on ethics and biotechnology we have three very distinguished speakers. But this has also been a conference on partnerships. We have been talking about partnerships a great deal, so I would like to quote this little poem from *Alice's Adventures in Wonderland* (Carroll 1865):

> I passed by his garden and marked,
> with one eye,
> How the Owl and the Panther
> were sharing a pie.
> The Panther took the pie-crust,
> and gravy, and meat,
> While the Owl had the dish
> for his share of the treat.
> When the pie was all finished,
> the Owl, as a boon
> Was kindly permitted to pocket
> the spoon:
> But the Panther obtained both the fork
> and the knife,
> So when he lost his temper, the Owl
> lost his life.
>
> *(Presenter's version)*

If we are involved in fostering partnerships, we should see to it that we do not have these kinds of partnerships—in which one stronger partner eats the other partner. This session is about partnerships between biotechnology and ethics. Hopefully, we will think of the panther and the owl as we go along.

It seems to me that the whole problem of science and technology—the way they have developed in the past 100 to 200 years—is that they have given human beings almost unlimited power and control over nature. But this has not taught humankind how to control itself. This lopsided development threatens the future of humanity; the battle for the survival of the human race must involve ethics and a concern for values of equity.

The early history of science and technology is steeped in violence. Scientists and technologists have used science for the domination of nature, and the domination of nature for people's use. The underlying social and cultural values sanctioned the exploitation of nature in any form, including the exploitation of women, for the benefit of humanity.

To illustrate my point, let me give you some quotations from Francis Bacon, one of the fathers of the scientific movement.1 "Nature has to be hounded in her wanderings," "bound into service," "made a slave," "put into constraint." The aim of science, Bacon said, is to "torture nature's secrets from her." Nature was female, and could therefore be exploited and violently dealt with. One can see the violence with which nature was to be dealt with by the way it was utilized for the benefit of humans. Science and technology also developed specialization to an extent that it is difficult to see people in society as a holistic part of nature anymore. This is what the ecological sciences are bringing us back to, what Captain

Cousteau was able to bring to us, a holistic vision of nature and its relations with living beings.

The yearning of mortals for prolonging life by biochemical processes and gene manipulation is creating moral and ethical questions. Death is no longer considered as a necessity belonging to the nature of life, but as an avoidable end, or at least one which can be postponed. How desirable is this for the individual and for the species? These questions involve the very meaning of our finiteness, the attitude toward death, and the balance of death and procreation.

The promised gifts of technology have raised questions of choice never raised before. These questions have to be dealt with ethically, not merely by greater scientific endeavors or by market benefits, but by greater partnerships between technology and ethics. With the growth of science and technology we are constantly confronted with issues and choices which require supreme wisdom. The length and reach of our actions in space and time put people's responsibility and their ethics in center stage.

Let us hear what wisdom our panel members have to suggest on this topic.

Editor's Note

1. In many cases in which Francis Bacon refers to "nature," his meaning is "human nature."

Reference

Carroll, L. 1865. *Alice's Adventures in Wonderland*.

Panelist's Remarks

Ismail Serageldin

Few technological changes have caused as much debate as the recent changes in biotechnology (Bt). Unfortunately, much of this debate has been dominated by the sensational and the visceral, and little coverage in the media has been truly deliberative, rigorous, or based on scientific evidence in framing the issues.

Defining the Problem

I would like to define the scope of the topic first by limiting it to agricultural biotechnology, that is, the bioengineering of crops, especially food crops, and livestock, fish and trees. These activities are distinct from the bioengineering of medicines for human health. Medical bioengineering does not seem to elicit the same criticism as agricultural bioengineering. Critics of biotechnology do not seem to address their critiques to medical research, on the grounds that the resulting medicines or treatments would help people in distress.

Nevertheless, it is important to remember that most people who do not object to medical uses of biotechnology, while objecting to its use in agriculture, take that position because they place a value on reducing human suffering and prolonging human life, which is held to be intrinsically worthwhile. This argument, which I believe emanates from a correct system of values (that is, one in which minimizing human suffering and prolonging human life is held to be positive), is important to retain as we move to the domain that we will discuss here, namely, agriculture, especially in developing countries. It is relevant to hold that thought because the issue of better food production in the developing world involves many of the same arguments, even though the debate in the North is largely among people whose most likely nutritional problem is obesity, not hunger. The hungry in the Northern industrial societies are largely the marginalized, and they do not participate in the debate to ban or not to ban genetically modified organisms (GMOs)!

The second delineation of the problem relates to what we mean by biotechnology. Biotechnology is a continuum of tools that has only recently evolved into the part that bothers critics: the transformation of the genetic makeup of organisms by recombinant techniques, especially when we introduce the genes of other species into the target species—for example, introducing the Bt gene from a bacterium into a plant.

Transforming the genetic makeup of a variety of plant through genetic transfer from another variety of the same species should not pose much of an ethical problem. In fact it would simply be an accelerated way of achieving by biotechnological means that which we could achieve through conventional breeding programs and therefore should not pose ethical or safety problems for anyone not opposed to the latter.

We might arguably extend this acceptance to the bioengineered product of a genetic transfer between closely related plants, such as wheat and barley. Here we are already tinkering with nature, but the boundary with the conventional "natural" breeding system is so close that, for many, that also would be acceptable. The result of such a gene transfer is unlikely to significantly modify or denature the plant. Triticale is such an interesting cross.

Beyond that we get on the slippery slope leading to the design of new plant types, based on the assemblage of desirable traits from individual plant species or even from other organisms. Are we now "playing God," with the likely results of the "sorcerer's apprentice"? That is part of this discussion.

The other, related problem that people have is with the idea of cloning, or the forced asexual reproduction of an organism that naturally reproduces sexually. This qualification is necessary because the critics of biotechnology generally, and of cloning specifically, obviously have no difficulty with the reproduction of plants through cuttings, a practice as old as civilization.

With the domain of the discussion delineated in this manner, the issues can be usefully grouped into ethical issues relating to:

- Tinkering with the natural order of things
- The likely risks associated with the new technology, which may well far transcend the actual users of the products of that technology
- The patenting of life forms.

Against this set of issues we must address the potential benefits that would be forgone if we do not use biotechnology to address the problems of the world today. This moral calculus must be undertaken if we are to chart an ethical course on this complex set of issues.

Tinkering with Nature

There is a profound distrust about people taking it upon themselves to change the natural order of things. One can argue, rightly, that by our very presence on this planet we are changing the natural order of things, and that our increasing numbers, ever-more powerful technology, and insatiable appetites for consumption and pollution are indeed affecting nature, mostly in negative and potentially dangerous ways. Witness global warming and biodiversity loss.

Yet, against this general proposition we must set the welfare of the human species. Any moral argument must include human welfare, regardless of whether one assumes that human beings are a privileged species or not. There is no reason to argue for the welfare of animals if one is not going to extend the same argument to human beings. Indeed, it is instructive that the first legislation to protect children against the abuses of child labor was sponsored by the Society for the Prevention of Cruelty to Animals!

It is difficult to argue that hunter-and-gatherer societies living "in harmony with nature" should be encouraged to stay as they are, even if that means enormous infant mortality rates and short life expectancies. Humane treatment would mean improving diet, education, and health. The resulting reduction in infant mortality and increases in consumption are likely to put pressure on the natural system. The questions then become how to handle that pressure, how to ensure that the patterns of development that are adopted are sustainable. Even arguing from a human-centric point of view, surely it does not make sense to undermine the ecosystems on which our long-term survival depends.

Biotechnology fits into the class of tools that humans are mastering for the potential benefit of humanity, and that holds both promise and perils that should be weighed intelligently, on the basis of the best available evidence, to determine whether, when, and how it should be used. Viewed thus, the matter becomes a simple calculus of the potential benefits and potential risks associated with the new technology.

However, let me add some qualifiers to the argument. We must recognize that the ethical issue of purposively changing the natural order of things is qualitatively different from trying to survive as best we can in this world in which we find ourselves. A course of action that tinkers with the natural order of things is equivalent if and only if it can be demonstrated that there is no alternative to pursuing that course, and that it has enough unique benefits in improved living conditions for human beings to outweigh the moral questions it raises.

Stated thus, the issues become propositions that can be elucidated by the best available scientific evidence about the issues of agriculture, poverty, food security, sustainable development, and the potential of alternative means to

reach the goals of food security for all in an ecologically sustainable world system. Here the evidence is mixed: the challenge of ensuring food
security is profound, and the likelihood of meeting it without recourse to the bioengineering of
crops is remote. Indeed, some authors, ranging
from Henry Kendall and David Pimentel to
Lester Brown and Hal Kane, have cast doubt on
the world's ability to feed its growing population in a sustainable fashion under any scenario.

However, I do not take that view and would
argue that we do have the chance to develop and
intensify agriculture to meet that challenge. I
would not argue that enhancing food security is
possible if the potential use of biotechnology in
this enterprise is prohibited. Remember that if
we fail to reach the goal of sustainable agriculture for food security in the developing countries, it implies enormous misery for an
enormous number of human beings. That dis-
tributive and income policies are equally important in ensuring food security does not in any
way diminish the need to have the production
side in hand. The production side is necessary
but not sufficient to meet the challenge of
hunger. Its absence makes discussion of income
or redistributive policies largely academic.

If this position is defensible, then the question becomes one of managing the safety and
other aspects of the technology, not proscribing
it a priori. On the other hand, if the goal of sustainable agriculture for food security in developing countries can be achieved by other means,
then the ethical argument against tinkering with
nature remains intact for those who support it.

We must always remember that not all that is
technologically feasible is ethically desirable.

Ethical Issues of Safety

In the case of biotechnology that would lead to
releasing genetically modified organisms into
nature, the issues of safety acquire a different
level of concern. Is there a risk that we would
affect the very ecosystems on which we all
depend? What if these scientific efforts produce
"super weeds" or "super viruses" that have a
broad impact on many? Again the question is
one of evaluating the scientific evidence and
assessing to the best of our ability the likely risks.

Clearly, it is not possible to entirely exclude
certain classes of risk, any more than one would
be able to exclude the risk of an asteroid hitting
the earth or of being struck by lightning. Yet
these risks are considered so remote that one
goes through life ignoring them. I am not saying that the potential risks of releasing genetically modified organisms into the environment
are in the same class of probability as asteroids
or lightning. However, the discussion should
not start with the premise that any potential
risk, no matter how remote, would automatically veto the potential application of a technology. After all, in a case much closer to everyday
life, we could ask whether people would be
willing to accept a technology that contributes
to global warming, kills about 50,000 people a
year and maims another 500,000 in the United
States alone, and adds nothing vital to our
lifestyles except the convenience of personal-
ized fast travel. Yet no one would be able to per-
suade the average person to agree to ban the
automobile.

So we come back to assess the real risks of
biotechnology in terms of how to ensure its safe
use so that its benefits can accrue safely to the
many who need it. This is the topic of a two-day
symposium, entitled "Biotechnology and Biosafety," starting tomorrow in which a large number of distinguished authorities will participate
(Serageldin and Collins 1998).

Patenting of Life Forms and Other Issues of Patenting

The third broad area of ethical issues involved in
biotechnology is that of patenting. One of the ethical questions raised is whether the patenting of
life forms is acceptable. There is no direct answer,
but the ownership of animals and plants, as well
as the right to own a particular breed, is recognized. It could be argued that allowing ownership rights to other life forms is a matter of degree.
After all, the varieties of flowers or livestock are
themselves owned and sold, and breeding of
horses and other show animals is recognized. So
what is more offensive in patenting, that is, establishing an ownership claim on, a gene or gene
sequence, than in asserting ownership of a whole
plant or animal or a variety thereof?

The difference lies in the idea of owning a "building block of life" rather than the living creature itself. The assumption is that the building block can then be part of many other living things. This is an issue that I still struggle with and cannot easily define to my satisfaction.

Nevertheless, the issue is one that affects many people, and we should strive to understand their qualms and to accommodate them. No legislature can function if it does not have the broad support of the majority of the population, and the views of the minority today could well be those of the majority tomorrow. However, such a transformation is best achieved by education and scientific evidence, not by assertive preemptive action by a vocal minority.

Why do I say this? Because the lessons of history teach us so. A comparison between the United States' experience of its failed banning of alcohol (prohibition) and its effective quasi banning of smoking is instructive. Efforts to reduce smoking benefited from a protracted education campaign that resulted in a significant shift in popular attitudes; the banning of alcohol did not. The substance of that education campaign was scientific evidence increasingly linking smoking to a plethora of health issues.

In the same spirit should we not marshal the resources of science to assess the substantive claims of the contrarian view, be it for or against the patenting of life forms, to explain the difference between that and outright ownership of animals and plants?

There is another side to the patenting story. It raises another set of ethical issues that I would like to put before this assembly. These include the progressive monopolization of knowledge and the increasing marginalization of the majority of the world's population. Concomitantly, selective focusing research and applications of new biotechnologies skew their benefits to the potential markets of the rich and exclude the concerns of the poor.

The issues operate at two levels:

- Privatization of the scientific research enterprise and the meaning of proprietary science in the coming century
- Proprietary aspects of biotechnology in terms of both process and product.

On the first, I am concerned by a growing gap in knowledge between the North and South, which is exacerbated by the privatization of the knowledge enterprise. Elsewhere, I have called this an emerging *scientific apartheid*.

But the problems posed by the new environment of proprietary knowledge are different. They lead to the hoarding of information, and they are changing the character of the scientific research enterprise, especially in the universities, with their claim of promoting the advance of knowledge and its diffusion. The race to publish is being replaced by the race to patent.

Increasingly, the proprietary climate that governs research on genome mapping and the patenting of genes and gene sequences has re-created the world of the mapmakers of the 15th and 17th centuries, eloquently evoked by Daniel Boorstin:

Geographic knowledge, a product of discovery, was a precious international currency, coveted by everyone, easily stolen, and valuable to hoard. Anybody's new bit of information about an easy passage or a treacherous shore could be added to anybody else's in the race for gold and glory....

In this grand universal enterprise of discovery, all scientists, explorers, and navigators were collaborating willy-nilly, intentionally or unintentionally. Collaboration, while necessary, was both desired and feared. All realized that they were working toward the same end, a more accurate map of the earth. And their efforts bore fruit. (1994, pp. 20–23)

In both examples the issue is not that the research efforts do not bear fruit, but that the climate of that research becomes more like the competitive and secretive climate of military research, and less like the open and participatory climate of the research university that we have come to know in this century. This proprietary research culture threatens the open partnerships of science that were established from the 18th century onward.

The emergence and rapid dominance of this proprietary science pose difficult issues for institutions of higher learning in countries such as the United States. Here the need to maintain a not-for-profit status and retain the 501c(3) tax deduction is at odds with the pursuit of lucrative and interesting research with the giants of the private sector. They also pose questions about ensuring the ready accessibility of knowledge, surely a function of the university.

Equally powerful is the claim of the private sector that if it is to mobilize and invest large sums in research, it must be able to recoup its investment. To do so, the protection of intellectual property rights (IPR) is the key. From the view of the investor simple justice would demand that intellectual property rights be respected.

So we have an ethical dilemma posed by the conflict between two desirable ends—two competing claims to a just and fair treatment. The way out of this dilemma is to recognize the domains of the claims more precisely. Public goods should be left to the public, and *the private goods that aid in achieving these public goods should be treated differently* than the private goods produced by the private sector directly for the end user.

This is a subtle argument, but an important one. In the past institutions such as the International Agricultural Research Centers (IARCs) supported by the Consultative Group for International Agricultural Research had access to the basic science and could apply it to the problems of the poor. The results were available to all for free, a public good. Today, this is no longer possible because the patenting of both process and product continue unabated.

I would not mind if private companies patented the products that they choose to sell. However, I do mind if their patents prevent the IARCs from using the same basic scientific processes to make products of interest to the poor—products that the private sector patenters are not going to make precisely because of their public goods nature. Surely, there is an ethical question here, not just a legal one.

Of course, this does not argue for abolishing patenting or nationalizing private research. It argues for an imaginative approach that recognizes the interests of the vast majority of the poor in the world today.

This is not a hypothetical question. Look at pharmaceuticals, an areas in which the private sector has dominated research for a long time and

patenting is increasingly enforced around the world through the trade-related intellectual property (TRIPs) agreements under the World Trade Organization (WTO) rules. What do we find?

Malaria today affects some 200–400 million human beings, severely affects some 10 million persons, and kills about a million people annually. Yet, there is no significant private sector research for a malaria vaccine. Why? Because malaria is not a disease of the industrial countries, and because the millions of people affected are poor and live in very remote areas, making them an unattractive market. Compare this to the research being done on AIDS. It is plentiful and, it is hoped, is leading to a real cure for this devastating disease. But the cure will cost at best between US$5,000 and US$10,000 per patient. With enormous luck the cost could be brought down to US$1,000 per patient. This is an enormous advance, but one that will leave the vast majority of very poor AIDS victims in such countries as India, Rwanda, and Uganda with no accessible treatment.

I do not say this to fault the private sector companies. They are doing what they are supposed to do. I fault the public bodies that use the enormous presence of the private sector in medical research to justify a retreat from the pursuit of what are essentially public goods in the classical economic definition of the term. Biotechnology in agricultural research poses many of the same problems. We should recognize the importance of public goods research to accompany and complement the massive private sector research. In this context we must reassess the ethical aspects of preemptive patents and the patenting of process as well as product. New ways of collaborating with the private sector while respecting its right to intellectual property rights protection must be found to access the process side of the biotechnology work for public goods research.

Envoi

I have argued for defining more narrowly the scope of the discussion, limiting it to the issues of biotechnology in agricultural research. I have tried, wherever possible, to isolate the issues that could be framed as scientific questions, allowing us to assess the evidence and make informed decisions based on a cost-benefit or risk assessment, from the issues where the problems are inherently normative and the arguments are based on values. The difference between these approaches is the same as that between an argument against surrogate motherhood based on religious or other ethical values and one based on the safety of the procedure for the mother or the fetus. The safety argument is one that can be resolved in scientific terms, subject to another set of decisions about how much risk is acceptable. The ethical is not debatable in the same terms. So it is with some of these questions of biotechnology and patenting.

Whatever the difficulties, the ethical debate is one that we must all join in seriousness and in depth. There are few technologies on the market today that are more transformative. There are few that pose as many serious questions for our consciences and our minds, even when we circumscribe the debate as narrowly as I have tried to do here.

So let us go forth into these new domains with open minds and sensitive hearts, combining skepticism with concern and compassion. Let us be firm in the determination to do good and to remember our responsibilities toward the poor and the marginalized and the future generations of human beings as well as other species. And let us adopt an inquisitive posture that will also remember that issues such as these are never settled, but must be constantly reviewed and weighed in the light of new developments and new evidence. Only in this way will we be able to tackle our problems and, perhaps, also fashion the wise constraints that will set us all free in the truest and most profound sense of the word.

Reference

Boorstin, Daniel J. 1994. *Cleopatra's Nose: Essays on the Unexpected.* New York: Vintage Books.

Serageldin, I., and W. Collins. 1998. *Biotechnology and Biosafety.* Proceedings of an Associated Event of the Fifth Annual World Bank Conference on Environmentally and Socially Sustainable Development, "Partnerships for Global Ecosystem Management: Science, Economics and Law," Washington, D.C.: World Bank.

Panelist's Remarks

Klaus Leisinger

I am going to talk about the risks and benefits of biotechnology and genetic engineering in the food crops of developing countries. First, it is important to remember what we have learned from the green revolution.

The original objective of the green revolution was to increase yields, and this it certainly accomplished. It did this by developing seed varieties that had several advantages: short vegetation periods, which allowed more than one harvest a year; the ability to turn high fertilizer inputs into high crop yields rather than stem and leaf growth; relative insusceptibility to fluctuation in daylight; resistance to or tolerance of plant diseases and animal pests; and tolerance to irregular irrigation, poor soils, and other stress factors. The result was substantial yield increases for rice, maize, and wheat ranging from 100 percent to 170 percent boosts in productivity.

The Green Revolution also had the welcome effect of improving the nutrition of the poor by moderating food prices. Where the new technologies allowed second or third harvests in a year, there was also an increase in employment and thus in income. At the same time the higher-yielding seed varieties proved to be a land-saving technology, providing at least temporary relief of some of the pressures on forests and biological diversity. As an illustration of this process, consider that if India had to produce today's harvest with the technology of the 1960s, it would need to use 208 million hectares of arable land, 116 million more than were available between 1961 and 1963. If the yield per hectare had not doubled, achieving the results recorded from 1991 to 1993 would have required doubling the land under cultivation—a sheer impossibility without causing an ecological disaster by destroying the last remaining forests and converting them to cropland.

Of course the Green Revolution also had negative impacts. The technologies themselves and the benefits of using them were not distributed equitably. When the new seeds were introduced, those who already had access to land, irrigation, or extension services were at a distinct advantage. The poor were left further behind. Another negative effect was the reduced use of biodiversity—as people gained access to the new, high-yielding varieties, they abandoned traditional ones.

Turning to genetic engineering and biotechnology, we can also see potential benefits for food crops and some possible negative impacts. First the benefits: as diagnostic aids, these technologies can help identify plant diseases; gene mapping allows the rapid identification of commercially and biologically interesting genetic material; most significantly, seeds can be created that have resistance to, or tolerance of, plant diseases and animal pests, as well as tolerance of stress factors. Soon we may be able to transfer genes that confer the ability to fix nitrogen to grain. Last but not least, the quality of food can be improved by overcoming vitamin or mineral deficiencies. To illustrate these likely benefits, we can look at rice, based on work by Ingo

Potrykus at the Federal Institute of Technology in Zurich:

- Fungal diseases destroy 50 million tons of rice a year; varieties resistant to fungi could be developed through the genetic transfer of proteins with antifungal properties.
- Insects cause the loss of 26 million tons of rice a year; the genetic transfer of proteins with insecticidal properties would mean an environmentally friendly insect control.
- Viral diseases devastate 10 million tons of rice a year; transgenes derived from the Tungro virus genome allow the plant to develop defense systems.
- Bacterial diseases cause comparable losses; transgenes with antibacterial properties are the basis for inbuilt resistance.
- Vitamin A deficiency causes health problems for more than 100 million children; transgenes can provide provitamin A with the rice diet.
- Iron deficiency in the diet is a health problem for more than 1 billion women and children; transgenes can supply sufficient iron in the diet.

Similar benefits can also be cited for cassava, also based on work by Ingo Potrykus at the Federal Institute of Technology in Zurich:

- The African Mosaic virus causes immense damages in cassava; transgenes interfering with the life cycle of the virus could lead to virus-resistent varieties.
- Cassava contains toxic cyanogenic glycosides; the integration of transgenes could inhibit their synthesis.
- Cassava roots store starch efficiently but do not contain protein; the transfer of genes for storage proteins would improve cassava's nutritional quality substantially.
- Cassava roots have a basic capacity for pro-vitamin A synthesis; transfer of appropriate genes could lead to regulated accumulation.

Most of these properties in rice and cassava can only be achieved through genetic engineering and biotechnology, not through traditional plant research.

Now let us look at the potential risks of these technologies. These include dangers to the environment and to public health, aggravation of the prosperity gap between North and South, growing disparities in the distribution of income and wealth within poor societies, and loss of biological diversity. It is imperative to distinguish here between risks that are inherent to a technology and those that transcend it—a distinction seldom made when the green revolution is discussed. There are major differences between these risks, and technology should not be blamed for problems that are part of the political and social environment of a country.

The risks inherent to technology are those potential hazards—unforeseeable problems or unwanted side effects—that might occur during the research, development, or implementation of a technology designed to improve an existing situation. Examples of these include the unexpected and harmful interaction of genetically engineered organisms with the environment, and the reduced use of biodiversity by farmers who now have access to higher-yielding varieties. (This does not mean, however, that the traditional varieties need be lost, for they can be kept in vitro or farmers could be offered an incentive to continue using them.)

In contrast, technology-transcending risks stem from the application of a technology in certain political and social circumstances. In developing countries today these risks arise from both the current course of the global economy and the specific situation in certain countries. Consider, for instance, the varying impact of introducing a new technology in a country that has policies that support small farmers (tenure reform, access to extension services) and in a country where 95 percent of the land is in the hands of 2 percent of the people and where the poor have no access to services.

Some of these risks can have the effect of aggravating the prosperity gap between North and South. The ability to produce tropical agricultural products in the laboratory or in temperate zones, for example, can have a significant impact on developing-country exports. The gap between North and South can also be widened when control of plant genetic resources is given free of charge.

The story of thaumatin illustrates both these trends. Some 10 years ago Nigerian researchers at the University of Ife identified the sweetener thaumatin in the berries of *Thaumatococcus danielli*, which is common in the forests of that part of Nigeria. At that time no industry was interested in using the fruit as a sweetener. With the advent of biotechnological possibilities, however, the gene for thaumatin—a protein that gram-for-gram is some 1,600 times sweeter than sugar—has been cloned and is now being used for the industrial production of sweetener in the confectionery industry. Patents on the process have been registered, but the people from whose lands the gene was obtained never received any compensation. And countries like Cuba or Mauritius, which depend on sugar cane for a decisive share of their export earnings, could find themselves extremely hard-pressed should the industrial manufacture of thaumatin or similar substances broadly supplant sugar cane.

Technology-transcending risks can also aggravate disparities in income and wealth in poorer countries themselves. For it is certainly true that where land ownership and tenancy systems, access to key services, and credit and marketing channels are governed by a power structure that favors only a small minority, technological progress cannot possibly be neutral in impact.

How can we manage these risks? Again, it is important to look at the two categories separately. First, risks inherent to technology. Biosafety risks are normally evaluated by specialists, controlled by good scientific practices and an appropriate regulatory framework. The only ethical risk here is if an institution supported by public funds used different standards of risk in the North and the South. We have an ethical duty to use the highest standards everywhere.

As a social scientist I am not qualified to pass judgment on biosafety risks, but I draw to your attention the comment of the U.S. National Academy of Sciences on this issue: "The safety assessment of a recombinant DNA-modified organism should be based on the nature of the organism and the environment into which it will be introduced, not on the method by which it was modified" (Persley 1990).

Management of technology-transcending risks is more difficult, for it involves more players. Political wishes, for example, cannot determine whether vanilla is produced in Madagascar, where it creates an income for 100,000 people, or in a laboratory in Switzerland or England. Or do we wish that to be controlled by politics. Market "logic" tells us that if "lab vanilla" or "lab sugar" (thaumatin) is cheaper or has some other edge—is healthier than the natural product, for example—then the innovation or substitution will simply happen.

Similarly, the price of copper is determined by the metal's electrical conductivity. Once electric current can be conducted cheaper and better by glass or carbon fibers, copper will in due course no longer be used for this purpose—with not surprising consequences for demand and thus price. The substitution will take place despite crumbling copper prices and rising unemployment in countries such as Chile and Zambia.

The discussion here should not be how we can prevent such a substitution from happening, but how to create an early warning system to find out what kinds of crops are vulnerable to substitution, and then help countries and communities to diversify. A larger allocation of international development funds to diversification efforts is therefore called for. A comprehensive risk-benefit analysis of the substitution of agricultural commodities from the tropics should also examine potential alternative uses of the land freed up in this way—for increasing local food production perhaps, or for reforestation.

There should also be fair compensation for the use of genetic resources. Suppose for instance, that a private seed company discovers a property in an Ethiopian barley strain that makes it resistant to certain plant diseases. The company transfers this property genetically to a wheat variety which is then commercialized in Ethiopia. Obviously, the farmers of Ethiopia have contributed something by selecting and preserving this variety for a long time, but without the research and development of the seed company this characteristic would not have been turned to use outside Ethiopia or in food grains other than barley. So both the farmers of Ethiopia and the seed company have contributed to the new wheat variety, and both have some kind of intellectual property right, and thus a right to compensation.

Although most industrial countries have signed the Convention on Biological Diversity, few national legislatures have ratified it. An important step in satisfying claims to compensation would be to work out binding national and international regulations. What especially needs unequivocal regulation is who should compensate whom for what, and how much the compensation should amount to. As a rough first approach, I have recommended for some time that the issue be dealt with through license agreements, with the price left to the mechanism of supply and demand. Those who benefit should pay the license fee to those who, over the centuries, helped preserve the varieties in question. It is crucial to ensure that remuneration, through whatever mechanism, does not land in the pockets of those who have ready access to it, while those the funds are meant to help end up empty-handed once again. As the Consultative Group on International Agricultural Research (CGIAR) already exists and does excellent work for the poor farmers of the world, no new institution need be created to address this problem. If license fees were funneled to CGIAR, the funds would go toward research on plants that improve the living circumstances in communities that are responsible for these crops.

In addition, to help with diversification and fair compensation for genetic resources, another way to avoid aggravating the North-South prosperity gap is to provide more publicly financed research for the South and in the South, where there are many excellent research capacities.

The second major technology-transcending risk described earlier is the growing disparity in the distribution of income and wealth within developing countries. Managing this risk requires good governance—a quality that is unfortunately in short supply lately. Take the case of Nigeria, to cite just one example. Nigeria has had an income from crude oil of hundreds of billions of dollars over the past 20 years. Have the multinationals wrecked this country? Or is it a lack of good governance? In giving these issues serious consideration, we must not release governments from their responsibility to do their job—serve their countries, not use them as illegitimate resources for private gain. Good gover-

nance in this case includes land reform, tenancy reforms, extension services for small farmers, appropriate credit and marketing systems, and so on. In short, the economic and social impact of genetic engineering and biotechnology can only be as good as the sociopolitical soil in which the resulting new varieties are planted.

One more point must be made about reducing disparities both between the North and the South and within countries. The private sector needs to be asked to cooperate further. For example Novartis, has made a gene of *Bacillus thuringiensis* available to the International Rice Research Institute. If the World Bank asked the five or six largest biotechnology companies to consider where private-sector research could be made available in poor countries—not in competing markets—they could surely come up with some useful recommendations.

In conclusion, when assessing the impact of genetic engineering and biotechnology on food security, we must live with ambivalence. It is intrinsic to every technical advance. But the existence of ambivalence and ethical dilemmas should not paralyze us. On the contrary, they must serve to clarify the course of action and expand our horizon of responsibility. There are both clear benefits and clear risks in this case. Balancing them will require a permanent political assessment process regarding what is acceptable under specific circumstances. Certainly there are no technical solutions to social or political problems, nor is there a silver bullet answer waiting to be discovered. Nevertheless underlying the political process should be the understanding that sustainable food security will not be achieved without better governance and a new dimension of solidarity between the "rich" and "poor" of this world. But it will also require new technologies, such as genetic engineering and biotechnology.

Reference

Persley, G. J. 1990. "Beyond Mendel's Garden: Biotechnology in the Service of World Agriculture." World Bank, Washington, D.C.

Panelist's Remarks

Miguel Altieri

For years academicians have assumed that agriculture poses no special problem for environmental ethics, despite the fact that human life and human civilization depend on the artificial use of nature for agricultural production. Even critics of the environmental impacts of pesticides and of the social implications of agricultural technology have failed to conceptualize a coherent environmental ethics applicable to agricultural problems (Thompson 1995). Most supporters of sustainable agriculture, driven by a technological determinism, do not understand the structural roots of the environmental degradation linked to capitalist agriculture. Therefore, by accepting the present socioeconomic and political structure of agriculture as a given, they are prevented from putting in place an alternative agriculture that challenges this structure (Levins and Lewontin 1985). This is worrisome, especially today, as profit motivations rather than environmental concerns shape the type of research and modes of agricultural production prevalent throughout the world (Busch and others 1990).

Here we contend that the key problem facing agroecologists is that modern industrial agriculture, today epitomized by biotechnology, is founded on philosophical premises that are fundamentally flawed. These premises are precisely the ones that need to be exposed and criticized in order to advance toward a truly sustainable agriculture. This is particularly relevant in the case of biotechnology, where there is an alliance of reductionist science and a multinational monopolistic industry. These jointly perceive agricultural problems as genetic deficiencies of organisms, treat nature as a commodity, and will take agriculture further down a misguided route (Levidow and Carr 1997).

This paper challenges the false promises made by the genetic engineering industry: that it will move agriculture away from a dependence on chemical inputs, that will increase productivity, as well as decrease input costs and help reduce environmental problems (OTA 1992). By challenging the myths of biotechnology we expose genetic engineering for what it really is; another "technological fix" or "magic bullet" aimed at circumventing the environmental problems of agriculture (which themselves are the outcome of an earlier technological fix), without questioning the flawed assumptions that gave rise to the problems in the first place (Hindmarsh 1991). Biotechnology develops single-gene solutions for problems that derive from ecologically unstable monoculture systems, designed on industrial models of efficiency. Such a unilateral approach was already proven ecologically unfit in the case of pesticides (Pimentel and others 1992).

Ethical Questions about Biotechnology

Environmentalists critical of biotechnology question the assumptions that biotechnological science is value free; that it cannot be wrong or misused, and call for an ethical evaluation of genetic engineering research and its products (Krimsky and Wrubel 1996). Supporters of biotechnology are perceived as having a utilitarian view of nature and as favoring the free trading of economic gains for ecological damage with indifference to the human consequences (James 1997). At the very heart of the critique are biotechnology's effects on social and economic conditions and religious and moral values giving rise to questions such as:

- Should we alter the genetic structure of the entire living kingdom in the name of utility and profit?
- Is there something sacred about life, or should life forms, including humans, be viewed simply as commodities in the new biotechnological marketplace?
- Is the genetic makeup of all living things the common heritage of all, or can it be appropriated by corporations and thus become the private property of a few?
- Who gave individual companies the right to the monopoly over entire groups of organisms?
- Do biotechnologists feel they are masters of nature? Is this an illusion constructed on scientific arrogance and conventional economics, blind to the complexity of ecological processes?
- Is it possible to minimize ethical concerns and reduce environmental risks while keeping the benefits?

There are also questions that arise specifically from the nature of the technology, while others such as the domination of agricultural research agendas by commercial interests, the uneven distribution of benefits, the possible environmental risks, and the exploitation of the poor nations' genetic resources by rich ones demand a deeper inquiry:

- Who benefits from the technology? Who looses?
- What are the environmental and health consequences?
- What alternatives have been sacrificed?
- To whose needs does biotechnology respond?
- How does the technology affect what is being produced, how it is being produced, and for what and for whom?

- What are the social goals and ethical criteria that guide research problem choices?
- What social and agronomic goals can be achieved by biotechnology?

Biotechnology Myths

The agrochemical corporations which control the direction and goals of agricultural innovation through biotechnology claim that genetic engineering will enhance the sustainability of agriculture by solving the very problems affecting conventional farming, and will spare farmers in developing countries from low productivity, poverty, and hunger (Molnar and Kinnucan 1989; Gresshoff 1996). By matching myth with reality the following section describes how and why current developments in agricultural biotechnology do not measure up to such promises and expectations.

Myth 1: Biotechnology Will Benefit Farmers in the United States and in the Industrial World.

Most innovations in agricultural biotechnology are profit driven rather than need driven, therefore, the thrust of the genetic engineering industry is not to solve agricultural problems as much as to create profitability. Moreover biotechnology seeks to further industrialize agriculture and to intensify farmers' dependence on industrial inputs, aided by a ruthless system of intellectual property rights which legally inhibits the right of farmers to reproduce, share, and store seeds (Busch and others 1990). By controlling the germplasm from seed to sale and by forcing farmers to pay inflated prices for seed-chemical packages, companies are determined to extract the most profit from their investment.

Because biotechnology is capital intensive, it will continue to deepen the pattern of change in U.S. agriculture, increasing the concentration of agricultural production in the hands of large corporate farms. Biotechnology increases productivity, and as with other labor-saving technology, tends to reduce commodity prices and set in motion a technology treadmill that forces out of business a significant number of farmers—especially small-scale farmers. The example of bovine growth hormone confirms the hypothesis that biotechnology will accelerate the foreclosure of small dairy farms (Krimsky and Wrubel 1996).

Myth 2: Biotechnology Will Benefit Small Farmers and Favor the Hungry and Poor of Developing Countries.

Green revolution technology bypassed small and resource-poor farmers, who will be further marginalized by biotechnology which is under corporate control and protected by patents. Biotechnology is expensive and inappropriate to the needs and circumstances of indigenous people (Lipton 1989). As biotechnology is primarily a commercial activity, this reality determines the priorities of investigation, application, and benefit. While the world may lack food and suffer from pesticide pollution, the focus of multinational corporations is profit, not philanthropy. This is why biotechnologists design transgenic crops for new marketable quality or for import substitution, rather than for greater food production (Mander and Goldsmith 1996). In general biotechnology companies are emphasizing a limited range of crops for which there are large and secured markets, targeted at relatively capital-intensive production systems. As transgenic crops are patented plants, indigenous farmers can lose rights to their own regional germplasm and not be allowed under the World Trade Organization (WTO) to reproduce, share, or store the seeds of their harvest (Crucible Group 1994). It is difficult to conceive how such technology will be introduced in developing countries to favor the masses of poor farmers. If biotechnologists are really committed to feeding the world, why is the scientific genius of biotechnology not turned to develop varieties of crops more tolerant to weeds rather than to herbicides? Or why are more promising products of biotechnology, such as nitrogen-fixing and drought-tolerant plants not being developed?

Biotechnology products will undermine exports from the developing countries, especially from small-scale producers. The development of a thaumatin product through biotechnology is just the beginning of a transition to alternative sweeteners, which will replace developing countries' sugar markets in the future (Mander and Goldsmith 1996). It is estimated that nearly 10 million sugar farmers in developing countries may face a loss of livelihood as laboratory-processed sweeteners begin invading world markets. Fructose produced by biotechnology has already captured over 10 percent of the world market and caused sugar prices to fall, throwing tens of thousands of workers out of jobs. But such foreclosures of rural opportunities are not limited to sweeteners. Approximately 70,000 vanilla farmers in Madagascar were ruined when a Texas firm produced vanilla in biotech labs (Busch and others 1990). The expansion of Unilever-cloned oil palms will substantially increase palm oil production with dramatic consequences for farmers producing other vegetable oils (groundnut in Senegal and coconut in the Philippines).

Myth 3: Biotechnology Will Not Transgress the Ecological Sovereignty of Developing Countries.

Ever since the North became aware of the vital role of biodiversity—of which the South is the major repository—developing countries have witnessed a "gene rush" as multinational corporations aggressively scour forests, crop fields, and coasts in search of the South's genetic gold (Kloppenburg 1988). Protected by the WTO, multinational companies freely practice "biopiracy," which the Rural Advancement Foundation estimates is costing US$5.4 billion a year through lost royalties from food and drug companies using indigenous farmers' germplasm and medicinal plants (Levidow and Carr 1997).

Clearly, indigenous people and their biodiversity are viewed as raw materials for the multinational companies, which have made billions of dollars on seeds developed in U.S. labs from germplasm that farmers in developing countries have carefully bred over generations (Fowler and Mooney 1990). Meanwhile peasant farmers go unrewarded for their millenary farming knowledge, while multinational companies stand to harvest royalties from developing countries estimated at billions of dollars. So far biotechnology companies offer no provisions to pay farmers from developing countries for the seeds they take and use (Kloppenburg 1988).

Myth 4: Biotechnology Will Lead to Biodiversity Conservation.

Although biotechnology has the capacity to create a greater variety of commercial plants, and thus contribute to biodiversity, this is unlikely to happen. The strategy of multinational companies is to create broad international seed markets for a single product. The tendency is toward uniform international seed markets (MacDonald 1991). Moreover the provisions of the patent system prohibiting farmers to reuse the seed yielded by their harvests—dictated by the multinational companies—will affect the possibilities of in situ conservation and on-farm improvements of genetic diversity.

The agricultural systems developed with transgenic crops will favor monocultures, which are characterized by dangerously high levels of genetic homogeneity leading to higher vulnerability to biotic and abiotic stresses (Robinson 1996). As the new bioengineered seeds replace the old, traditional varieties and their wild relatives, genetic erosion will accelerate in developing countries (Fowler and Mooney 1990). Thus the push for uniformity will not only destroy the diversity of genetic resources, but will also disrupt the biological complexity that underlines the sustainability of traditional farming systems (Altieri 1994).

Myth 5: Biotechnology Is Ecologically Safe and Will Launch a Period of Chemical-Free Sustainable Agriculture.

Biotechnology is being pursued to patch up the problems that have been caused by previous agrochemical technologies (pesticide resistance, pollution, soil degradation, and so on) which were promoted by the same companies now leading the biorevolution. Transgenic crops developed for pest control follow closely the pesticide paradigm of using a single control mechanism, which has proven to fail over and over again with insects, pathogens, and weeds (National Research Council 1996). Transgenic crops are likely to increase the use of pesticides and to accelerate the evolution of "super weeds" and resistant insect pests strains (Rissler and Mellon 1996). The "one gene-one pest" resistant

approach has proven to be easily overcome by pests, which are continuously adapting to new situations and evolving detoxification mechanisms (Robinson 1996).

There are many unanswered ecological questions regarding the impact of the release of transgenic plants and micro-organisms into the environment. Among the major environmental risks associated with genetically engineered plants are the unintended transfer to plant relatives of the "transgenes" and the unpredictable ecological effects (Rissler and Mellon 1996).

Given the above considerations, agroecological theory predicts that biotechnology will exacerbate the problems of conventional agriculture, and by promoting monocultures will also undermine ecological methods of farming such as rotation and polycultures (Hindmarsh 1991). As presently conceived, biotechnology does not fit into the broad ideals of a sustainable agriculture (Kloppenburg and Burrows 1996).

Myth 6: Biotechnology Will Enhance the Use of Molecular Biology for the Benefit of All Sectors of Society.

The demand for the new biotechnology did not emerge as a result of social demands, but it emerged out of changes in patent laws and the financial interests of chemical companies in linking seeds and pesticides. The supply emerged out of breakthroughs in molecular biology and the availability of venture capital as a result of favorable tax laws (Webber 1990). The danger is that the private sector is influencing the direction of public sector research in ways unprecedented in the past (Kleinman and Kloppenburg 1988). As more universities enter into partnerships with corporations, serious ethical questions emerge about who owns the results of research and what research is carried out. The trend toward secrecy by university scientists involved in such partnerships raises questions about personal ethics and conflicts of interest. In many universities a professor's ability to attract private investment is often more important than his academic qualifications, taking away the incentives for scientists to be socially responsible. Fields such as biological control and agroecology which do not attract corporate sponsorship are being phased out and this not in the public interest (Kleinman and Kloppenburg 1988).

Conclusions

In the late 1980s Monsanto issued a statement indicating that biotechnology would revolutionize agriculture in the future with products based on nature's own methods, making farming more environmentally friendly and more profitable for the farmer (Office of Technology Assessment 1992). Moreover, plants would be provided with built-in defenses against insects and pathogens. Since then many others have promised several more valuable rewards that biotechnology can bring through crop improvement. The ethical dilemma is that many of these promises are unfounded, and many of the advantages or benefits of biotechnology have not, or may not, be realized. Although clearly biotechnology holds promise for an improved agriculture, given its present orientation it mostly holds promise for environmental harm, for the further industrialization of agriculture, and for the intrusion of private interests too far into public interest sector research. Until now the economic and political domination of the agricultural development agenda by multinational companies has thrived at the expense of the interests of consumers, farm workers, small family farms, wildlife, and the environment.

It is urgent for society to have earlier entry points and broader participation in technological decisions so that corporate interests do not dominate scientific research. National and international public organizations such as the Food and Agriculture Organization of the United Nations (FAO) and the Consultative Group for International Agricultural Research (CGIAR) will have to monitor carefully and control the provision of applied, nonproprietary knowledge to the private sector, to make sure that such knowledge will continue in the public domain for the benefit of rural societies. Regulatory regimes which are publicly controlled must be developed and used to assess and monitor the environmental and social risks of biotechnological products (Webber 1990).

Finally, the trends toward a reductionist view of nature and agriculture—set in motion by contemporary biotechnology—must be reversed by a more holistic approach to agriculture, to ensure that agroecological alternatives are not neglected and that only ecologically sound aspects of biotechnology are researched and developed. The time has come to counter effectively the challenge and the reality of genetic engineering. As it has been with pesticides, biotechnology companies must feel the impact of environmental, farm labor, animal rights', and consumers'lobbies, so that they start reorienting their work for the overall benefit of society and nature. The future of biotechnology-based research will be determined by power relations; farmers and the public in general, if sufficiently empowered, could influence the direction of biotechnology toward sustainable agriculture.

References

Altieri, M.A. 1994. *Biodiversity and Pest Management in Agroecosystems*. New York: Haworth Press.

Busch, L., W.B. Lacy, J. Burkhardt, and L. Lacy. 1990. *Plants, Power and Profit*. Oxford: Basil Blackwell.

Crucible Group. 1994. *People, Plants and Patents*. Ottawa: IDRC.

Fowler, C., and P. Mooney. 1990. *Shattering: Food, Politics and the Loss of Genetic Diversity*. Tucson: University of Arizona Press.

Gresshoff, P.M. 1996. *Technology Transfer of Plant Biotechnology*. Boca Raton, Fla.: CRC Press.

Hindmarsh, R. 1991. "The Flawed 'Sustainable' Promise of Genetic Engineering." *The Ecologist* 21: 196–205.

James, R.R. 1997. "Utilizing a Social Ethic toward the Environment in Assessing Genetically Engineered Insect-Resistance in Trees." *Agriculture and Human Values* 14: 237–49.

Kleinman, D.L., and J. Kloppenburg. 1988. "Biotechnology and University-Industry Relations: Policy Issues in Research and the Ownership of Intellectual Property at a Land Grant University." *Policy Studies Journal* 17: 83–96.

Kloppenburg, J., and B. Burrows. 1996. "Biotechnology to the Rescue? Twelve Reasons Why Biotechnology Is Incompatible with Sustainable Agriculture." *The Ecologist* 26: 61–7.

Kloppenburg, J.R. 1988. *First the Seed: The Political Economy of Plant Technology*. Cambridge: Cambridge University Press.

Krimsky, S., and R.P. Wrubel. 1996. *Agricultural Biotechnology and the Environment: Science, Policy and Social Issues*. Urbana: University of Illinois Press.

Levidow, L., and S. Carr. 1997. "How Biotechnology Regulation Sets a Risk/Ethics Boundary." *Agriculture and Human Values* 14: 29–43.

Levins, R., and R. Lewontin. 1985. *The Dialectical Biologist.* Cambridge, Mass.: Harvard University Press.

Lipton, M. 1989. *New Seeds and Poor People.* Baltimore: The Johns Hopkins University Press.

MacDonald, D.F. 1991. "Agricultural Biotechnology at the Crossroads." NABC Report 3. Union Press of Binghamton.

Mander, J., and E. Goldsmith. 1996. *The Case against the Global Economy.* San Francisco: Sierra Club Books.

Molnar, J.J,. and H. Kinnucan. 1989. *Biotechnology and the New Agricultural Revolution,* Boulder, Col.: Westview Press.

National Research Council. 1996. *Ecologically Based Pest Management.* Washington D.C.: National Academy of Sciences.

Office of Technology Assesment. 1992. *A New Technological Era for American Agriculture.* Washington, D.C.: U.S. Government Printing Office.

Pimentel, D., and others. 1992. "Environmental and Economic Costs of Pesticide Use." *Bioscience* 42: 750–60.

Rissler, J., and M. Mellon. 1996. *The Ecological Risks of Engineered Crops.* Cambridge, Mass.: MIT Press.

Miguel Altieri *to Reduce Pesticide Resistance.* Davis, Calif.: AgAccess.

Thompson, P.B. 1995. *The Spirit of The Soil: Agriculture and Environmental Ethics.* London: Routledge.

Webber, D.J., ed. 1990. *Biotechnology: Assessing Social Impacts and Policy Implications.* Westport, Conn.: Greenwood Press.

Discussion

Ismail Serageldin: Klaus Leisinger said some very important things that I hope we will focus on. One was that if we are concerned about the inadequacy of public resources, one of the ways to tackle that is to increase public investment in research that the private sector is not going to do. There is a balance between the two: there are some things that the public sector will do, and there are some things that the private sector needs to do.

Miguel Altieri highlighted the set of what he referred to as the kinds of biotechnology that should be done, and he was happy that the Novartis Foundation is funding some of that, working in the Sahel. But we cannot expect that the Novartis, which is a profit-making institution, would necessarily invest its money in doing that kind of research, except through the removal from commercial considerations.

The second point of concern is that we need to try to resolve the degrees of risks that really are associated with that question. Over the next two days some very distinguished people will be addressing that. Professor Werner Arber, the president of the International Council of Scientific Unions and a Nobel Prize winner for research in enzymes, will be our opening speaker tomorrow, and Henry Kendall, of the Union of Concerned Scientists, and a Nobel Laureate in physics, also will be speaking. The question of just how much risk there is, and how we can guard against it—that is a separate set of issues which we can also address. But it will take time, and we have two whole days for that, tomorrow and the day after.

Audience comment: I was very interested in the comment on how Ciba-Geigy is handling this issue of licensing, allowing the Consultative Group on International Agricultural Research access to licenses. I have experience with a somewhat different system, which we have practiced within the Biofocus Foundation. Many private companies with which we have been in touch have accepted it without hesitation. We favor patenting, but we also say that the license fee should be tied to the GNP per capita in the country where the intellectual property right is practiced. That may be a variety of the same approach that you take.

Pat Mishey: I am taken by the question that you raised of the biotechnology being driven by market forces, rather than concern for the common good of poverty and hunger alleviation. I would like that addressed. And the question of who is responsible and accountable when things go wrong? And what about the precautionary principle, to prevent harm? How can we hold companies accountable for the prevention of harm? Is the burden on the people to deal with a disaster after it happens, or is the burden on the companies to show, in advance of applying the technology, that it will do no harm?

Audience comment: It is not the companies that are responsible for the mess that we are in, or the multinationals, but rather our whole economic system, which is incompatible with ecological well-being.

Gabby Balsheart: I have two questions. First, do consumers want genetically manipulated organisms in their food? Second, do small farmers in developing countries want the seeds that they cannot use any way they want to?

Klaus Leisinger: On the last questions first, I am very much in favor of open labeling, because then consumers have the choice. If they want to buy a tomato, they should be able to see whether it is a "normal" one or a flavor-saver, and then they can make the choice.

Do the farmers in the developing countries want genetically engineered varieties? They want varieties that bring them an economic benefit. If a farmer with one or two hectares can feed his or her family with one variety and cannot feed his family with the other variety, his choice will be obvious, and he will not care about whether that variety was modified by traditional methods or by genetic engineering.

Miguel Altieri, I can give you, for free, the results of our 12 years' research on striga. If you intercrop with cowpeas, the striga goes down by 85 percent without any chemicals being used. The choice is not between the most modern biotechnology and traditional technologies. There must be technological pluralism. The right mix very much depends on the circumstances. It depends on the time. Ten years from now more than 50 percent of the people in developing countries will be urban people who cannot produce food for themselves. Then we might have to look at a dual agriculture, where part of the food is mass produced, and we have to do anything that is possible to help the marginal farmer to survive. And to bring up this Manichean picture—it is either bad or good—this is simply not my perception of the world. Do farmers buy things they do not benefit from? Is the propaganda of the multinationals so powerful that they can overcome the economic judgment of farmers? If so they must be very different from the farmers we have in Switzerland or Germany.

Last but not least, and I do not want to be unfriendly or politically incorrect, but I have heard a lot of this diffused uneasiness about our economic system not being fit for the survival of humanity. Well, about eight years ago we had another system collapse. So there are not too many alternatives. The political task is to make the market economy socially compatible and ecologically sustainable. There are no instant solutions. For many countries this will be a matter of trial and error, which is going to be developed over many years. One element that was mentioned by Ismail in the morning session will produce a lot of progress—let us try anything to make prices tell the ecological truth. Once it is no longer possible to externalize ecological costs, then all of a sudden it will be the consumers' choice.

Last, if we put the burden of proof about risks on those who innovate, we will not have any more innovation. Because we can never guarantee that we have not missed a risk during the research stage. We have to use the best available knowledge to minimize the probability that severe risks may emerge. That is the precautionary principle today. Most companies cease producing products that show ecological incompatibility in the early stages.

Lori Thrupp: I found it very interesting that both Dr. Serageldin and Dr. Leisinger pointed to the fact very lucidly that, to use your exact words, "there are no technological solutions to social and political problems." And that was preceded by a very strong point which many of us have acknowledged for many years, that the root of food insecurity is largely related to social and political factors. Food production, therefore, is not sufficient, we acknowledge that.

Yet it seems ironic that we come back repeatedly to funding, to investing tremendous amounts of funds from the private sector and the public sector in purely technological solutions. If we are looking at issues that are largely related to distributional questions, to ensuring sustainability over the long term, which requires a change in paradigm, of production, related to the sort of model of science and of society that Miguel alluded to, then why do we come back repeatedly to look for technological solutions? I am not denying that there is a food insecurity issue, or that we do not need more production. But I think that we are looking for the wrong solution by investing huge sums of money into largely technological solutions. I wonder if some of you might want to address that?

Ismail Serageldin: This discussion is focusing on biotechnology because that is the issue before this panel. The issue of biotechnology as a technology raises many issues of a visceral nature, of an ethical nature. This is not to say that other issues are not important: the bulk of the World Bank's investments in agriculture, which are running at US$3.5 billion a year, in support of maybe a total of US$7 billion of spending by the developing countries, is largely not in technology. Out of that there may be a couple of hundred million that are going to technological improvements. The bulk of it is going to issues from land reform to rural roads to agricultural credit to access—a whole range of issues, changing the prices that you were talking about.

Second, and I tried to emphasize this point, the fact that we recognize that the distributional issues are absolutely essential does not remove the fact that the production side is extremely important. Everybody agrees on the demand side—that we will need roughly twice as much production of food on this planet within a generation and a half, partly due to population growth, partly due to income growth. Before we worry about the distributional aspects, if we do not have the overall balances, we know who is going to be squeezed out. It will not be the rich who will go hungry, it will be the poor. That was Amartya Sen's major observation: that people who focus only on the production side and who say that if the balances are in place then everything takes care of itself are not correct, a point that Norman Myers reminded us of.

This conversation is not a total picture, but it is focusing on one subset of it. In that light we are not denying the importance of all these other aspects.

PART III. BIOENGINEERING OF CROPS
Report of the World Bank Panel on Transgenic Crops

About the Authors

Roger Beachy
Scripps Family Chair, Scripps Research Institute; full member, Department of Cell Biology; Head, Division of Plant Biology. Co-director, International Laboratory of Tropical Agricultural Biotechnologies. Fellow, American Association for the Advancement of Science. Received 1991 Commonwealth Award for Science and Invention. Member, National Academy of Sciences.

Thomas Eisner
Schurman Professor of Chemical Ecology and director, Cornell Institute for Research in Chemical Ecology, Cornell University Fellow, National Academy of Sciences, and several other nations' academies of science. Awarded 1994 National Medal of Science.

Fred Gould
Reynolds Professor of Entomology, North Carolina State University. Research areas: integrated pest management, population ecology and genetics, evolutionary biology. Consultant, International Rice Research Institute. Received U. S. Award for Excellence in Integrated Pest Management.

Robert Herdt
Director, agricultural sciences, Rockefeller Foundation, with responsibility for the foundation's agricultural work throughout the world. Agricultural economist, International Rice Research Institute, 1973-83. Faculty member, University of Illinois, and science adviser, World Bank, 1983-86. Fellow, American Association for the Advancement of Science.

Henry W. Kendall
J. A. Stratton, Professor of Physics, Massachusetts Institute of Technology Chair, Union of Concerned Scientists. Awarded 1990 Nobel Prize in Physics.

Peter H. Raven
Director, Missouri Botanical Garden. Professor of botany, Washington University. Home secretary, National Academy of Sciences. Fellow, thirteen other national academies of science. Awarded numerous honorary degrees and other awards, including the Japan International Prize for Biology, and jointly received the Sasakawa Prize, the Volvo Prize, and the Prize of the Institut de la Vie.

lozef S. Schell
Director, Department of Genetic Principles of Plant Breeding, Max Planck Institut für Züchtungsforschung. Professor, plant molecular biology, Collège de France. Member, ten national academies, including the Deutsche Akademie der Naturforscher Leopoldina, the National Academy of Sciences, and the Royal Swedish Academy of Sciences. Winner of numerous awards and distinctions, including the Wolf Prize, the Sir Hans Krebs Medal, and the Australia Prize.

M. S. Swaminathan
UNESCO Professor in Ecotechnology and chair, M.S. Swaminathan Research Foundation, Madras, India. Fellow, Royal Society of London. Foreign associate, National Academy of Sciences, and several other nations' academies of science. Awarded numerous honorary degrees and other awards, including the World Food Prize.

Acknowledgments

This volume was prepared for the World Bank and the Consultative Group on International Agricultural Research. The authors wish to express their thanks to Ismail Serageldin, vice president for Environmentally and Socially Sustainable Development (ESSD), World Bank, for initiating this study and supporting it throughout its course. Robert T. Watson, Director of the World Bank's Environment Department, provided aid and advice that advanced the project.

A number of thoughtful people reviewed the manuscript. Their comments provided an array of additional checks on the work and raised important issues, leading to useful changes in the paper. We are grateful for their help, although the authors of the report remain solely responsible for its content. The reviewers were Nina Fedoroff, Pennsylvania State University; Rebecca Goldberg, Environmental Defense Fund; Mardi Mellon, Union of Concerned Scientists; Per Pinstrup-Andersen, International Food Policy Research Institute; Alison G. Power, Cornell University; and Virginia Walbot, Stanford University.

We also wish to thank Barbara Corbisier for her work in preparing and maintaining the Web site that proved so useful during our work.

Introduction

The primary objectives of the World Bank Group are to alleviate poverty, malnutrition, and human misery in developing nations while encouraging and supporting a transition to environmentally sustainable activities. The issue of providing adequate food, based on sustainable agricultural practices, looms large in gaining these objectives, for failure in this area will virtually guarantee failure to meet other objectives. Moreover, failure will make certain continued misery for many of our fellow human beings. Agricultural systems are already under stress, and they will become more stressed as populations continue to swell and the need for food supplies increases.

The World Bank has made important contributions to the alleviation of hunger and malnutrition through its programs that aid agriculture in the developing world. Its aid was a major factor in making India self-sufficient in food production in the difficult time after World War II. Similarly, its support to the Consultative Group on International Agricultural Research (CGIAR) was instrumental in enabling the CGIAR to be a major player in introducing the Green Revolution, which contributed so much to economic growth in the developing world.[1] But despite contributions by the Bank and other organizations and by nations, the need to enhance food security in much of the developing world will remain a critical problem for many years to come.

Among the numerous approaches to expanding food supplies in the developing world in environmentally benign ways is the bioengineering of crops. Bioengineering has much to contribute, but it is a novel system and possible risks need to be evaluated carefully. Opposition to bioengineering research and its application has already arisen, not all of it carefully thought out. As the World Bank has recognized, a considered and technically competent understanding of both the potential and the perceived risks of bioengineered crops is a requisite to their successful development and use. Public perceptions that genetically engineered crops and animal products pose specific dangers must be carefully considered and addressed if such products are to reach widespread use.

In 1996 Ismail Serageldin, the World Bank's vice president for Environmentally and Socially Sustainable Development and chairman of the CGIAR, initiated a study panel to assess the potential of crop bioengineering as well as the inherent risks. The panel was to provide the Bank with guidance in its activities, including its support to the CGIAR. This is the panel's report. In what follows we review the status of world food supplies and the prospects and needs for the future with emphasis on the developing world. We then describe bioengineering technology and the potential contributions that transgenic crops might make to the alleviation of problems of food security. After that we deal with possible risks from the widespread deployment of genetically altered crops. Finally, we offer some conclusions and recommendations.

Note

1. Henry Owen, "The World Bank: Is 50 Years Enough?" Foreign Affairs 73 (September/October 1994): 99.

CHAPTER 1

World Food Supplies

Current and future demands for food and the pressures and stress on the world's agricultural sector generate the need to set priorities among a cluster of problems and available solutions, including the bioengineering of crops.[1] This section of the report sets out and assesses the challenges as they stand today and evaluates what the future may bring.

Current Circumstances

We are now facing the following challenges.

Population

The world's population stands at 5.8 billion and is growing at about 1.5 percent a year. The industrial, wealthy nations, including Japan and the nations of Europe and North America, have about 1.2 billion people. These nations are growing at a slow rate, roughly 0.1 percent a year.

Population in the developing world is 4.6 billion and is expanding at 1.9 percent a year, a rate that has been decreasing somewhat in the past decade. The least developed nations, with a total population of 560 million, are growing at 2.8 percent a year. If they continue to grow at this rate, their population will double in twenty-four years. At present about 87 million people are added to the world's population each year.

Food: Nutrition and Malnutrition

The wealthy nations have high levels of nutrition and little problem supplying all their citizens with adequate food when they wish to do so. Indeed, well over one-third of world grain production is fed to livestock to enhance the supply of animal protein, which is consumed most heavily in the industrial world.

In the developing world, matters are different. More than 1 billion people do not get enough to eat on a daily basis and live in what the World Bank terms "utter poverty"; about half of that number suffer from serious malnutrition. A minority of nations in the developing world are markedly improving their citizens' standard of living: in some fifteen countries 1.5 billion people have experienced rapidly rising incomes over the past twenty years. But in more than a hundred countries 1.6 billion people have experienced stagnant or falling incomes. Since 1990 incomes have fallen by a fifth in twenty-one countries of eastern Europe.

Had the world's food supply been distributed evenly in 1994, it would have provided an adequate diet of about 2,350 calories a day per person for 6.4 billion people, more than the actual populations.[2]

In addition to the food shortages suffered by many in developing' countries, there are widespread deficiencies in certain vitamins and minerals. Vitamin A appears to be lacking from many diets, especially in Southeast Asia, and there is deficiency in iron, which contributes to widespread anemia among women in the developing world.[3]

Food prices have been declining over the past several decades, and some observers have argued that the decline is a sign that adequate food for all is now available. But those in utter poverty do not have the resources to purchase adequate food, even at today's prices. More recently, food prices have risen, while grain stocks have fallen to their lowest level in thirty years.[4]

Agriculture

About 12 percent of the world's total land surface is used to grow crops, about 30 percent is forest or woodland, and 26 percent is pasture or meadow. The remainder, about one-third, is used for other human purposes or is unusable because of climate or topography. In 1961 the amount of cultivated land supporting food production was 0.44 hectares per capita. Today it is about 0.26 hectares per capita, and based on population projections, it will be in the vicinity of 0.15 hectares per capita by 2050.[5] The rate of expansion of arable land is now below 0.2 percent a year and continues to fall. The bulk of the land best suited to rainfed agriculture is already under cultivation, and the land that is being brought into cultivation generally has lower productivity.

Urbanization frequently involves the loss of prime agricultural land, because cities are usually founded near such land. Losses of prime land are often not counterbalanced by the opening of other lands to production because the infrastructure that is generally required for market access is frequently lacking on those lands.

Irrigation plays an important role in global food production. Of the currently exploited arable land, about 16 percent is irrigated, producing more than one-third of the world crop. Irrigated land is, on balance, over two and a half times more productive than rainfed land.

The situation in India and China is particularly acute because their people account for nearly half of the developing world's population. Both countries have expanding populations and diminishing per capita arable land and water resources. The average farm size in both countries is one hectare or less. Agriculture, including crop and animal husbandry, forestry, and fisheries, has been a way of life and a means to achieve a livelihood for several thousand years. Expansion in population and increases in purchasing power, coupled with the diversion

of prime farm land for nonfarm uses, make it essential for these two countries to adopt ecologically sustainable, intensive, and integrated farming systems (see appendix).

In China land is communally owned but individually cultivated under the country's Household Responsibility System. In India land is individually owned and agriculture constitutes the largest private-sector enterprise in the country. India's population of 950 million is growing at about 1.9 percent annually, while China's stands at 1.22 billion and is growing at 1.1 percent a year. China has nearly 50 percent of its cultivated land under irrigation, while less than 30 percent of India's cultivated area is irrigated.[6]

Agriculture in both countries must provide not only more food but also more employment and income. Modern industry is frequently associated with economic growth, but growth without adequate expansion of employment. Modern agriculture can foster job-led economic growth. Therefore, farming cannot be viewed in either country as merely a means of producing more food and other agricultural commodities; instead, it must be looked upon as the very foundation of a secure livelihood. New technologies, such as biotechnology, information and space technologies, and renewable energy, are pivotal to building vibrant agricultural sectors, to producing more from less land and water, and to strengthening local economies.

Pressures on Agricultural Systems

Widespread injurious agricultural practices, in both the industrial and the developing worlds, have damaged the productivity of land, in some cases severely.[7] These practices have led to water- and wind-induced erosion, salination, compaction, waterlogging, overgrazing, and other problems. For example, the estimated loss of topsoil in excess of new soil production is estimated to be about 0.7 percent of the total topsoil each year; this loss amounts to some 25 billion tons, equivalent to the total in Australia's wheat growing area. An additional 0.7 percent annual loss occurs from land degradation and the spread of urbanization. Erosion has made a billion hectares of soil unusable for agriculture over past years.[8] Asia has the highest percentage of eroded land, nearly 30 percent, but in all major regions the percentage exceeds 12.[9] It is estimated that 17 percent of all vegetated land was degraded by human activity between 1945 and 1990.

The effects of erosion on crop yield are not well documented because researching such effects is difficult and expensive and because degradation can be masked for short periods of time by more intensive agricultural practices. However certain data are available.[10] Erosion can ultimately destroy the land's productive capacity by stripping off all of the soil, as has occurred in Haiti. "Haiti suffers some of the world's most severe erosion, down to bedrock over large parts of some regions, so that even farmers with reasonable amounts of land cannot make a living."[11]

Irrigation practices continue to contribute to salinization and other forms of land damage. For example, more than half of all irrigated land is in dry areas, and 30 percent of that land is moderately to severely degraded. Salinization is a serious problem in Australia, Egypt, India, Mexico, Pakistan, and the United States. Some 10 percent of the world's irrigated land suffers from salinization.

There are also serious problems with supplies of water-much of the world is in short supply.[12] Worldwide, nations with some 214 river or lake basins and 40 percent of the world's population now compete for water.[13] Much irrigation depends on "fossil" underground water supplies, which are being pumped more rapidly than they are being recharged.[14] This problem affects portions of Africa, China, India, the United States, and several countries in the Middle East, especially Israel and Jordan. The human race now uses 26 percent of the total terrestrial evapotranspiration and 54 percent of the fresh water runoff that is geographically and temporally accessible. Most land suitable for rainfed agriculture is already in production.[15]

It is now clear that agricultural production is currently unsustainable. Indeed, human activities, as they are now conducted, appear to be approaching the limits of the earth's capacity These unsustainable activities, like all unsustainable practices, must end at some point. The end will come either from changes that establish a basis for a humane future or from partial or complete destruction of the resource base, which would bring widespread misery

The Future

In future years we are likely to face the following challenges.

Population

Although fertility has been declining worldwide in recent decades, it is not known when it will decline to replacement level. There is broad agreement among demographers that if current trends are maintained, the world's population will reach about 8 billion by 2020, 10 billion by 2050, and possibly 12 to 14 billion before the end of the next century Virtually all of the growth in coming decades will occur in the developing world.

Food Demand

To provide increased nutrition for a growing world population, it will be necessary to expand food production faster than the rate of population growth. Studies forecast a doubling in demand for food by 2025-30.[16] Dietary changes and the growth in nutritional intake that accompany increased affluence will contribute to making food demand larger than the projected increase in population.

Asia, which has 60 percent of the world's population, contains the largest number of the world's poor; 800 million people in Asia live in absolute poverty and 500 million live in extreme poverty. Projections by the United Nations Food and Agriculture Organization (FAO), the World Bank, and the International Food Policy Research Institute show that the demand for food in Asia will exceed the supply by 2010.[17] China, the world's most populous nation, has more than 1.2 billion people and an annual growth rate of 1.1 percent a year. The country will face considerable challenges in years ahead from stress resulting from major environmental damage, shortages of water, and diversion or degradation of arable lands.[18] Animal protein has increased in the Chinese diet from about 7 percent in 1980 to more than 20 percent today, aggravating the country's food challenges. Most of the water available in China is used for agriculture, and heavy use of fertilizers has polluted much of the water supply.

Lester Brown and Hal Kane have argued that by 2030 India will need to import 45 million tons of food grain annually and China 216 million tons to feed their growing populations.[19] The widening gap between grain production and consumption in the two countries, caused by increases in population and purchasing power, will lead to the need for such imports. Brown and Kane have pointed out that while demand will grow, production prospects are not bright owing to stagnation in applying yield-enhancing technologies and growing damage to the ecological foundations essential for sustainable advances in farm productivity. It is apparent that without substantial change there will not be enough grain to meet the needs of the two countries, a conclusion that at least some Chinese scholars agree with.[20]

Latin America, which is economically and demographically advanced compared with Africa and Asia, appears to enjoy a relatively favorable situation with respect to food supplies and food security. Some regions are, however, under stress because of economic problems and continuing high rates of population increase. Bolivia, northeast Brazil, Peru, much of Central America, and parts of the Caribbean, especially El Salvador, Guatemala, Haiti, and Honduras, face important challenges. Latin America's population is expected to increase from 490 million to nearly 680 million by 2025, and it is possible that more than a quarter of the area's annual cereal consumption will be imported by 2020. The major countries in the region, including Argentina, Brazil, Chile, Colombia, and Mexico, appear to have the resources necessary to meet their projected food needs, but doing so will require maintaining stable populations and implementing successful land management programs.[21]

Countries in the Middle]East and North Africa have seen demand for food outpace domestic production. Differences in oil wealth and agricultural production determine differences in ability to import grains and livestock products.[22] The greatest challenges will be faced by nations that lack the capacity for substantial oil exports or other sources of wealth with which to purchase food imports. These nations include Afghanistan, Cyprus, Egypt, Jordan, Lebanon, Mauritania, Somalia, Tunisia, and Yemen, whose combined population exceeded 125 million in 1994. Food self-sufficiency is unattainable for most of these countries. Oil exporting nations will, as their oil resources dwindle, join this less fortunate group.

Sub-Saharan Africa is the region whose prospective food supplies generate the greatest concern; since 1980 agriculture there has grown at 1.7 percent a year, while population, now at 739 million, has grown at 2.9 percent a year.[23] Some twenty years ago, Africa produced food equal to what it consumed; today it produces only 80 percent of the food it consumes.[24] With a population growth rate of close to 3 percent a year, Sub-Saharan Africa cannot close its food gap. The gap will likely grow, requiring increased imports of food to prevent growing malnutrition and increased risk of famine. If present worldwide decreases in foreign aid persist, these imports may not be forthcoming.

Agriculture and Irrigation

As described above, the current rates of injury to arable land are troubling. Since 1950, 25 percent of the world's topsoil has been lost, and continued erosion at the present rate will result in the further irreversible loss of at least 30 percent of the global topsoil by the middle of the next century. A similar percentage may be lost to land degradation, a loss that can be made up only with the greatest difficulty through conversion of pasture and forest, themselves under pressure. In Asia 82 percent of the potentially arable land is already under cultivation. Much of the land classed as potentially arable is not available because it is of low quality or easily damaged.

The FAO has projected that over the next twenty years arable land in the developing countries could be expanded by 12 percent at satisfactory economic and environmental costs, although such expansion would inflict major damage to the world's remaining biodiversity.[25] The yields per hectare on this land would be less than on the land already in production. This expansion is to be compared with the 61 percent increase in food demand that is expected to occur in these countries during the same period, according to a scenario discussed by the FAO. The last major frontiers that can potentially be converted to arable land are the acid soil areas of the Brazilian cerrado, the Ilanos of Colombia and Venezuela, and the acid soil areas of central and southern Africa. Bringing these unexploited, potentially arable lands into agricultural production poses formidable but not insurmountable challenges.[26]

The prospects for expanding irrigation, so critical to the intensification of agricultural productivity, are also troubling. The growth of irrigated land has been slowing since the 1970s, owing to the problems discussed above as well as to "siltation" of reservoirs and the environmental problems and related costs that arise from the construction of large dam systems. The problems can include the spread of disease.

An important "wild card" in any assessment of future agricultural productivity is climatic change resulting from anthropogenic emissions of greenhouse gases. The consequences of such change touch on a wide range of technical issues that will not be summarized here.[27] However, the Intergovernmental Panel on Climate Change (IPCC) concluded in its second assessment report that the balance of evidence suggests that there is a discernable human influence on climate and that a global warming of about two degrees Celsius, with a range of uncertainty from one to three and a half degrees Celsius, will occur by 2100. The consequences of a two-degree warming would include regional and global changes in climate and climate-related parameters such as temperature, precipitation, soil moisture, and sea level. These changes could in turn give rise to regional increases in "the incidence of extreme high temperature events, floods, and droughts, with resultant consequences for fires, pest outbreaks and ecosystem composition, structure and functioning, including primary productivity."[28] According to the IPCC:

> Crop yields and changes in productivity due to climate change will vary considerably across regions and among localities, thus changing the patterns of

production. Productivity is projected to increase in some areas and decrease in others, especially the tropics and subtropics. . . . There may be increased risk of hunger and famine in some locations; many of the world's poorest people—particularly those living in subtropical and tropical areas and dependent on isolated agricultural systems in semi-arid and arid regions—are most at risk of increased hunger. Many of these at-risk populations are found in Sub-Saharan Africa; South, East, and Southeast Asia; and tropical areas of Latin America, as well as some Pacific island nations.[29]

Further deleterious changes may occur in livestock production, fisheries, and global supplies of forest products. Salt intrusion into coastal area aquifers, many of which supply water for irrigation, can occur as a result of rising sea levels. While important uncertainties about climatic change and its consequences will remain for some years, the matter must be considered in assessing the prospects for expanding nutrition in the developing world.

Prospects

Today, there are hundreds of millions of people who do not get enough food. Given the circumstances described above, it appears that over the next quarter century grave problems of food security will almost certainly affect even more people, as a number of observers have pointed out.[30]

> Given present knowledge, therefore, maximum realization of potential land, and water, supplies at acceptable economic and environmental costs in the developing countries still would leave them well short of the production increases needed to meet the demand scenarios over the next twenty years.[31]

The task of meeting world food needs to 2010 by the use of existing technology may prove difficult, not only because of the historically unprecedented increments to world population that seem inevitable during this period but also because problems of resource degradation and mismanagement are emerging. Such problems call into question the sustainability of the key technological paradigms on which much of the expansion of food production since 1960 has depended.[32]

As is the case now, those in the lower tier of the developing countries will continue to be most affected by shortfalls in food production. The industrial nations and the developing nations whose economies continue to improve will face acceptable costs in providing their citizens with adequate nutrition. The extent of deprivation and economic and environmental costs remains the subject of controversy between optimists and pessimists.[33]

Meeting the Challenges

The main challenge is to expand agricultural production at a rate exceeding population growth in the decades ahead so as to provide food to the hungry new mouths to be fed. This goal must be accomplished in the face of a fixed or slowly growing base of arable land offering little expansion, and it must involve simultaneous replacement of destructive agricultural practices with more benign ones. Thus the call for agricultural sustainability.[34] Owing to the daunting nature of this challenge, every economically, ecologically, and socially feasible improvement will have to be carefully exploited. A list of potential improvements includes:

- Introducing energy-intensive farming, including, in some areas, increased fertilizer use
- Conserving soil and water, with special priority given to combating erosion
- Maintaining biodiversity
- Improving pest control
- Expanding irrigation and making it more efficient
- Improving livestock management
- Developing new crop strains with increased yield, pest resistance, and drought tolerance
- Reducing dependency on pesticides and herbicides.

The application of modem techniques of crop bioengineering could be a key factor in implementing many of these improvements. These techniques are a powerful new tool with which to supplement pathology, agronomy, plant breeding, plant physiology, and other approaches that serve us now.

If crop bioengineering techniques are developed and applied in a manner consistent with ecologically sound agriculture, they could decrease reliance on broad spectrum insecticides, which cause serious health and environmental problems. This reduction could be accomplished by breeding crop varieties that have specific toxicity to target pests but do not affect beneficial insects. Furthermore, bioengineering techniques could assist in the development of crop varieties that are resistant to currently uncontrollable plant diseases. At their best bioengineering techniques are highly compatible with the goals of sustainable agriculture because they offer surgical precision in combating specific problems without disrupting other functional components of the agricultural system.

While it is feasible to use biotechnology to improve the ecological soundness of agriculture, well-informed decisions must be made regarding which specific biotechnology projects are encouraged and which are discouraged. For example, ten years ago, when crop bioengineering was being introduced in the United States, some projects were focused on engineering crops for tolerance against a dangerous herbicide. The projects were dropped after environmental groups protested. Projects targeted for developing countries will have to be scrutinized to make sure that their long-term impacts are beneficial.

Not all challenges to sustainable and productive agriculture can be addressed with biotechnology. For example, improving soil and water conservation, maintaining biodiversity, and improving irrigation techniques must be dealt with by other means.

We must emphasize that the improvements in agriculture described in this report, while badly needed, do not address all of the difficulties faced by the lower tier of developing nations. There is almost no dispute that careful planning and selection of priorities, coupled with substantial commitments from both industrial and developing nations, will be required to provide the food supplies that the future will demand, to move to sustainable agricultural practices, and to alleviate hardship in now-impoverished nations.

Notes

1. See H. W. Kendall and David Pimentel, "Constraints on the Expansion of the Global Food Supply," AMBIO 23 (May 1994):198-205.

2. Norman E. Borlaug, "Feeding the World: The Challenges Ahead," in *Meeting the Challenges of Population, Environment, and Resources: The Costs of Inaction*, H. W. Kendall and others. (Washington, D.C.: World Bank, 1996).

3. Robert W. Herdt, "The Potential Role of Biotechnology in Solving Food Production and Environmental Problems in Developing Countries," in *Agriculture and Environment: Bridging Food Production and Environmental Protection in Developing Countries*, ed. Anthony S.R. Juo and Russell D. Freed, American Society of Agronomy Special Publication 60 (Madison, Wis., 1995),33-54.

4. Per Pinstrup-Andersen and James L. Garrett, *Rising Food Prices and Falling Grain Stocks: Short-Run Blips or New Trends?* 2020 Brief (Washington, D.C.: International Food Policy Research Institute, 1996).

5. Robert Engelman and Pamela LeRoy, *Conserving Land: Population and Sustainable Food Production* (Washington, D.C.: Population Action International, 1995).

6. World Resources Institute, *World Resources 1994-95* A Report of the World Resources Institute (Washington, D.C., 1995).

7. See especially D. Norse and others, "Agriculture, Land Use, and Degradation," in An *Agenda of Science for Environment and Development into the 21st Century*, ed. J. C. I. Dooge and others (Cambridge, U.K.: Cambridge University Press).

8. Food and Agriculture Organization of the United Nations, *Agriculture towards 2010* (Rome, 1993).

9. Robert W. Herdt, "The Potential Role of Biotechnology in Solving Food Production and Environmental Problems in Developing Countries," 33-54; World Resources Institute, *World Resources 1992-93* (New York: Oxford University Press, 1993).

10. David Pimentel and J. Krummel, "Biomass Energy and Soil Erosion: Assessment of Resource Costs," *BioScience* 14 (1987): 15-38.

11. World Commission on Environment and Development, Our *Common Future* (New York: Oxford University Press, 1987).

12. Sandra Postel, "Water and Agriculture," in *Water in Crisis, A Guide to the World's Fresh Water Resources*, ed. Peter H. Gleick (New York: Oxford University Press, 1993), 56-62.

13. World Resources Institute, *World Resources 1992-93* (Washington, D.C., 1995).

14. Lester R. Brown, "Future Supplies of Land and Water Are Fast Approaching Depletion," in *Population and Food in the Early Twenty-First Century: Meeting Future Food Demand of an Increasing Population*, ed. Nurul Islam (Washington, D.C.: International Food Policy Research Institute, 1995).

15. Sandra Postel, Gretchen Daily, and Paul Ehrlich, "Human Appropriation of Renewable Fresh Water," *Science*, 9 February 1996, 785-88.

16. Donald L. Plucknett, "Prospects of Meeting Future Food Needs through New Technology," in *Population and Food in the Early Twenty-First Century*, 207-08; Borlaug, "Feeding the World: The Challenges Ahead."

17. Kirit Parikh and S. M. Dev, "Comments: Asia," in *Population and Food in the Early Twenty-First Century*, 117-18.

18. Vaclav Smil, "Comments: Asia," in *China's Environmental Crisis—An Inquiry into the Limits of National Development* (Armonk, N.Y: M. E. Sharpe, 1993).

19. Lester R. Brown and Hal Kane, *Full House: Reassessing the Earth's Population Carrying Capacity* (New York: W. W. Norton, 1994); Lester R. Brown, *Who Will Feed China? Wake-Up Call for a Small Planet* (New York: W. W. Norton, 1995).

20. "Malthus Goes East," *Economist*, 12 August 1995,29.

21. Tim Dyson, *Population and Food* (London and New York: Routledge, 1996).

22. Thomas Nordblom and Farouk Shomo, "Comments: Middle East/North Africa," in *Population and Food in the Early Twenty-First Century*, 131.

23. World Bank, *Rural Development: From Vision to Action* (Washington, D.C., 1997).

24. J. Cherfas, *Science*, 1990, 1140-41.

25. Food and Agriculture Organization of the United Nations, *Agriculture: Towards 2010*; Pierre Crosson, in *Population and Food in the Early Twenty-First Century*, 143-59.

26. Borlaug, 'Feeding the World: The Challenges Ahead."

27. Intergovernmental Panel on Climate Change (IPCC), *Radiative Forcing of Climate Change—The 1994 Report of the Scientific Assessment Working Group of IPCC* (New York: IPCC, World Meteorological Organization, and United Nations Environment Programme, 1994); John Houghton, *Global Warming—The Complete Briefing* (Oxford: Lion Publishing, 1994).

28. IPCC, *Summary for Policymakers: Impacts, Adaptation, and Mitigation Options*, The Second Assessment Report of Working Group II (Washington, D.C., 1995).

29. IPCC, *Summary for Policymakers*. See also ADB (Asian Development Bank), *Climate Change in Asia: Executive Summary* (Manila, 1994); David W. Wolfe, "Potential Impact of Climate Change on Agriculture and Food Supply" (Paper presented at the Center for Environmental Information's Conference on

Sustainable Development and Global Climate Change, Arlington, Va., 4-5 December 1995).

30. Klaus M. Leisinger, *Sociopolitical Effects of New Biotechnologies in Developing Countries,* Food, Agriculture, and the Environment Discussion Paper 2 (Washington, D.C.: International Food Policy Research Institute, 1995).

31. Crosson, in *Population and Food in the Early Twenty-First Century, 157.*

32. Peter A. Oram and Behjat Hojjati, in *Population and Food in the Early Twenty-First Century,* 167.

33. See John Bongaarts, "Can the Growing Human Population Feed Itself?" *Scientific American,* March 1994, 18; Alex F. McCalla, "Agriculture and Food Needs to 2025: Why Should We Be Concerned?" (Consultative Group on International Agricultural Research, Sir John Crawford Memorial Lecture, Washington, D.C., 27 October 1994).

34. D. L. Plucknett and D. L. Winkelmann, "Technology for Sustainable Agriculture," *Scientific American,* September 1995, 182-86.

CHAPTER 2

Bioengineering Technology

Plant scientists can now transfer genes into many crop plants and achieve stable intergenerational expression of new traits. "Promoters" (deoxyribonucleic acid [DNA] sequences that control the expression of genes, for example) can be associated with transferred genes to ensure expression in particular plant tissues or at particular growth stages. Transformation can be achieved with greater efficiency and more routinely in some dicots (for example, tomatoes, potatoes) than in some monocots (for example, rice and wheat), but with determined effort nearly all plants can or will be modified by genetic engineering.

Gene Transformation

Genetic transformation and other modern crop breeding techniques have been used to achieve four broad goals: to change product characteristics, improve plant resistance to pests and pathogens, increase output, and improve the nutritional value of foods.

Genetic modification to alter product characteristics is illustrated by the Flavr Sarv™ tomato, one of the first genetically engineered plants to receive approval from the U.S. Food and Drug Administration and to be made available for general consumption by the public; the fruit ripening characteristics of this variety were modified to provide a longer shelf life.[1] Biotechnology has also been used to change the proportion of fatty acids in soybeans, modify the composition of canola oil, and change the starch content of potatoes.[2]

Natural variability in the capacity of plants to resist damage from insects and diseases has long been exploited by plant breeders. Biotechnology provides new tools to the breeder to expand plant capacity. In the past crop breeders were generally limited to transferring genes from one crop variety to another. In some cases they were able to transfer useful genes to a variety from a closely related crop species or a related native plant. Genetic engineering now gives plant breeders the power to transfer genes to crop varieties independent of the gene's origin. Thus bacterial and even animal genes can be used to improve a crop variety.

Bacillus thuringiensis (Bt), a bacterium that produces an insect toxin particularly effective against lepidoptera (such as caterpillars and moths), has been applied to crops by gardeners for decades. It is also effective against mosquitoes and certain beetles. Transformation of tomato and tobacco plants with the gene that produces Bt toxin was one of the first demonstrations of how biotechnology can be used to enhance a plant's ability to resist damage from insects.[3] Transgenic cotton that expresses Bt toxin at a level providing protection against cotton bollworm has been developed, and a large number of Bt-transformed crops, including corn and rice, are currently being field tested.[4] Other strategies to prevent insect damage include using protein coding genes of plant origin, such as lectins, amylase inhibitors, protease inhibitors, and cholesterol oxidase, that retard insect growth.[5]

Genes that confer resistance to viral diseases have been derived from the viruses themselves, most notably with coat protein mediated resistance (CP-MR). Following extensive field evaluation, a yellow squash with CP-MR resistance to two plant viruses was approved for commercial production in the United States.[6] Practical resistance to fungal and bacterial pathogens has been more elusive, although genes encoding enzymes that degrade fungal cell walls or inhibit fungal growth are being evaluated. More recently, natural genes for resistance to pathogens have been cloned, modified, and shown to function when transferred to susceptible plants.[7]

While protecting plants against insects and pathogens promises to increase crop yield by saving a higher percentage of present yield, several strategies seek to increase the potential crop yield. These strategies include exploiting hybrid vigor, delaying plant senescence, and inducing plants to flower earlier and to increase starch production.

Several strategies to produce hybrid seeds in new ways will likely contribute to increasing yield potential. Cytoplasmic male sterility was widely used long before the age of biotechnology, but strategies to exploit male sterility require biological manipulations that can only be carried out using tools from molecular biology; several of these strategies are well advanced.[8] Some of the strategies entail suppressing pollen formation by changing the temperature or day length. Delayed senescence or "stay-green" traits enable a plant to continue producing food beyond the period when a nontransformed plant would, thereby potentially producing a higher yield.[9] Potatoes that produce higher starch content than nontransformed control potatoes have been developed.[10]

Plants have been modified to produce a range of lipids, carbohydrates, pharmaceutical polypeptides, and industrial enzymes, leading to the hope that plants can be used in place of microbial fermentation.[11] One of the more ambitious of such applications is the production of vaccines against animal and human diseases. The hepatitis B surface antigen has been expressed in tobacco, and the feasibility of using the purified product to elicit an immune response in mice has been demonstrated.[12]

Gene Markers

Far-reaching possibilities for identifying genes have been made possible through various molecular marker techniques with exotic names such as restriction fragment length polymorphism (RFLP), random amplified polymorphic DNA (RAPD), and microsatellites. These techniques allow scientists to follow genes from one generation to the next, adding to the tools at the disposal of plant breeders. In particular, the techniques enable plant breeders to combine several resistance genes, each of which may have different modes of action, leading to longer-acting or more durable resistance against pathogens. Marking also makes it possible for the breeder to combine several genes, each of which may individually provide only a weakly expressed desirable trait but in combination have higher activity.

Ongoing Research

Research continues to improve the efficiency and reduce the costs of developing transgenic crops and using genetic markers. As this research succeeds, it will be applied to different plants and genes.

By far the greatest proportion of current research in crop biotechnology is being conducted in industrial countries on the crops of economic interest in those countries. Plant biotechnology research in the fifteen countries of the European Union is probably a fair reflection of current global research in plant biotechnology Almost 2,000 projects are under way, 1,300 of them actually using plants (as opposed to plant pathogens, theoretical work, and the like). About 210 of the projects using plants are on wheat, barley, and other cereals; 150 of the projects are on the potato; 125 are on oilseed rape; and about 90 are on maize.[13]

The worldwide record of field trials reflects the focus of research activities, and the record shows that work on cereals was started somewhat later than work on other plants. Some 1,024 field trials were conducted worldwide through 1993; 88 percent of those trials were in Organization for Economic Cooperation and Development (OECD) countries, with 38 percent in the United States, 13 percent in France, and 12 percent in Canada. Belgium, the Netherlands, and the United Kingdom each hosted about 5 percent of the total number of field trials. Argentina, Chile, China, and Mexico led in numbers of trials in developing countries, but none had more than 2 percent of the total.[14]

The largest number of field trials was conducted on the potato (19 percent). Oilseed rape accounted for 18 percent of the field trials, while tobacco, tomatoes, and maize each accounted for about 12 percent. There were more than ten trials each on alfalfa, cantaloupe, cotton, flax, sugar beet, soybean, and poplar. Nine tests were done on rice, and fewer than nine on wheat, sorghum, millet, cassava, and sugarcane, the crops that, aside from maize, provide most of the food to most of the world's people, who live in the developing countries.

Herbicide tolerance has been the most widely tested genetically engineered trait, accounting for 40 percent of the field trials for agronomically useful transgenes. Twenty-two percent of tests were conducted on ten different types of modified product quality, including delayed ripening, modified processing characters, starch metabolism, and modified oil content.[15] About 40 percent of field trials in developing countries were for virus resistance. Twenty-five percent of the trials were for crops modified for herbicide resistance, and another 25 percent were for insect resistance, with the balance for product quality, fungal resistance, or agromatic traits.[16]

Although much of the biotechnology research in agriculture has focused on bioengineering (that is, gene transfer), the techniques of biotechnology extend beyond this approach. The techniques involved in tissue culture have been advanced and refined over the past decade. These techniques can be used to regenerate plants from single cells and have proven especially useful in producing disease-free plants that can be propagated and distributed to farmers. The use of these plants has resulted in significant yield improvements in crops as diverse as potato and sugarcane.

Another use for biotechnology is in developing diagnostic techniques. Too often, poorly performing crops have observable symptoms that are so general that the farmer cannot determine the specific cause. For example, Tungro disease in rice produces symptoms that match those of certain nutrient deficiencies. Biotechnology

techniques can be used to develop easy-to-use kits that can alert the farmer to the presence of deoxyribonucleic acid (DNA) from the Tungro virus in rice plants. Such knowledge can decrease the frustration and money spent on solving the wrong problem.

Current Efforts

Most biotechnology research in industrial countries is being conducted on human health issues rather than on agriculture. Government spending for biotechnology research in the United States is about $3.3 billion a year, with $2.9 billion going to health issues and $190 million to agricultural issues.[17] It is estimated that between 1985 and 1994 $260 million was contributed in the form of grants to agricultural biotechnology in the developing world; another $150 million was contributed in the form of loans. An average of perhaps $50 million a year has been contributed in more recent years.[18] At least a third and perhaps half of these funds have been used to establish organizations designed to help bring the benefits of biotechnology to developing countries.

Maize is the focus of much crop biotechnology work in the United States. Most of this work on maize is directed toward making it better suited for production or more capable of resisting the depredations of the pests in industrial countries. The International Wheat and Maize Improvement Center sponsors the largest international effort directed at identifying traits of maize that could be improved using biotechnology, but the center spends barely $2 million a year on those efforts.

There are, at present, only four coherent, coordinated programs directed specifically at enhancing biotechnology research on crops in developing countries, one supported by the U.S. Agency for International Development (USAID), one by the Dutch government, one by the Rockefeller Foundation, and one by the McKnight Foundation.

The USAID-supported project, Agricultural Biotechnology for Sustainable Productivity (ABSP), is headquartered at Michigan State University and implemented by a consortium of U.S. universities and private companies. It is targeted at five crop/pest complexes: the potato and the potato tuber moth, the sweet potato and the sweet potato weevil, maize and the stem borer, the tomato and the tomato yellow leaf virus, and cucurbits and several viruses. The ABSP is an outgrowth of an earlier USAID-supported project on improving tissue culture techniques for crops. It builds on the network of scientists associated with that earlier project and draws on other scientists as well.

The cassava biotechnology network, sponsored by the Netherlands Directorate General for International Cooperation, held its first meeting in August 1992. Its goals include using the tools of biotechnology to modify cassava to better meet the needs of small-scale cassava producers, processors, and consumers. More than 125 scientists from 28 countries participated in the first network meeting. Funding to date has been about $2 million. An important initial activity is a study of farmers' needs for technical change in cassava. The study will be based on a field survey of cassava producers in several locations in Africa.

Another important initiative, the International Laboratory of Tropical Agricultural Biotechnology, is being developed at the Scripps Institute in La Jolla, California. It is jointly administered by the institute and by L'Institut français de recherche scientifique pour le développement en coopération (ORSTOM), a French governmental development agency. Funding for research in the control of diseases of rice, cassava, and tomato through applications of biotechnology is provided in grants from ORSTOM, the Rockefeller Foundation, the ABSP, and USAID. Most of the research is carried out by fellows, students, and other trainees from developing countries.

The Rockefeller Foundation began to support rice biotechnology in the developing world in 1984. The foundation's program has two objectives: (1) to create biotechnology applicable to rice to produce improved rice varieties suited to developing country needs and (2) to ensure that scientists in developing countries know how to use biotechnology techniques and are capable of adapting the techniques to their own objectives. Approximately $50 million in grants have been made through the program.

About two hundred senior scientists and three hundred trainee scientists are participating in the program. The scientists are spread throughout all the major rice-producing countries of Asia and a number of industrial countries. Researchers from the group transformed rice in 1988, a first for any cereal. Transformed rice has been field-tested in the United States. A significant number of lines transformed with agronomically useful traits now exist and are being developed for field tests. RFLP maps, that is "road maps" that allow breeders to follow genes, are being used to assist breeding, and some rice varieties developed by advanced techniques not requiring genetic engineering are now being grown by Chinese farmers.

The McKnight Foundation recently established its Collaborative Crop Research Program, which links researchers in less developed countries with U.S. plant scientists in order to strengthen research in selected countries and to focus the work of U.S. scientists on food needs in the developing world. The program is being funded at $12 to $15 million for the first six years. While crop engineering is not the sole research tool supported by the program, it plays an extremely important role.

Early in the effort to apply bioengineering to crop improvement, there was great hope placed in the potential to engineer the capacity for nitrogen fixation into crops without it. After the investment of millions of dollars in public and venture capital and many years of research, it has become apparent that the genetic machinery involved in nitrogen fixation by legumes is extremely complex and beyond our current capacity for gene transfer and expression. At some point in the future nitrogen fixation may be transferred to crops such as corn and rice, but such an achievement must be seen as a far-off goal.

It is unlikely that the budgets of these four focused crop biotechnology efforts, taken together, come to more than $20 million annually. Total agricultural biotechnology research in the developing world may not greatly exceed $50 million annually.[19] Brazil, China, Egypt, India, and a few other countries have a reasonable base for biotechnology, but most developing countries will find it difficult to develop useful biotechnology products without sharply directed assistance. Little attention will be paid to crops of importance in the developing world or to the pests, diseases, and stresses that afflict them unless the crops are also important to the more advanced countries. That is, while the gains in fundamental knowledge that apply to all organisms will be available, the programs may not produce applications in the form of transformation techniques, probes, gene promoters, and the like.

Potential Contributions of Transgenic Crops

Transgenic crops have the potential to contribute to increased production and food quality, environmental well-being, and human health.

Potential Applications to Improved Production and Food Quality

How will the developments of molecular biology contribute to solving the food production problems in developing countries in the years ahead? Contributions may come through two different paths: (1) research in molecular biology directed specifically at food needs in the developing world or (2) "spillover" innovations directed at issues in industrial countries but also beneficial to food production in developing countries.

The preceding section shows that the resources directed at food crop production in developing countries are small, especially when compared with those directed at crops in the industrial world. Still, some important contributions should come from the resources being applied to developing countries. Training of scientists in developing countries under various programs means that there is a small cadre of plant molecular biologists in a number of developing countries. The Rockefeller Foundation's support for rice biotechnology should begin to pay off in two to five years in the form of new varieties available to some Asian farmers. In China varieties produced through anther culture, a form of biotechnology, are now being grown on thousands of hectares by farmers in rural areas near Shanghai. The speed with which varieties get into farmers' hands depends largely on national conditions—the closeness of

links between biotechnologists and plant breeders; the ability of scientists to identify the constraints and the genes that overcome them; the ability of scientists to get those genes into good crop varieties; and the success of plant scientists and others in crafting meaningful biosafety regulations.

It is likely that efforts to improve the rice yield in Asia through biotechnology will result in a production increase of 10 to 25 percent over the next ten years. The increase will come from improved hybrid rice systems in China; in other Asian countries it will come from rice varieties transformed with genes for resistance to pests and diseases. These transformed rice varieties will raise average yields by preventing crop damage, not by increasing yield potential. The reason is simple: few strategies are being pursued to directly raise yield potential because few strategies have been conceived. The use of hybrid rice is one exception. Potential ways to raise yield potential revolve around increasing "sink" size and "source" capacity. Adding to sink size involves increasing the number of grains or the average grain size; increasing source capacity means improving the capacity of the plant to fill these grains with carbohydrate. Both improvements are desired, but there are only a few investigators thinking about how biotechnology might help to achieve these improvements, especially in rice crops. While there is a community of scientists working to understand basic plant biochemistry, including photosynthesis, this work as yet offers no hints about which genes can be manipulated to advantage using the tools of molecular biology and genetic engineering.

Maize yields in developing countries may be affected by biotechnology if genes useful in tropical countries are discovered in the course of the great amount of research on maize under way in the United States. Although most of the maize research is being carried out by private firms, some discoveries may be made available for applications in developing countries either at no cost or at low enough cost to make them commercially feasible. Biotechnology applications beneficial to cassava are further in the future, as are those on the smallholder banana and other crops of importance in the developing world.

Herbicide resistance is potentially the simplest of traits to incorporate into a plant, because application of the herbicide is an ideal way to select a modified individual cell. A population of cells exposed to DNA that confers herbicide resistance can quickly be screened. A number of different herbicides are available, and there is a strong self-interest on the part of herbicide manufacturers to encourage farmers to use herbicides. Thus a number of pressures are at work to ensure that transgenic crops with herbicide resistance are produced. Given that weeds currently constrain crop yields in developing countries, crop yields may rise if herbicide use increases. In addition, proper regulatory activities may lead to increased use of herbicides that are less damaging to the environment (biodegradable herbicides, for example). In impoverished countries cash-poor farmers typically do not have access to such herbicides, especially the expensive ones such as glyphosphate, for which resistance is being engineered. Thus herbicide resistance may not benefit the average farmer in impoverished countries unless the cost of herbicides is reduced. It should be noted that prices are decreasing as patent protection is lost.

Prospects for incorporating pest and disease resistance into developing country crops are more favorable than prospects for increasing yields. Pest and insect problems are much simpler to address, and much of the effort in biotechnology is focused on these problems. Many of the genes that resolve insect and disease problems in temperate crops may also be effective in tropical crops. If they are, problems related to gaining access to the genes and transforming plants with them will remain, because most of the genes have associated intellectual property rights. In one case Monsanto made available to Mexico, without cost, the genes that confer resistance to important potato viruses and trained Mexican scientists in plant transformation and other skills needed to make use of the genes.. The transformed potatoes are now being field-tested in Mexico. Monsanto has also worked with USAID and KARI to develop and donate a similar virus control technology to Kenya and Indonesia for virus control in the sweet potato. These cases are, however, exceptional.

Drought is a major problem for nearly all crop plants, and the prospect of a "drought resistance gene" has excited many scientists. However, plant scientists recognize that many traits contribute to drought tolerance or resistance: long, thick roots; thick, waxy leaves; the ability to produce viable pollen when under drought stress; the ability to recover from a dry period; and others. Some of these traits can undoubtedly be controlled genetically, but little progress has been made thus far in identifying the genes that control them. Salt tolerance is often discussed along with drought tolerance because salt conditions and drought cause plants to react in similar ways. Unfortunately, some of the genes that confer drought tolerance may be useless for salty conditions and vice versa. Some early workers held that fusing cells of plants tolerant to drought with nontolerant plants would result in a useful combination, but that has not been demonstrated despite considerable effort.

The possibility of increasing the starch content of crops through genetic manipulation that modifies the biosynthetic pathways of the plant is enticing. Some success has been demonstrated in the case of the potato. This success holds out the hope that it may be possible to achieve the goal of a significant increase in production potential in the potato and other root and tuber crops such as cassava, yams, and sweet potatoes.[20]

Prospects for achieving this goal may depend on two factors: (1) the extent to which there are alternative metabolic routes to the same product and (2) the extent to which control of plant metabolism is shared among the component reactions of individual pathways.[21] "There may well be short pathways in plant metabolism where control is dominated by one or two steps, but the current evidence suggests that this is not so for the longer pathways. This conclusion has far-reaching effects on our ability to manipulate plant metabolism."[22]

Potential Applications to Environmental Problems

Genetic engineering holds out the possibility that plants can be designed to improve human welfare in ways other than by improving crop properties or yields. For example, a biodegradable plastic can be made from the bacterial storage product polyhydroxbutyrate, and the bacterial enzymes required to convert acetyl-CoA to polyhydroxbutyrate have been expressed in the model plant *Arabidopsis thaliana.* This accomplishment demonstrates the possibility of developing a plant that can accumulate appreciable amounts of polyhydroxbutyrate.[23] The optimization of such a process in a plant that will produce the substance in commercial quantities has not yet been achieved.

At present 80 percent of potato starch is chemically modified after harvest. If starch modification could be tailored in the plant, costs might be lower, and the waste disposal problems associated with chemical modification would be reduced.[24]

The observation that certain plants can grow in soils containing high levels of heavy metals such as nickel or zinc without apparent damage suggests the possibility of deliberately removing toxic substances using plants. Plants with the ability to remove such substances (hyperaccumulators) typically accumulate only a single element and grow slowly. In addition, most have not been cultivated, so their seeds and production techniques are poorly understood. One way around these limitations might be to genetically engineer crop plants to hyperaccumulate toxic substances. Some increased metal tolerance has been obtained in transgenic *Arabidopsis plants*.[25] The use of plants for decontamination of soil, water, and air is still at a early stage of research and development. "No soil has been successfully decontaminated yet by either phytoextraction or phytodegradation."[26]

Potential Applications to Human Health Problems

As a result of biotechnology, compounds that were previously available only in limited quantities or from exotic plant species or other organisms can now be produced in domesticated crops. It has already proved feasible to produce carbohydrates, fatty acids, high-value pharmaceutical polypeptides, industrial enzymes, and biodegradable plastics.[27] Production of proteins and peptides has been demonstrated, and it has been shown that plants have several potential advantages over microbial fermentation systems. Bacterial fermentation requires significant capital investment and often results in the production of insoluble aggregates of the desired material that require resolubization before use. Plant production of such proteins would avoid the capital investment and would in most cases produce soluble materials. However, the cost involved in extracting and purifying proteins from plants may be significant and may offset lower production costs, although the economics of purifying proteins from plant biomass has not been evaluated extensively.[28] This disadvantage can to some extent be offset by expressing the protein in the seed at a high level.[29]

Plants can potentially be used as the producers of edible vaccines. The hepatitis B surface antigen has been expressed in tobacco, and the feasibility of oral immunization using transgenic potatoes has been demonstrated.[30] The challenges involved in the design of specific vaccines include optimizing the expression of the antigenic proteins, stabilizing the expression of proteins in the post-harvest process, and enhancing the oral immunogenicity of some antigens.[31] There are even greater challenges to developing effective protocols for immunization.

Notes

1. R. G. Fray and D. Grierson, "Molecular Genetics of Tomato Fruit Ripening," *Trends in Genetics* 9 (1993): 438-43.

2. T. A. Voelker, and others, *Science* 257 (1992): 72-74; D.M. Strak, K. P. Timmerman, G. R Barry, J. Preiss, and G. M. Kishore, *Science* 258 (1992): 287-92.

3. F. J. Perlak and D. A. Fishoff, "Advanced Engineered Pesticides," in *Advanced Engineered Pesticides,* ed., Leo Kim (New York: Marcel Dekker, 1993),199-211.

4. F. J. Perlak and others, "Insect Resistant Cotton Plants," *Bio/Technology* 8 (1990): 939-43; see also www.aphis.usda.gov/bbep/bp, a U.S. Department of Agriculture site which provides biotechnology field test information.

5. D. M. Shah, C. M. T. Rommens, and R. N. Beachy, "Resistance to Diseases and Insects in Transgenic Plants: Progress and Applications to Agriculture," *Trends in Biotechnology* 13 (1995): 362-68.

6. Shah, Rommens, and Beachy, "Resistance to Diseases and Insects in Transgenic Plants: Progress and Applications to Agriculture."

7. W. Y. Song, G. L. Wang, and P. Ronald, "A Receptor Kinase-Like Protein Encoded by the Rice Disease Resistence Gene," *Science* 270 (1995): 1804-06.

8. M. E. Williams, "Genetic Engineering for Pollination Control," *Trends in Biotechnology* 13 (1995): 344-49.

9. S. Gan and R. M. Amasino, "Inhibition of Leaf Senescence by Autoregulated Production of Cytokinin," *Science* 270 (1995): 1986-88.

10. D. M. Stark, K. P. Timmerman, and G. F. Barry, "Regulation of the Amount of Starch in Plant Tissues by ADP Glucose Pyrophosphorylase," *Science 258* (1992):287-92.

11. 0. J. M. Goddijn and Jan Pen, "Plants as Bioreactors," *Trends in Biotechnology* 13 (1995): 379-87.

12. Y. Thonavala and others, in *Proceedings of the National Academy of Sciences,* USA 92 (1995): 3358-61.

13. L. P. Meredith Lloyd-Evans and Peter Barfoot, "EU Boasts Good Science Base and Economic Prospects for Crop Biotechnology," *Genetic Engineering News 16* (1996). For a description of field testing being carried on in the United States, see A. A. Snow and P. M. Palma, "Commercialization of Transgenic Plants: Potential Ecological Risks," *BioScience* 47 (February 1997): 86-96.

14. P. J. Dale, "R&D Regulation and Field Trailling of Transgenic Crops," *Trends in Biotechnology* 13 (1995): 398-403.

15. Dale, "R&D Regulation and Field Trailling of Transgenic Crops."

16. A. F. Krattinger, *Biosafety for Sustainable Agriculture* (Ithaca, N.Y.: Stockholm Environmental Institute and International Service for the Acquisition of Agri-Biotechnological Applications, 1994).

17. Office of the President, *Budget of the United States* (Washington, D.C.: U.S. Government Printing Office, 1992).

18. Carliene Brenner and John Komen, "International Initiatives in Biotechnology for Developing Country Agriculture: Promises and Problems," in *Organisation for Economic Co-operation and Development Technical Paper* 100 (Organisation for Economic Co-operation and Development Center, 1994).

19. Brenner and Komen, "International Initiatives in Biotechnology for Developing Country Agriculture: Promises and Problems."

20. Stark, Timmerman, and Barry, "Regulation of the Amount of Starch in Plant Tissues by ADP Glucose Pyrophosphorylase."

21. Tom ap Rees, "Prospects of Manipulating Plant Metabolism," *Trends in Biotechnology* 13 (1995): 375-78.

22. Brenner and Komen, "International Initiatives in Biotechnology for Developing Country Agriculture: Promises and Problems."

23. Y. Poirier, Y. Nawrath, and C. Somerville, "Production of Polyhydroxyalkanoates, A Family of Biodegradable Plastics and Elastomers, in Bacteria and Plants," *Bio/Technology* 13 (1995): 142-50.

24. Goddijn and Pen, 'Plants as Bioreactors.'

25. R. B. Meagher and others, *Abstract of the 14th Annual Symposium on Current Topics in Plant Biochemistry, Physiology, and Molecular Biology* (University of Missouri, 1995), 29-30.

26. Scott D. Cunningham, William R. Berti, and Jianwei W. Huang, "Phytoremediation of Contaminated Soils," *Trends in Biotechnology* 13 (1995): 393-97.

27. Goddijn and Pen, "Plants as Bioreactors."

28. Goddijn and Pen, "Plants as Bioreactors."

29. E. Krebbers and J. van de Kerckhove, "Production of Peptides in Plant Seeds," *Trends in Biotechnology* 8 (1990): 1-3.

30. T. A. Haq, H. S. Mason, and C. J. Arntzen, "Oral Immunization with a Recombinant Bacterial Antigen Produced in Transgenic Plants," *Science* 268 (1995): 714-16.

31. Hugh S. Mason and Charles J. Arntzen, "Transgenic Plants as Vaccine Production Systems," *Trends in Biotechnology* 3 (1995): 388-92.

CHAPTER 3

Possible Problems

All new technologies must be assessed in terms of benefits and costs. This section outlines a number of potential costs or problems that may be associated with developing and using the new tools of biotechnology in developing countries. Some of the problems associated with biotechnology for crop improvement are not new. Indeed, some of the problems that were faced thirty years ago during the Green Revolution must be addressed once again to safeguard the use of agricultural biotechnology. The new tools of biotechnology give us more power to make positive or negative impacts on the environment than was the case with conventional plant breeding, technologies used during the Green Revolution. Thus it is essential that we review critically the potential problems that have been raised by scientists and environmentalists.[1] Our intention here is to present a balanced review of current knowledge concerning risks and problems.

Gene Flow in Plants: Crops Becoming Weeds

In most groups of plants related species regularly form hybrids, and the transfer of genes between the differentiated populations that such hybridization makes possible is a regular source of enhancement for the populations involved. Thus all white oaks and all black oaks (the two major subdivisions of the genus, including all but a few of the North American species) are capable of forming fertile hybrids. Some of the species and distinct races that have evolved following such hybridization occupy wide ranges in nature and can be recognized as a result of their distinctive characteristics. The characteristics of corn, wheat, and many other crops were enhanced during the course of their evolution as a result of hybridization with related species or weedy or cultivated strains that were nearby; those related, infertile, and sometimes weedy strains have also been enhanced genetically, in some instances following hybridization with the cultivated crop to which they are related.

In view of these well-known principles, studied for well over fifty years, it is clear that any gene that exists in a cultivated crop or plant, irrespective of how it got there, can be transferred following hybridization to its wild or semidomesticated relatives. The transfer would occur selectively if the gene or genes being transferred enhanced the competitive abilities of the related strains, and the weedy properties of some kinds of plants might be enhanced in particular instances as a result of this process. If so, those new strains might need special attention in controlling such plants, just as the many thousands of weedy strains of various plants that have developed over the history of cultivation need control.

Because most crops, such as corn and cotton, are highly domesticated, it is unlikely that any single gene transfer would enable them to become pernicious weeds. Of greater concern is the potential for less domesticated, self-seeding crops (alfalfa, for example) and commercial tree varieties (pines, for example) to become problems. These plants already have the capacity to survive on their own, and transgenes could enhance their fitness in the wild. For example, a pine tree engineered for resistance to seed-feeding insects might gain a significant advantage through decreased seed destruction, potentially allowing it to outcompete other indigenous species. If this happened, forest communities could be disrupted.

Gene Flow in Plants: From Transgenic Crops to Wild Plants

Crop varieties are often capable of breeding with the wild species from which they were derived. When the two plant types occur in the same place, it is possible for transgenes, like other genes in the domesticated plant, to move into the wild plants. In some cases these crop relatives are serious weeds (wild rices and Johnson grass, for example). If a wild plant's fitness was enhanced by a transgene, or any other gene, that gave it protection from naturally occurring diseases or pests, the plant could become a worse pest, or it could shift the ecological balance in a natural plant community. Wild relatives of crops suffer from diseases and insect attack, but there are few studies that enable us to predict whether the development of resistance to pests in wild plants would result in significant ecological problems. Weeds often evolve resistance to diseases by natural evolutionary processes. However, in some cases, gene transfer from crops could speed up this process by hundreds of years.

Wild rices are especially important weeds in direct-seeded rice (direct seeding of rice is an agricultural practice that is becoming more widely used in Asia). It has been shown that genes are often naturally transferred between domesticated rice and weedy wild rices. If a herbicide tolerance gene was engineered into a rice cultivar, it would be possible to control the wild rice in commercial rice fields with the herbicide until the wild rice acquired the herbicide tolerance gene from the cultivar. Once the wild rice obtained this gene, the herbicide would become useless. The wild rice would not become a worse weed than it was before genetic engineering as a result of acquiring the herbicide tolerance gene. However, this natural gene transfer would make the investment in the engineering effort much

less sustainable. Therefore, it is important to consider such gene transfer before investing in specific biotechnology projects. Weeds can evolve resistance to some herbicides without gene transfer, but the process takes much longer. For example, herbicides such as glyphosate (Round-Up) from Monsanto are difficult for plants to resist with their normally inherited genes. (It should be noted, however, that the intensive use of glyphosate has led to weed resistance in Australia.)

Development of New Viruses from Virus-Containing Transgenic Crops

Viral diseases are extremely destructive to plant productivity, especially in the tropics. Consequently, the genetic modification of plants to resist viruses has been an important objective of conventional breeding. Over the past decade biotechnology has made possible the more rapid and precise production of individual strains resistant to particular viruses as a result of the ability to move particular genes into specific crop strains. One of the goals of genetic engineering has been to identify novel virus-resistant genes that can be rapidly transferred to many types of crops, thus easing the problems of the plant breeder and meeting the needs of the farmer. As has always been the case with such efforts, the major challenge is to find virus-resistant genes that cannot be overcome easily by the action of natural selection of the virus. Now, however, we have the potential to react more efficiently to this challenge than before.

One potential advantage of genetic engineering is that it may make possible the transfer of multiple genes for disease resistance that affect the disease organism by different mechanisms. In many cases such a transfer would make adaptation by the disease organism more difficult. Engineering multiple genes for disease resistance into crops requires advanced technical effort, and the benefits of such an effort will only be seen years after the varieties are commercialized. Therefore, it is important that genetic engineers be given a mandate to develop genes that will protect crops for extended periods of time.

Pathogen-Derived Resistance

To date the most widely applied genetic engineering technology for controlling plant viruses has been the use of genes derived from the plant viruses themselves. When transferred to plants, a set of genes called viral coat protein genes inhibit replication of the virus. (Other virus-derived genes can have a similar impact when they are transferred to plants in an appropriate manner.)

Transgenes encoding a variety of viral genes have been tested in transgenic plants over the past ten years with a range of effects. Plants that produce viral coat proteins have been tested the most widely, and some of these plants have received approval for commercial sale in the United States and China. In 1995 the U.S. Department of Agriculture proposed a rule that would substitute a notification requirement for the permit requirement now in effect for most field tests of selected genetically engineered crops. If this rule is formalized, researchers will only have to notify the department, not obtain a permit, before field-testing certain genetically engineered plants, including those that express viral coat protein genes. Some have found this proposed rule controversial.[2] The U.S. Environmental Protection Agency also ruled that coat proteins are not pesticidal and are safe for environmental release. The U.S. Food and Drug Administration has approved for sale and consumption foods derived from transgenic plants that contain viral coat proteins.

Concerns about Release of Plants Containing Genes Encoding Viral Sequences

As research and development of plants that exhibit pathogen-derived resistance moved from the lab to the field, several concerns were voiced about the release of plants that encode viral sequences, including the following:

- Virus proteins may trigger allergic reactions if included in foods. This concern has been largely abandoned, in part because many foods are infected with plant viruses and have been consumed for many years without known deleterious effects.

- Virus-resistant plants may have a competitive advantage in the field, and outcrossing with weed species may confer increased competition and weediness. As indicated above, we lack data on how important this problem can be.

- The presence of transgenic viral sequences in large crops would increase the likelihood of creating novel viruses because of recombination between the transgenes and other viruses that infect the plant. While it is known that many crops are simultaneously infected by multiple plant viruses, there are few examples of confirmed genetic recombination between different viruses. And, while there is evidence of recombination between like viruses or virus strains, there is no evidence that this recombination would occur with greater frequency in transgenic plants than in typical situations of virus infection. In conclusion there is little evidence for the contention that virus recombination will cause ecological problems.

- Virus coat proteins produced by transgenic crops could combine with natural viruses and produce more harmful strains. It has been concluded that while such an occurrence is theoretically possible, the risk of it is too low to be considered in assessing the impacts of transgenic crops.

- Virus genes other than coat protein genes could elicit greater safety concerns. Genes encoding ribonucleic acids (RNAS) that do not produce proteins yet provide resistance are likely to receive approval because there is no scientific expectation of risk. However, it is unclear whether or not other genes will receive approval. Viral genes that have the capacity to decrease infection by one virus but increase the chance of infection by another virus will probably not receive approval unless they are mutated and made to act only in a protective manner.

Effects of Plant-Produced Insecticides on Unintended Targets

In terms of plant-produced insecticides the only insecticidal compounds that are currently commercialized are proteins that are naturally produced by *Bacillus thuringiensis* (Bt). These proteins are highly specific in their toxic effects. One group of these proteins affects only certain species of caterpillars *(lepidoptera)*, while others affect only a restricted set of beetle species. None of these proteins has been shown to have a significantly disruptive effect on predators of pest species (beneficial insects). The proteins degrade rapidly when exposed to sunlight and have been shown to degrade even when protected by being inside crop residues. Monsanto presented data to the Environmental Protection Agency that confirm the safety of the protein. Studies with enzymes from the human digestive system indicated that these Bt proteins are quickly digested and are unlikely to cause harmful effects.

Ecosystem Damage

Unfortunately little is known about the flow of genetic information from plants to microorganisms, making it difficult to assess the risk of genes spreading from plants to soil organisms. It is a fact that soil organisms, especially bacteria, are able to take up DNA from their environment and that DNA can persist when bound to soil particles. Although one can speculate about a gene-flow situation in which plant DNA is released from plant material, bound to soil particles, and subsequently taken up by soil bacteria, such a scenario is highly unlikely. Any potential risks of such a transfer can be eliminated by making transgenes that bacteria are unable to use (those with introns, for example). It is even more speculative to consider the possible transfer of genes to soil-dwelling funguses (molds), since gene transfer to funguses is generally much more difficult than gene transfer to bacteria.

Assessing the Cost-Benefit Ratio of Genetically Engineered Crops

Two questions that must be addressed before investing in a project to engineer a crop cultivar are (1) will the gene being transferred serve an important function in the targeted geographical area and (2) how long will the gene continue to serve its function?

Will the Gene Being Transferred Serve an Important Function in the Targeted Geographical Area?

The pests of a specific crop, such as cotton or corn, vary from one geographical region to another. For example, the caterpillars of two insect species, the cotton bollworm and the budworm, are major pests to the cotton grown in the southern United States. A variety of cotton developed by Monsanto contains a specific protein derived from Bacillus thuringiensis that is highly toxic to these two closely related pests. In Central America the major insect pest species that affect cotton are the fall armyworm and the boll weevil. Since the toxins in the cotton developed by Monsanto have no impact on these pests, investing in the transfer of these seeds to Central America would be futile. Instead, it would be better to invest resources in finding more appropriate genes that would truly control Central American cotton pests.[3]

A number of companies have engineered corn varieties that tolerate herbicide sprays. At this point the commercial corn varieties that possess herbicide tolerance are developed by crossing a parent corn line that contains the transgene for herbicide resistance with another line that does not contain the gene. Therefore, all of the commercially sold corn seeds contain one copy of the herbicide-resistance gene and are resistant to the herbicide. In the United States farmers buy hybrid corn seed every year and plant it only once so that all of their plants are tolerant of the herbicide spray. While this system works well in the United States and other similar economies, it will not work well in agricultural settings in most developing countries unless changes are made. For example, in El Salvador many farmers buy hybrid corn seed only once every three years, because it is very expensive. The first year they plant the commercial seed, and the next two years they plant the offspring from the plants. Because of genetic segregation in the offspring, only three-quarters of the corn plants in the second and third year have the herbicide-resistance gene, so the farmer kills half of the crop by applying the herbicide. It has proven too difficult for seed companies to put the gene in both parents of the plant. Clearly, an agricultural plan that works in a developed country may not work in a developing country

It is often said that biotechnology is a transferable technology because "the technology is all in the seeds." It is important to recognize that the interface between seed traits and worldwide crop production is not always simple. As indicated above, sending herbicide-resistant corn seed to El Salvador without educating farmers about the problem of using the second generation seed could lead to immediate economic losses, and it could also lead to rejection of the new technology. Similarly, breeding a corn variety in the United States and then sending it to West Africa would be useless if the corn was resistant to U.S. pests but not to West African pests. It should be noted that corn pests are not even the same in all West African countries, so varieties must be developed by tailoring them to specific problems.

Once a variety is matched with local pest problems, the technology may be transferable simply by supplying the seed, although doing so does not mean that the seed will provide a sustainable solution to the pest problem. There is abundant evidence indicating that pests will overcome genes for pest and disease resistance, regardless of whether the genes have come through biotechnology or classical plant breeding, unless seeds are used properly. Getting farmers to use seeds properly will require educational efforts.

How Long Will the Gene Continue to Serve Its Function?

Insects, disease-causing organisms, and weeds are known to adapt to most pesticides and crop varieties that contain resistant genes. In some cases adaptation occurs within one or two years. Some insect strains have evolved the ability under laboratory and field conditions to tolerate high concentrations of the toxins derived from the *Bacillus thuringiensis* that are produced by transgenic cotton and corn sold commercially in the United States. Considerable theoretical and empirical research has assessed whether certain insect pests will overcome the effects of transgenic crops that produce these insecticidal proteins. If major crops, such as corn, cotton, and rice, that produce insecticidal proteins are planted intensively over wide areas, the chance for insect adaptation is high unless care is taken in developing and deploying the insect-resistant varieties.

The U.S. Environmental Protection Agency has put restrictions on the sale of cotton containing *Bacillus thuringiensis* to ensure that every U.S. farm has some fields planted with varieties that do not produce the Bt proteins. These restrictions are an example of the kinds of strategies that can be employed to "conserve resistance." The fields planted with non-Btproducing varieties act as refuges for individual pests that are susceptible. The insects produced in these refuges will mate with resistant insects emerging from fields where the transgenic varieties are planted, diluting the frequency of insects that are resistant to the Bt proteins and leading to more sustainable resistance. Instituting such practices in developing counties would probably be difficult. Furthermore, the refuge strategy works best if the transgenic variety produces enough Bt protein to kill close to 100 percent of the susceptible insects that feed on it. A variety developed to kill 100 percent of the pest individuals of a species that occurs in Mexican corn may kill only 80 percent of the insects in a Nigerian cornfield. Therefore, attempts to build one transgenic corn type to fit the needs of a number of countries may be misguided.

Adaptation problems similar to those described for insects may affect crops engineered for resistance to disease and tolerance of herbicides. Although there are some types of herbicides, such as glyphosate (Round-Up), that are considered "immune" to weed adaptation, it is not clear that this immunity will hold up when there is intensive use of the herbicides.[4]

When investing in biotechnology for crop protection, it is important to consider the global effectiveness of the protection and how long it will last. The same is true of agriculture in general. Improved strains of any kind of crop or domestic animal, regardless of how the genetic modification was attained, must be carefully managed to be as productive as possible. Integrated systems involving the best and most sustainable practices of soil preparation; the most conservative and appropriate use of water, fertilizers, and pesticides (if pesticides are used);

and the selection of the best and most appropriate strains of a particular crop are the key to success in agriculture. These practices are important to all agricultural systems, and they are necessary for improving systems, regardless of the exact methods used to genetically modify the crop strains being grown.

Investments in new and improved crop strains must also be judged by their global effectiveness, irrespective of how the strains were produced. The Green Revolution succeeded in enhancing productivity in many areas because of the system of cultivation that was built up around the new strains of crops, not solely because of the properties of those strains. The design of plantings has a great deal to do with the longevity of resistance to particular diseases and pests, but design has not always been carefully considered in efforts to introduce genetically engineered strains or other novel strains. The design of plantings may need special attention in developing countries with respect to the particular conditions found there.

As mentioned above, biotechnologies other than bioengineering can be used to improve agriculture in developing countries. But use of such technologies can also have drawbacks for developing countries. For example, tissue culture can be used to produce disease-free plants and to help increase the productivity of farms in developing countries. But tissue culture can also be used to shift the production center for specialty agricultural products from developing to industrial countries. Vanilla is typically considered a tropical product, but recent work with tissue culture allows its production in the laboratory. If such innovations in tissue culture proliferate, it is possible that other tropical products will be manufactured in the laboratory as well.

Notes

1. A. A. Snow and P. M. Palma, "Commercialization of Transgenic Plants: Potential Ecological Risks," *BioScience* 47 (February 1997).

2. Personal communication.

3. N. Strizhov and others, "A Synthetic cryIC Gene, Encoding a *Bacillus Thuringiensis* D-Endotoxin, Confers *Spodoptera* Resistance in Alfalfa and Tobacco," in *Proceedings of the National Academy of Sciences USA* (forthcoming).

4. J. Gressel, "Fewer Constraints Than Proclaimed to the Evolution of Glyphosate-Resistant Weeds," *Resistant Pest Management* 8 (1996): 2-5; B. Sindel, "Glyphosate Resistance Discovered in Annual Ryegrass," *Resistant Pest Management* 8 (1996): 5-6.

CHAPTER 4

Conclusions and Recommendations

The panel's recommendations to the World Bank are based on its members' belief that urgent priority must be assigned to the expansion of agriculture and to increased production of food in the developing world. It is critically important that increases in food production outpace population growth. Damaging agricultural practices must be replaced with lower-impact, sustainable activities so that the global capacity to produce food does not decline. Only by these means will it prove possible to lessen hunger and improve food security in the poorest nations in the years ahead.

Because transgenic technology is so powerful, it has the ability to make significant positive or negative changes in agriculture. Transgenic crops are not in principle more injurious to the environment than traditionally bred crops. This report has outlined a number of criteria that can be used to determine whether a specific biotechnology program is likely to enhance or detract from ecologically sound crop production. Transgenic crops that are developed and used wisely can be very helpful, and may prove essential, to world food production and agricultural sustainability. Biotechnology can certainly be an ally to those developing integrated pest management (IPM) and integrated crop management (ICM) systems.

The recommendations to the World Bank follow.

Support of Developing World Science

The Bank should direct attention to the need for liaison with and support of the developing world's agri-
cultural science community.

It is of the greatest importance to the development of sound agriculture, based on the best environmental principles, to enhance the capabilities of science and scientists in the developing world. A specific and urgent need is the training of developing world scientists in biotechnology methods so that each nation will have a cadre of scientists to assist it in setting and implementing its own policies on biotechnology research and biosafety.

The education of farmers can be greatly facilitated with the aid of scientists from their own nations. These scientists can contribute to the success of newly introduced crop strains and help to implement early warning systems to identify any troubles that arise during the introduction of new crops or new agricultural methods.

Research Programs

The Bank should identify and support high-quality research programs whose aim is to exploit the favorable potential of genetic engineering for improving the lot of the developing world.

As noted earlier in this report, not all of the research in progress in the industrial nations will, even if successful, prove beneficial to the developing world. Research should be planned so that key needs are met. Much of the necessary research will need to be done in advanced laboratories in industrial countries in conjunction with laboratories in developing countries. Research priorities should focus on promoting sustainable agriculture and higher yields in the developing world as well as on decreasing the variation in food production arising from, for example, environmental stresses.

Variance in production can result in food shortages with numerous attendant complications. Crops with resistance to insects and diseases, including crops developed by genetic modification, can decrease production variance if the crops are developed and deployed in ways that minimize the ability of pests and diseases to overcome the resistance factors in the crop. A poorly conceived strategy for developing and deploying crops can have the opposite effect if pests or diseases adapt to resistant cultivars. If farmers are taught to depend solely on a crop's ability to ward off pests and diseases, the farmers will not be prepared to use alternative means of control when pests become adapted to the resistance factors in the crop.

Surveillance and Regulation

The Bank should support the implementation of formal, national regulatory structures in its client nations by seeing to it that these structures retain their vigor and effectiveness through the years and by providing scientific and technical support to the client nations as requested.

Effective regulatory structures will prove critical should problems arise during the introduction of transgenic crops or, indeed, of other tools of industrialized agriculture, including chemical inputs, some of which may be promoted in conjunction with genetically engineered herbicide-tolerant crops. These tools can all pose problems for developing countries. Effective, comprehensive regulatory structures appear to exist in few nations, if any, including the United States. To provide the basis for a strong national regulatory structure, there must be a designated agency with a clear mandate to protect the environment and the economy from risks associated with the uncritical application of new methods, including inappropriate new strains of crops or animals that may pose special risks for the environment. The agency must have the technical capacity to develop competent risk assessment and the power to enforce its decisions.

The Bank should support, in each developing country, the deployment of an early warning system to identify any troubles that may arise and to introduce improvements in adapting new strains.

As an early warning system helped to identify troubles, it would also spot unexpected success, so that gains could be exploited and duplicated elsewhere. The system would also provide feedback to speed up and optimize the introduction of new plant varieties.

Investment in International Agricultural Research Centers

The Bank should increase its support of research in biotechnology and related areas at international agricultural research centers because these centers are in the best position to ensure that high-quality, environmentally sustainable agricultural products and processes are developed and transferred to developing countries.

International agricultural research centers are well placed to assist in the implementation of many of our recommendations. Investment in biotechnology research at these centers is marginally low. Although some of the centers have healthy but small programs in place, most of them lack the infrastructure and personnel needed to conduct high-quality biotechnology research. The Bank should determine how best to invest in infrastructure and personnel at each site. The Bank should adopt a broad perspective on biotechnology research that includes support for marker-assisted breeding, development of transgenic plants, development of molecular-based but farmer-friendly diagnostics, and genetic analysis of crop pests and pathogens. Research should emphasize development of agricultural products and processes that are unlikely to be provided by the private sector, such as those that would alleviate problems specific to subsistence farmers. Any increased investment in new agricultural technology must be accompanied by significant investment in ecological and sociological research to ensure that new products and processes support safe and sustainable food production.

In implementing Bank support for international agricultural research centers, two matters are important. The first is for the Bank to ensure that leaders of research organizations are aware of the potential and importance of supporting biotechnology research. The second is for the Bank to ensure that the recommendations—to focus on liaison and to identify and support high-quality research—are adopted in the implementation of a program of enhanced support for international agricultural research centers. Increases in funding for agricultural biotechnology should involve cooperation with scientists from developed countries, and any facilities that may be built at the centers should match the scientific capabilities that are to be maintained over the long term.

The Agricultural Challenge

The Bank should continue to give high priority to all aspects of increasing agricultural productivity in the developing world while encouraging the necessary transition to sustainable methods.

While genetically engineered crops can play an important role in meeting the goal of improved food security, their contribution alone will not suffice. Their use must be accompanied by numerous other actions, as we have noted in preceding sections of this report. These actions include:

- Increasing priority on conventional plant breeding and farming practices

- Ensuring that adequate energy and water become available and that procedures for their efficient use are made known and adopted
- Ensuring the introduction of modern means of controlling pests, including the use of integrated pest management systems, safe chemicals, and resistant crops
- Supporting the transition to sustainable activities and the reduction of waste and loss in all elements of the agriculture enterprise
- Providing the necessary education to farmers so that they can implement the array of new techniques that are needed (integrated pest management, for example)
- Ensuring that the changes in agriculture will provide the employment opportunities that will be needed in the developing world.

The scale and importance of the challenge that the Bank faces in the agricultural sector are formidable. We have concluded that the Bank should establish a permanent technical and scientific advisory group to deal broadly with the goal of improving food security while ensuring the transition to sustainable agricultural practices. The group should deal with all the elements that comprise a successful program and provide the required liaison to the scientific communities in the target nations.

APPENDIX

Integrated Intensive Farming Systems

Intensive Farming

China and India, as well as numerous other developing nations, must achieve the triple goals of more food, more income, and more livelihoods from their land and water resources. One approach that can be adopted is the integrated intensive farming systems methodology (IIFS).

The M. S. Swaminathan Research Foundation has designed a bio-village program to convert IIFS from a concept into a field-level reality. By making living organisms both the agents and beneficiaries of development, the bio-village serves as a model for human-centered development. The pillars of the IIFS methodology follow.

Soil Health Care

Soil health care is fundamental to sustainable intensification of agriculture. The IIFS approach affords the opportunity to include stem-nodulating legumes such as *Sesbania rostrata* in the farming system and to incorporate *Azolla*, or blue-green algae, and other sources of symbiotic and nonsymbiotic nitrogen fixation. Vermiculture constitutes an essential component of IIFS. IIFS farmers maintain a soil health card to monitor the impact of farming systems on the physical, chemical, and microbiological components of soil fertility.

Water Harvesting, Conservation, and Management

IIFS farm families include in their agronomic practices measures to harvest and conserve rainwater so that it can be used in conjunction with other sources of water. Where water is the major constraint, technologies that can help to optimize income and jobs from every liter of water must be chosen and adopted. Maximum emphasis should be placed on efficient on-farm water use and on the use of techniques such as drip irrigation to help optimize the benefits from the available water.

Crop and Pest Management

Integrated nutrient supply (INS) and integrated pest management (IPM) systems form important components of IIFS. The precise composition of the INS and the IPM systems should be chosen on the basis of the farming system and the agro-ecological and soil conditions of the area. Computer-aided extension systems should be developed to provide farm families with timely and precise information on all aspects of land, water, pest, and postharvest management.

Energy Management

Energy is an important and essential input. In addition to the energy-efficient systems of land, water, and pest management described above, every effort should be made to harness biogas, biomass, solar, and wind energies to the maximum extent possible. Solar and wind energy can be used in hybrid combinations with biogas for farm activities such as pumping water and drying grains and other agricultural produce.

Postharvest Management

IIFS farmers should not only adopt the best available threshing, storage, and processing measures, but should also try to produce value-added products from every part of the plant or animal. Postharvest technology assumes particular importance in the case of perishable commodities such as fruits, vegetables, milk, meat, eggs, fish, and other animal products. A mismatch between production and postharvest technologies adversely affects both producers and consumers. As this report has noted, growing urbanization leads to a diversification of food habits. This diversification will increase demand for animal products and processed food. Agro-processing industries can be promoted on the basis of an assessment of consumer demand. Such food-processing industries should be promoted in villages in order to increase employment opportunities for rural youth.

Investment in sanitary and phyto-sanitary measures is important to providing quality food for domestic consumers and for export. To assist the spread of IIFS, governments should make major investments in storage facilities, roads, communication, and sanitary and phyto-sanitary measures.

Choice of Crops and Other Components of the Farming System

In IIFS it is important to give careful consideration to the composition of the farming system. Soil conditions, water availability, agro- climatic features, home needs, and above all, marketing opportunities have to determine the choice of crops, farm animals, and aquaculture systems. Small and large ruminants have a particular advantage among farm animals since they can live largely on crop biomass. IIFS farming has to be based on both land-saving agriculture and grain-saving animal husbandry.

Information, Skills, Organization, and Management

To succeed, IIFS farms need a meaningful and effective information and skill empowerment system. Decentralized production systems have to be supported by a few key centralized services, such as the supply of seeds, biopesticides, and diagnostic and control methods for plant and animal diseases. Ideally, an "information shop" should be set up by trained local youth in order to give farm families timely information on meteorological, management, and marketing factors. Organization and management are key elements to success, and depending on the area and farming system, steps have to be taken to provide to small producers advantages of scale in processing and marketing. IIFS farming is best developed through participatory research between scientists and farm families. This approach helps to ensure economic viability, environmental sustainability, and social and gender equity in IIFS villages. The starting point is to learn from families who have already developed successful IIFS procedures.

It should be emphasized that IIFS will succeed only if centered on humans; a mere technology-driven program will not work. The essence of IIFS is the symbiotic partnership between farming families and their natural resource endowments of land, water, forests, flora, fauna, and sunlight. Without appropriate public policy support in areas such as land reform, security of tenure, rural infrastructure, input and output pricing and marketing, small farm families will find it difficult to adopt IIFS.

The eco-technologies and public policy measures needed to make IIFS a mass movement should receive concurrent attention. The program will fail if it is based solely on a technological quick-fix approach. On the other hand the HFS program can trigger an "ever-green revolution" if mutually reinforcing packages of technology, training, techno-infrastructure, and trade are introduced.

Appendix A
Program

Biotechnology and Biosafety
An Associated Event of the Fifth World Bank Conference
on Environmentally and Socially Sustainable Development

Held at the World Bank, Washington, D.C.
October 9–10, 1997

SESSION I: Setting the Stage
     Chair: Thomas E. Lovejoy, The Smithsonian Institution
     Introductory Remarks and Stating the Problem
         Ismail Serageldin, World Bank Group
     The Scientific Scene
         Werner Arber, International Council of Scientific Unions
     The Special Case of Agricultural and Food Biotechnology
         Henry W. Kendall, Union of Concerned Scientists
     Discussion

SESSION II: The Promise and the Perils
     Chair: Roger N. Beachy, Scripps Research Institute
     Overview
         Christopher R. Somerville, Carnegie Institution of Washington
     The Opportunities and the Risks
         Robert B. Horsch, Monsanto Company
         Miguel A. Altieri, University of California at Berkeley
     Discussion
     Regulatory Framework Issues
         Chair: Hamdallah Zedan, United Nations Environment Programme
         Desmond Mahon, Convention on Biological Diversity
         Timothy Roberts, Roberts and Company
     Discussion

SESSION III: Reviewing the Evidence
     Chair: Michel Petit, World Bank Group
     Panel 1: *Are the Opportunities of Genetically Modified Organisms Being Fully Exploited?*
         George Tzotzos, UNIDO
     Discussants: Gabrielle Persley, AusBiotech Alliance
              Carlienne Brenner, Consultant, Science, Agriculture and Technology

Panel 2: *Are the Risks of Developing and Releasing Genetically Modified Organisms Being Adequately Evaluated and Assessed?*
Rita R. Colwell, Biotechnology Institute, University of Maryland
Discussants: L. Val Giddings, Biotechnology Industry Organization
Rebecca Goldburg, Environmental Defense Fund
Discussion

SESSION IV: Role of International Agricultural Research
Chair: Louise O. Fresco, FAO
The Consultative Group on International Agricultural Research
Timothy G. Reeves, CIMMYT
The Global Forum
Fernando Osorio Chaparro, COLCIENCIAS
Perspectives from National Agricultural Research Systems
Maria José A. Sampaio, EMBRAPA
Magdy Madkour, AGERI
Discussion

SESSION V: Role of Public Policy
Chair: Per Pinstrup-Andersen, IFPRI
Vernon W. Ruttan, University of Minnesota
Michel Dron, CIRAD
George A. Lloyd, Zambian Grain Growers and Marketing Association
Discussion

SESSION VI: Recommendations for Action
Chair: Alexander F. McCalla, World Bank Group
Synopsis of Sessions
Wanda Collins, CGIAR
Discussion
Wrap-up and Next Steps
Ismail Serageldin

Appendix B
Presenters and Chairs

Miguel A. Altieri
SANE General Coordinator
University of California, Berkeley
College of Natural Resources
Center for Biological Control
1050 San Pablo Avenue
Albany, CA 94706, USA
Tel: 510/642-9802
Fax: 510/642-0875
Email: agroeco3@nature.berkeley.edu

Werner Arber
President
International Council of Scientific Unions
c/o Biocentre
University of Basel
Basel CH-4056, Switzerland
Tel: 41-61/267-2130
Fax: 41-61/267-2118

Roger N. Beachy
Head, Division of Plant Biology, BCC 206
The Scripps Research Institute
10550 No. Torrey Pines Road
La Jolla, CA 92037, USA
Tel: 619/784-2550
Fax: 619/784-2994
Email: beachy@scripps.edu

Carlienne Brenner
4, Allé du Bord de l'eau
Paris 75016, France
Tel: 33-1/4651-9700
Fax: 33-1/4651-9700
Email: brenner@oecd.fr

Fernando Osorio Chaparro
Director General
COLCIENCIAS
Transversel 9A, No. 133-28
Apartado Aéreo 051580
Santafé de Bogotá, DC, Colombia
Tel: 571/216-9800
Fax: 571/625-1788
Email: info@colciencias.gov.co

Wanda Collins
Deputy Director General for Research
International Potato Center
Apartado 1558
Lima 12, Peru
Tel: 51-1/349-5779
Fax: 51-1/349-5638
Email: W.Collins@cgnet.com

Rita R. Colwell
President
University of Maryland Biotechnology Institute
4321 Hartwick Road, Room 550
College Park, MD 20740, USA
Tel: 301/403-0501
Fax: 301/454-8123
Email: colwell@umbi.umd.edu

Michel Dron
Centre de Coopération Internationale en
   Recherche Agronomique pour le
   Développement (CIRAD)
42, rue Scheffer
Paris 75116, France
Tel: 33-1/53-70-2035
Fax: 33-1/5370-2133
Email: mdron@cirad.fr

Louise O. Fresco
Director
Research, Extension, and Training Division (SDR)
Food and Agriculture Organization
Sustainable Development Department
Viale delle Terme di Caracalla, D-446/7
Rome 00100, Italy
Tel: 39-6/5705-3363
Fax: 39-6/5705-5246
Email: louise.fresco@fao.org

L. Val Giddings
Vice President for Food and Agriculture
Biotechnology Industry Organization (BIO)
1625 K Street, NW, Suite 1100
Washington, DC 20006-1604, USA
Tel: 202/857-0244
Fax: 202/857-0237
Email: lvg@bio.org

Rebecca Goldburg
Biologist
Environmental Defense Fund
257 Park Avenue South
New York, NY 10010, USA
Tel: 212/505-2100
Fax: 212/505-2375

Robert B. Horsch
Director of Technology, General Manager
Monsanto Company
8520 University Green
Middletown, WI 53562, USA
Tel: 608/836-7300
Fax: 608/836-9710
Email: robert.b.horsch@monsanto.com

Henry W. Kendall
Chairman of the Board
Union of Concerned Scientists
c/o 24-514 MIT
Cambridge, MA 0139, USA
Tel: 617/253-7584
Fax: 617/253-1755
Email: hkendall@mit.edu

George A. Lloyd
Chairman
Zambian Grain Growers and Marketing
   Association
PO Box 50960, 8537 Mwembeshi Road
Heavy Industrial Area
Lusaka, Zambia
Tel: 260-1/286-619
Fax: 260-1/291-717, 254-283
-or-
33 Lime Gardens
West End
Southampton SO30 3RG, United Kingdom
Tel: 44-1703/471-748
Fax: 44-1703/471-748

Thomas E. Lovejoy
Counselor to the Secretary for Biodiversity
   and Environmental Affairs
The Smithsonian Institution
1000 Jefferson Drive, SW, Suite 317
Washington, DC 20560, USA
Tel: 202/786-2263
Fax: 202/786-2304

Magdy Madkour
AGERI
Agricultural Research Center
9 Gamaa Street
Giza 12619, Egypt
Tel: 20-2/
Fax: 20-2/568-9519
Email: madkour@ageri.sci.eg

Desmond Mahon
Senior Program Officer
Convention on Biological Diversity
World Trade Center
393 St. Jacques, Suite 300
Montréal, Québec H2Y 1N9, Canada
Tel: 514/287-7023
Fax: 514/288-6588
Email: desmond.mahon@biodiv.org

Peter J. Matlon
Chief, Food Security and Agriculture Programme
Sustainable Energy and Environment Division
United Nations Development Programme
304 E. 45th Street, 10th Floor
New York, NY 10017, USA
Tel: 212/906-6408
Fax: 212/906-6973
Email: peter.matlon@undp.org

Alexander F. McCalla
Director
Rural Development
World Bank Group
1818 H Street, NW, Room S 8-055
Washington, DC 20433, USA
Tel: 202/458-5028
Fax: 202/522-3207
Email: amccalla@worldbank.org

Gabrielle Persley
National Manager, Biotechnology
Australian Trade Commission
Level 13, 145 Eagle Street
GPO Box 1061
Brisbane, Qld 4000, Australia
Tel: 61-7/3365-4939
Fax: 61-7/3365-7093
Email: g.persley@mailbox.uq.edu.au

Michel Petit
Director
Agricultural Research Group (ESDAR)
Rural Development
World Bank Group
1818 H Street, NW, Room MC 4-113
Washington, DC 20433, USA
Tel: 202/473-0340
Fax: 202/522-3246
Email: mpetit@worldbank.org

Per Pinstrup-Andersen
Director General
International Food Policy Research Institute
1200 17th Street, NW, Suite 200
Washington, DC 20036-3006, USA
Tel: 202/862-5600
Fax: 202/467-4439
Email: P.Pinstrup-Andersen@cgnet.com

Timothy G. Reeves
Director General
CIMMYT
Lisboa 27, Apartado Postal 6-641
Mexico, D.F. 06600, Mexico
Tel: 52-5/726-9091
Fax: 52-5/726-7585
Email: username@alphac.cimmyt.mx

Timothy W. Roberts
Roberts and Co.
13, Spring Meadow
Bracknell
Berks RGR 2JP, United Kingdom
Tel: 44-1344/422-902
Fax: 44-1344/869-059
Email: twr@compuserve.com

Vernon W. Ruttan
Regents Professor
Applied Economics Department
University of Minnesota
332 C Classroom Office Building
2381 Commonwealth Avenue
St. Paul, MN 55108, USA
Tel: 612/625-4701, 2729, 6245
Fax: 612/625-1222

Maria José Amstalden Sampaio
EMBRAPA
Department of Research and Development
SAIN - Parque Rural - Final AV.
W/3 Norte - Ed. Sede, PO Box 04.0315
Brasilia - DF CEP70770-901, Brazil
Tel: 55-61/348-4433
Fax: 55-61/347-1041

Ismail Serageldin
Vice President
Special Programs
World Bank Group
1818 H Street, NW, Room MC 4-123
Washington, DC 20433, USA
Tel: 202/473-4502
Fax: 202/473-3112
Email: iserageldin@worldbank.org

Christopher R. Somerville
Director
Carnegie Institution of Washington
290 Panama Street
Stanford, CA 94305-4102, USA
Tel: 650/325-1521, x203
Fax: 650/325-6857
Email: CRS@andrew.stanford.edu

George Tzotzos
Biotechnology Programme Coordinator, ITPD/TS
United Nations Industrial Development
    Organization
PO Box 300 A-1400
Vienna, Austria
Tel: 43-1/21131-4336
Fax: 43-1/21131-6810
Email: george@binas.unido.org

Hamdallah Zedan
United Nations Environment Programme
Chief, Biodiversity Unit
PO Box 30552
Nairobi, Kenya
Tel: 254-2/623-260
Fax: 254-2/624-300 or 226-890

Appendix C

Cosponsors

American Association for the Advancement of Science (AAAS)
Rita R. Colwell
President
University of Maryland Biotechnology Institute
4321 Hartwick Road, Room 550
College Park, MD 20740
Tel: 301/403-0501
Fax: 301/454-8123
Email: colwell@umbi.umd.edu

The Conservation Fund
Lawrence A. Selzer
Vice President, Sustainable Programs
The Conservation Fund
PO Box 1746
Sheperdstown, WV 25443
Tel: 304/876-2815
Fax: 304/876-0739

Consultative Group on International Agricultural Research (CGIAR)
Alexander von der Osten
Executive Secretary
Consultative Group on International
Agricultural Research
1818 H Street, NW, J 4-073
Washington, DC 20433
Tel: 202/473-8918
Fax: 202/473-8110
Email: avonderosten@worldbank.org

Food and Agriculture Organization of the United Nations (FAO)
Louise O. Fresco
Director, Research, Extension, and Training Division (SDR)
Food and Agriculture Organization
Sustainable Development Department
Viale delle Terme di Caracalla, D-446/7
Rome 00100, Italy
Tel: 39-6/5705-3363
Fax: 39-6/5705-5246
Email: louise.fresco@fao.org

International Council of Scientific Unions (ICSU)
ICSU Secretariat
51 Boulevard de Montmorency
75016 Paris, France
Tel: 33-1/4525-0329
Fax: 33-1/4288-9431
Email: icsu@lmcp.jussieu.fr
http://www.lmcp.jussieu.fr/icsu/

The Smithsonian Institution
Thomas E. Lovejoy
Counselor to the Secretary for Biodiv. &
Environmental Affairs
Smithsonian Institution
1000 Jefferson Drive, SW
Suite 317
Washington, D.C. 20560
Tel: 202/786-2263
Fax: 202/786-2304

Third World Academy of Sciences (TWAS)
M.H.A. Hassan, Executive Director
Third World Academy of Sciences
c/o International Centre for Theoretical Physics
Strada Costiera 11
P.O. Box 586
34100 Trieste, Italy
Tel: 39-40/224-0327
Fax: 39-40/224-559
Email: twas@ictp.trieste.it

Union of Concerned Scientists (UCS)
Henry W. Kendall
Chairman of the Board
Union of Concerned Scientists
c/o 24-514 MIT
Cambridge, MA 0139
Tel: 617/253-7584
Fax: 617/253-1755
Email: hkendall@mit.edu

United Nations Development Programme (UNDP)
Peter J. Matlon
Chief, Food Security and Agriculture
Programme
Sustainable Energy and Environment Division,
UNDP
304 E. 45th Street, 10th Floor
New York, NY 10017
Tel: 212/906-6408
Fax: 212/906-6973
Email: peter.matlon@undp.org

United Nations Educational, Scientific and Cultural Organisation (UNESCO)
Professor Indra K. Vasil
Chairman
Laboratory of Plant, Cell,and Molecular
Biology
University of Florida
PO Box 110690, Bldg. 885
Gainesville, FL 32605-3498
Tel: 352/392-1193
Fax: 352/392-9366
Email: ikv@gnv.ifas.ufl.edu

United Nations Environment Programme (UNEP)
Hamdallah Zedan
United Nations Environment Programme
Biodiversity Unit
PO Box 30552
Nairobi, Kenya
Tel: 254-2/623-260
Fax: 254-2/624-300 or 226-890

United Nations Industrial Development Organization (UNIDO)
George Tzotzos
Biotechnology Programme Coordinator,
ITPD/TS
United Nations Industrial Development
Organization
PO Box 300 A-1400
Vienna, Austria
Tel: 43-1/21131-4336
Fax: 43-1/21131-6810
Email: george@binas.unido.org

U.S. National Academy of Sciences (NAS)
2100 C Street, NW
Washington, DC 20418
Tel: 202/334-2000
http://www.nas.edu/

World Bank Group
Ismail Serageldin
Vice President for Special Programs
World Bank Group
1818 H Street, NW, MC 4-123
Washington, D.C. 20433
Tel: 202/473-4502
Fax: 202/473-3112
Email: iserageldin@worldbank.org

The World Conservation Union (IUCN)
David McDowell, Director General
28 Rue Mauverney, 1196 Gland
Switzerland
Tel: 41-22/999-0001
Fax: 41-22/999-0002
Email: mail@hq.iucn.org
http://www.iucn.org

Appendix D
Consultative Group on International Agricultural Research Secretariat and Centers

Consultative Group on International Agricultural Research

Chair: Ismail Serageldin
Vice President Special Programs
The World Bank
1818 H Street, NW
Washington, DC 20433, USA
    Phone: (1-202) 473-4502
    Cable: INTBAFRAD
    Fax: (1-202) 473-3112

CGIAR Secretariat

Executive Secretary: Alexander von der Osten
701 18th Street, NW
Room J-4073
Washington, DC 20433, USA
    Phone: (1-202) 473-8918/8919
    E-mail: avonderosten@worldbank.org
              a.von-der-osten@cgnet.com

Secretariat:
    Phone: (1-202) 477-1234 (IBRD Operator)
              (1-202) 473-8951 (Secretariat)
    Fax: (1-202) 473-8110
    E-mail: cgiar@cgnet.com
    Website: http://www.cgiar.org

Mailing Address:
The World Bank
CGIAR Secretariat
1818 H Street, NW
Washington, DC 20433, USA

Science Advisor: Manuel Lantin
    Phone: (1-202) 473-8912
    E-mail: m.lantin@cgnet.com

Finance Team: Ravi Tadvalkar
    Phone: (1-202) 473-8894
    E-mail: r.tadvalkar@cgnet.com

Information Team: Shirley Geer
    Phone: (1-202) 473-8930
    E-mail: sgeer@worldbank.org

Management Team: Selçuk Özgediz
    Phone: (1-202) 473-8937
    E-mail: s.ozgediz@cgnet.com

Documents/Information Center: Danielle Lucca
    Phone: (1-202) 473-8949
    E-mail: dlucca@worldbank.org

Public Awareness Campaign for Agriculture

Director of Operations: Barbara Alison Rose
701 18th Street, NW
Room J-4029
Washington, DC 20433, USA
    Phone: (1-202) 473-4734
    Fax: (1-202) 473-8110
    E-mail: brose@worldbank.org
              b.rose@cgnet.com

Mailing Address:
Public Awareness Campaign for Agriculture
The World Bank
1818 H Street NW
Room J-4029
Washington, DC 20433, USA

Projects Assistant: Geralynn Batista
    Phone: (1-202) 473-3553
    E-mail: gbatista@worldbank.org
                 g.batista@cgnet.com

CGIAR Centers

CIAT

Centro Internacional de Agricultura Tropical
Apartado Aereo 6713
Cali, Colombia
    Phone: (57-2) 445-0000 (CIAT Headquarters)
                 (1-415) 833-6625 (USA direct)
    Fax: (57-2) 445-0073 (CIAT Headquarters)
                 (1-415) 833-6626 (USA direct)
    E-mail: ciat@cgnet.com
    Internet: http://www.ciat.cgiar.org

Chair: Robert D. Havener
2859 Stadium Drive
Solvang, California 93463, USA
    Phone: (1-805) 688 3204
    Fax: (1-805) 688 4574
    E-mail: R.Havener@cgnet.com

Director General: Grant M. Scobie
    Phone: (57-2) 445 0027
    Fax: (57-2) 445 0099
    E-mail: g.scobie@cgnet.com

Information Officer: Nathan Russell
    E-mail: n.russell@cgnet.com

Librarian: Elizabeth Goldberg
    E-mail: ciat-library@cgnet.com

Regional Offices:

Brazil (Cassava)
EMBRAPA
Centro Nacional de Pesquisa de Mandioca
    e Fruticultura Tropical (CNPMF)
Caixa Postal 007
CEP 44380-000 Cruz das Almas-BA, Brazil
    Phone: (55-75) 7212534
    Fax: (55-75) 7212534
    E-mail: ospina@cnpmf.embrapa.br

Ecuador (Beans Andean Project/PROFRIZA)
MAG/INIAP/CIAT
Avn. Eloy Alfaro y Amazonas
Edificio MAG Piso 4
Quito, Ecuador
    Phone: (593-2) 567-645 (INIAP)
    Phone: (593-2) 524-238 (IICA)
    Fax: (593-2) 500-316

Guatemala (Beans)
Regional Network for Beans in Central
America (PROFRIJOL)
Apartado Postal 231-A
IICA Office
Primera Avenida 8-00
Zona 9
Guatemala, Guatemala, C.A.
    Phone: (502) 3610925
    Fax: (502) 3316304
        E-mail: profrijol@guate.net

Honduras (Hillsides)
IICA/CIAT
Apartado Aéreo 410
Edificio Palmira, 2 piso
Frente Hotel Honduras Maya
Tegucigalpa, Honduras
    Phone: (504) 321-862
    Fax: (504) 391-443
    E-mail: ciathill@hondutel.hn

Malawi (Beans)
CIAT-Malawi
Chitedze Research Station
P.O. Box 158
Lilongwe, Malawi
   Phone: (265) 822-851
   Fax: (265) 782-835
   E-mail: v.aggarwal@cgnet.com

Nicaragua (Hillsides)
CIAT-Nicaragua
Apdo. Postal LM-172
Managua, Nicaragua
   Phone: (505-2) 663010/667328/669155
   Fax: (505-2) 784089
   E-mail: r.vernooy@cgnet.com

Philippines (Tropical Forages)
Forage for Smallholder Project
AUSAID/CIAT/CSIRO
IRRI/CIAT
Los Baños, Laguna
c/o P.O. Box 933
1099 Manila, The Philippines
   Phone: (63-2) 818-1926 or 844-3351
   Fax: (63-2) 891-1292 or 817-8470
   E-mail: w.stur@cgnet.com

Tanzania (Beans)
SADCC/CIAT Regional Program on Beans
   in Southern Africa
Selian Agricultural Research Institute
P.O. Box 2704
Arusha, Tanzania
   Phone: (255-57) 2268
   Fax: (255-57) 8558/8264
   E-mail: ciat-tanzania@cgnet.com

Thailand (Cassava)
CIAT Regional Office for Asia
Field Crops Research Institute
Department of Agriculture
Chatuchak, Bangkok 10900 Thailand
   Phone: (66-2) 579-7551
   Fax: (66-2) 940-5541
   E-mail: ciat-bangkok@cgnet.com

Uganda (Beans)
Regional Program on Beans in Eastern Africa
Kawanda Agricultural Research Institute
P.O. Box 6247
Kampala, Uganda
   Phone: (256-41) 567-670
   Fax: (256-41) 567-635
   E-mail: ciat-uganda@imul.com

CIFOR

Center for International Forestry Research
Jalan CIFOR
Situ Gede, Sindangbarang
Bogor Barat 16680, Indonesia

Mailing Address:
P.O. Box 6596 JKPWB
Jakarta 10065, Indonesia
   Phone: (62-251) 622 622 (operator)
   Phone: (62-251) 622 070 (direct extension)
   Fax: (62-251) 622 100
   E-mail: cifor@cgnet.com
   Internet: http://www.cgiar.org/cifor

Chair: Gill Shepherd
Research Fellow
Overseas Development Institute
Forestry Research Programme
Portland House, Stag Place
London SW1E 5DP, United Kingdom
   Phone: (44-171) 393-1600
   Fax: (44-171) 393-1699
   E-mail: g.shepherd@odi.org.uk

Director General: Jeffrey Sayer
   E-mail: j.sayer@cgnet.com

Director of Information Services: Michael Ibach
   E-mail: m.ibach@cgnet.com

Director of Communications: Sharmini Blok
   E-mail: s.blok@cgnet.com

Librarian: Yuni Soeripto
   E-mail: y.soeripto@cgnet.com

CIMMYT

Centro Internacional de Mejoramiento de Maiz
  y Trigo
Lisboa 27
Apartado Postal 6-641
06600 Mexico, D.F. Mexico
  Phone: (52-5) 726-9091
  Telex: 1772023 CIMTME
  Fax: INTL (52-595) 54425
  E-mail: cimmyt@cimmyt.mx
            cimmyt@cgnet.com
            username@cimmyt.mx
  Internet: http://www.cimmyt.mx

Chair: Wally Falcon
Director, Institute for International Studies
Stanford University
200 Encina Hall
Stanford, CA 94305-6055, USA
  Phone: (415) 725 1496
  Telex: 372871 Stanuniv
  Fax: (415) 725 2592
  E-mail: Wally.falcon@forsythe.stanford.edu

Director General: Timothy Reeves
  Fax: (52-5) 726-7585
  E-mail: treeves@cimmyt.mx

Director of External Relations: Tiffin D. Harris
  Fax: (52-5) 726-7536
  E-mail: tharris@cimmyt.mx

Library, Head: Corinne de Gracia
  E-mail: cdgracia@cimmyt.mx

Publications, Head: Kelly Cassaday
  E-mail: kcassaday@cimmyt.mx

Regional Offices:

Bangladesh
CIMMYT
P.O. Box 6057, Gulshan
Dhaka-1212, Bangladesh
  Phone: (880-2) 89 30 64
  Fax: (880-2) 88 35 16
  E-mail: cm@cimmyt.bdmail.net

Bolivia
CIMMYT
c/o ANAPO
Casilla 2305
Santa Cruz, Bolivia
  Phone: (591-3) 423011/423030
  Fax: (591-3) 427194
  E-mail: cimmyt@mitai.nrs.bolnet.bo

Colombia
CIMMYT
c/o CIAT
Apartado Aereo 67-13
Cali, Colombia
  Phone: (57-2) 4450-025
            (57-2) 4450-495
  Fax: (57-2) 4450 025
  E-mail: cdeleon@cgnet.com

Costa Rica
CIMMYT
Apartado 55
2200 Coronado
San Jose, Costa Rica
  Phone: (506-2) 292457
  Fax: (506-2) 292457
  E-Mail: gsain@iica.ac.cr

Ethiopia
CIMMYT
P.O. Box 5689
Addis Ababa, Ethiopia
  Phone: (252-1) 613215/615017
  Fax: (252-1) 611 892
  E-Mail: cimmyt-ethiopia@cgnet.com

Guatemala
CIMMYT
12 Calle 1-25 Zona 10
Edificio Geminis
Torre Norte, 16 Nivel, Of. 1606
Apartado Postal 231-A
Guatemala, Guatemala
  Phone: (502) 335 3418
            (502) 335 3428
  Fax: (502) 335 3407
  E-mail: cimmyt@ns.guate.net

Honduras
CIMMYT
CIAT-Laderas
c/o IICA-Honduras
Apdo. Postal 1410
Tegucigalpa, DC 11101 Honduras
  Phone: (504) 321862/322502
  Fax: (504) 315472
  E-mail: "ciathill@hondutel.hn"

Kenya
CIMMYT
P.O. Box 25171
Nairobi, Kenya
  Phone: (254-2) 632054/632206/
           630165
  Fax: (254-2) 631 499/630 164
  E-mail: cimmyt-kenya@cgnet.com

Nepal
CIMMYT
P.O. Box 5186
Kathmandu, Nepal
  Phone: (977-1) 417 791, 422 773
  Fax: (977-1) 414 184
  E-mail: phobbs@cimmyt.mos.com.np

Syria
CIMMYT
Cereal Improvement Program
ICARDA
P.O. Box 5466
Aleppo, Syria
  Phone: (963-21) 213 433 ext. 510
  Fax: (963-21) 213 490
  E-mail: m.nachit@cgnet.com

Thailand
CIMMYT
P.O. Box 9-188
Bangkok 10900, Thailand
  Phone: (66-2) 579 05 77
           (66-2) 579 48 58
  Fax: (66-2) 561-4057
  E-mail: bangkok@cimmyt.mx

Turkey
CIMMYT
P.K. 39 Emek
06511 Ankara, Turkey
  Phone: (90-312) 287 35 95/96/97
  Fax: (90-312) 287-8955
  E-mail: cimmyt-turkey@cgnet.com

Uruguay
CIMMYT-Uruguay
CC 1217
Montevideo, Uruguay
  Phone: (598-2) 928 522/923 630
  Fax: (598-2) 928 522/923 633
  E-mail: cimmyt@inia.org.uy

Zimbabwe
CIMMYT
P.O. Box MP163
Mount Pleasant
Harare, Zimbabwe
  Phone: (263-4) 30 18 07
  Fax: (263-4) 30 13 27
  E-mail: cimmyt-zimbabwe@cgnet.com

CIP

Centro Internacional de la Papa
Apartado 1558
Lima 12, Peru
  Phone: (51-1) 349-6017
  Fax: (51-1) 349-5638
  E-mail: cip@cgnet.com
            cip@cipa.org.pe
  Internet: http://www.cgiar.org/cip

Street Address:
Avenida La Universidad 795
La Molina, Lima 12, Peru

Chair: David R. MacKenzie
NERA
0106 Symons Hall
University of Maryland
College Park, MD 20742-5580 USA
  Phone: (1-301) 405-4928
  Fax: (1-301) 405-5825
  Email: dm184@umail.umd.edu

Director General: Hubert Zandstra
    Phone: (51-1) 349-2124
    Fax: (51-1) 349-5638
    E-mail: cip-dg@cgnet.com

Information Officer: Steven Kearl
    E-mail: s.kearl@cgnet.com

Regional Offices:

Peru
Latin American and Caribbean
Apartado 1558
Lima 12, Peru
    Phone: (51-1) 349-6141
    Fax: (51-1) 349-5638
    E-mail: f.ezeta@cgnet.com

Bolivia CIP Project/PROINPA
Casilla Postal 4285
Cochabamba, Bolivia
    Phone: (591-42) 49506 and 49013
    Fax: (591-42) 45708
    E-mail: proinpa@papa.bo
             devaux@papa.bo

Ecuador
Estacion Experimental INIAP Santa Catalina
Km 14, Panamericana Sur
Quito, Ecuador
    Phone: (593-2) 690-362/63
             (593-2) 690-990
    Fax: (593-2) 692-604
    E-mail: cip-quito@cgnet.com

Kenya
Sub-Saharan Africa Regional Office
P.O. Box 25171
Nairobi, Kenya
    Phone: (254-2) 632-054/632-206
    Fax: (254-2) 630-005/632-151 (ILRI)
    Telex: 22040
    Cable: CIPAPA Nairobi
    E-mail: cip-nbo@cgnet.com

Cameroon Office
BP 279
c/o Delegation of Agriculture, North West
Province
Bamenda, Cameroon
    Phone: (237) 362289
    Telex: 58442 (NWDA)
    Fax: (237) 363921/363893/363284

Uganda
PRAPACE/Uganda (Network)
P.O. Box 22274
Kampala, Uganda
    Phone: (256-41) 223-445
    Fax: (256-41) 341242
    E-mail: iita-uganda@imul.com
             iita-uganda@cgnet.com
             nbluta@imul.com

Uganda Liaison Office
P.O. Box 7878
Kampala, Uganda
    Phone: (256-41) 241-554
    Fax: (256-41) 236-918
    E-mail: iita-uganda@imul.com
             iita-uganda@cgnet.com
             n.smit@imul.com

Nigeria Liaison Office
c/o IITA
PMB 5320
Ibadan, Nigeria
    Phone: (234-22) 400-300/318
             871-145-4324
    Fax: 871-145-4325 via INMARSAT
             Satellite or (234-22) 412-21
    Telex: TROPIB NG (903) 31417/31159
    Cable: TROPFOUND,IKEJA
    E-mail: iita@cgnet.com

Egypt
Middle East and North Africa Regional Office
P.O. Box 17
Kafr El Zayat, Egypt
    Phone: (20-40) 586-720
    Fax: (20-40) 580-800
    Telex: (927) 23605 PBTNA UN
    E-mail: cip-egypt@cgnet.com

India
South and West Asia Regional Office
c/o International Potato Center
IARI Campus
New Delhi 110012, India
    Phone: (91-11) 574-8055
               (91-11) 573-1481
    Telex: 3173140 FI IN
               3173168 EIC IN
    Cable: CIPAPA, New Delhi
    E-mail: cip-delhi@cgnet.com

Indonesia
East and Southeast Asia
  and the Pacific Regional Office
c/o CRIFC, Jalan Merdeka 147, Bogor 16111
or
P.O. Box 929
Bogor 16309, West Java, Indonesia
    Phone: (62-251) 317951/313687
    Fax: (62-251) 316264
    E-mail: cip-bogor@cgnet.com

Philippines Office
c/o IRRI
P.O. Box 933
Manila, The Philippines
    Phone: (63-94) 536-1662, 536-0235,
               536-0015
    Fax: (63-2) 845-0606
    E-mail: cip-manila@cgnet.com

Liaison Office Philippines
UPWARD Network
c/o IRRI
P.O. Box 933
Manila, The Philippines
    Phone: (63-94) 536-0235
    Fax: (63-94) 536-1662

Indonesia
Lembang Liaison Office:
P.O. Box 1586
Bandung 40391, Indonesia
    Phone: (62-22) 278-8151
    Fax: (62-22) 278-6025
    E-mail: cip-indonesia@cgnet.com

China Office
c/o The Chinese Academy of Agricultural
  Sciences
Bai Shi Qiao Road No. 30
West Suburbs, Beijing
People's Republic of China
    Phone: (86-10) 6217-9141
    Fax: (86-10) 6217-9135
    Telex: (716) 222720 CAASCN or 22233
    Cable: AGRIACA
    E-mail: cip-china@cgnet.com

ICARDA

International Center for Agricultural Research
  in the Dry Areas
P.O. Box 5466
Aleppo, Syrian Arab Republic
    Phone: Tel Hadya (963-21)
               213433/213477/225112/225012
               DG Office (963-21) 210741
    Fax: Tel Hadya (963-21) 213490
               DG Office (963-21) 225105
    Telex: (492) 331208,331263 ICARDA SY
    E-mail: icarda@cgnet.com
    Internet: http://www.cgiar.org/icarda

City Office:
    Phone: (963-21) 743104, 746807, 748964
    Fax: (963-21) 744622
    Telex: (492) 331206 ICARDA SY

Chair: Alfred Bronnimann
Director
Swiss Federal Research Station for Agroecology
  and Agriculture
Reckenholzstrasse 191
8046 Zurich, Switzerland
    Phone: (41-1) 3777 111
    Fax: (41-1) 3777 201

Director General: Adel El-Beltagy
    Phone: (963-21) 225517
    E-mail: a.el-beltagy@cgnet.com

Head, Information Services: Surendra Varma
    Phone: (963-21)213433 ext.260
    E-mail: s.varma@cgnet.com

Damascus Office
ICARDA
Hamed Sultan Building, 1st Floor
Abdul Kader Gazairi Street
Abu Rommaneh - Malki Circle
P.O. Box 5908
Damascus, Syrian Arab Republic
    Phone: (963-11) 3331455/3320482
    Telex: 492 412924 ICARDA SY
    Fax: (963-11) 3320483
    E-mail: icarda-damascus@cgnet.com

Abdul Karim El Ali
Barze, Bldg. no. 6
Apt. 3, 3rd Floor
Damascus
    Phone: 5118414 (home)

Lebanon
ICARDA
Dalia Bldg. 2nd Floor
Rue Bashir El Kassar
P.O. Box 114/5055
Beirut, Lebanon
    Phone: (961-1) 813303/804071
    Telex: 494 22509 ICARDA LE
    Fax: (961-1) 804071

Anwar Agha
Ramlet-El Baida
Saniyah Habboub Street
Sea Star Bldg, 8th Floor
Beirut, Lebanon
    Phone: 802415 (home)

Terbol Station
ICARDA
Beka'a Valley
Terbol, Lebanon
    Phone: (961-3) 211553
    Fax: (961-3) 598008
    E-mail: icarda-terbol@destination.com.lb

Regional Offices:

Nile Valley and Red Sea Regional Program

Egypt
ICARDA
15 G. Radwan Ibn El-Tabib Str.
P.O. Box 2416
Cairo, Egypt
    Phone: (20-2) 5725785/5735829/5724358
    Telex: 91 21741 ICARD UN
    Fax: (20-2) 5728099
    E-mail: ICARDA-CAIRO@cgnet.com

Nagwa Lotfi
Cairo
    Phone: 3363272 (home)

North Africa Regional Program

Tunisia
mailing address:
ICARDA Tunis Office
B.P. 435
El-Menzah 1004
Tunis, Tunisia
    Phone: (216-1) 232207, 767829
    Fax: (216-1) 75166
    Telex: (409) 14066 ICARDA TN
    E-mail: icarda-tunis@cgnet.com

Building address:
8 rue Ibn Khaldoun
1004 El-Menzah 1
B.P. 84
Tunis, Tunisia

Abderrezak Belaid
57 avenue Salah Ben-Youssef
2092 El-Menzeh 9A
Tunis, Tunisia
    Phone: 883276 (home)

Morocco
ICARDA Office
Station Experimentale INRA (Guich)
B.P. 6299
Rabat-Instituts, Rabat, Morocco
    Phone: (212-7) 682909
    Telex: 407 36212 ICARDA M
    Fax: (212-7) 675496

West Asia Regional Program

Jordan
ICARDA
P.O. Box 950764
Amman 11195, Jordan
    Phone: (962-6) 825750, 817561
    Telex: 493 23278 ICARDA JO
    Fax: (962-6) 825930
    E-mail: ICARDA-Jordan@cgnet.com

Habib Halila
Amman, Jordan
    Phone: 5513963 (home)

Highland Regional Program

Turkey
Mailing address:
ICARDA
P.K. 39 Emek
Ankara 06511, Turkey
    Phone: (90-312) 2873595/96/97
    Telex: (607) 44561 CIMY TR
    Fax: (90-312) 2878955
    E-mail: icarda-turkey@cgnet.com

Building address:
ICARDA
Eskisehir Yolu, 10km
Lodumlu
Ankara, Turkey

S.P.S. Beniwal
41/13, Cayhane Sokak
Ghazi Osman Pasa
Ankara 06700, Turkey
    Phone: 4470371 (home)
    Fax: 4463002 (home)

Iran
Agricultural Research Education & Extension
Organization (AREEO)
Ministry of Agriculture
Tabnak Avenue, Evin
P.O. Box 111, Tehran 19835, Iran
    Phone: (98-21) 2400094
    Fax: (98-21) 2401855
    E-mail: icarda-iran@cgnet.com

Mr. Tahir
House 34
Street 21, Velenjak
Tehran, Iran
    Phone: 2404533 (home)

Arabian Peninsula Regional Program

United Arab Emirates
ICARDA-APRP
P.O. Box 13979
Dubai, U.A.E.
    Phone: (971-4)230338
    Fax: (971-4) 247501
    E-mail: j.peacock-t@cgnet.com
             icdub@emirates.net.ae

Building address:
Room 602
Ministry of Agriculture & Fisheries Bldg.
124, 40c Street
Opp. Al-Riqa Rost Office
Nr Clock Tower Roundabout
Dubai, UAE

John Peacock
    Phone: (971-50) 6521385 (mobile)

Yemen
ICARDA-AREA - Yemen Program
P.O. Box 87334
Dhamar, Republic of Yemen
    Phone: (967-6) 500768, 500684
    E-mail: icarda@y.net.ye
             aprp-yemen@cgnet.com

Sana'a
    Phone: (967-1) 417556
    Fax: (967-6) 509414/509418

S.V.R. Shetty, Team Leader, Dhamar
    Phone: 506854 (home)

Latin America Regional Program

Mexico
ICARDA
c/o CIMMYT
Lisboa 27
P.O. Box 6-641
Mexico 06600, D.F., Mexico
    Phone: (52-5) 726 9091
    Telex: 22 1772023 CIMTME
    Fax: (52-5) 726 7559/7558
    E-mail: cimmyt@cgnet.com
              cimmyt@cimmyt.mx

ICLARM

International Center for Living Aquatic
    Resources Management
MC P.O. Box 2631 Makati Central Post Office
0718 Makati City, The Philippines
    Phone: (63-2) 812-8641 to 47
              (63-2) 818-0466
    Fax: (63-2) 816-3183
    E-mail: iclarm@cgnet.com
    Internet: http://www.cgiar.org/iclarm

Chair: Kurt J. Peters
Department of Animal Breeding in the Tropics
Institute of Applied Animal Sciences
Humboldt University of Berlin
Lentzeallee 75
D-14195 Berlin (Dahlem), Germany
    Phone: (49-30) 31471100
              (49-30) 31471339
    Fax: (49-30) 31471422
    E-mail: k.peters@cgnet.com

Director General: Meryl J. Williams
    Phone: (63-2) 812-8641 to 47
              (63-2) 818-0466
              (63-2) 815-3873 (home)
    Fax: (63-2) 816-3183
              (63-2) 812-3798 (direct)
    E-mail: m.j.williams@cgnet.com

Information and Training Division:
    Joanna Kane-Potaka, Leader
    Phone: (63-2) 818-0466 ext. 222
    E-mail: j.kane@cgnet.com

Library and Information Services Unit:
    Rosalinda M. Temprosa, Manager
    Phone: (63-2) 818-0466 ext. 101
    E-mail: l.temprosa@cgnet.com

Outreach Offices:

Solomon Islands
ICLARM
Coastal Aquaculture Centre
P.O. Box 438
Honiara, Solomon Islands
    Phone: (677) 29255
    Fax: (677) 29130
    E-mail: iclarm@welkam.solomon.com.sb

Bangladesh
ICLARM Bangladesh Office
House 75, Road 7
Block-H, Banani Model Town
Dhaka, Bangladesh
    Phone: (880-2) 871151/873250
    Fax: (880-2)871151
    E-mail: iclarm@dhaka.agni.com

Malawi
ICLARM Malawi Project Office
P.O. Box 229
Zomba, Malawi
    Phone: (265) 531-274/531-215
    Fax: (265) 522-733
    E-mail: rbrummett@cgnet.com

British Virgin Islands
ICLARM Caribbean/Eastern Pacific Office
P.O. Box 3323, Road Town
Tortola, British Virgin Islands
    Phone: 1-809-494 5681
    Fax: 1-809-494-2670
    E-mail: j.munro@cgnet.com

Regional Office:

Egypt
ICLARM Research Center for Africa
   and West Africa
P.O. Box 2416 Cairo, Egypt
1st floor, 15 G Radwan Ibn El Tabib
Giza, Egypt

Deputy Director-General Africa-West Asia:
Roger Rowe
    Phone: (202) 572-5785
              (202) 573-5829 ext. 21
              (202) 572-4358
    Fax: (202) 572-8099
    E-mail: iclarmca@intouch.com

ICRAF

International Centre for Research in
   Agroforestry
United Nations Avenue
P.O. Box 30677
Nairobi, Kenya
    Phone: (254-2) 521450
    Telex: (987) 22048
    Fax: (254-2) 521001
    E-mail: icraf@cgnet.com
    Internet: http://www.cgiar.org/icraf

Chair: Yemi M. Katerere
IUCN Rosa
No. 6 Lanark Road, Belgravia
P.O. Box 745
Harare, Zimbabwe
    Phone: (263-4) 728266/7
    Fax: (263-4) 720738
    E-mail: yek@iucnrosa.org.zw

Director General: Pedro A. Sanchez
    Phone: (254-2) 521003
    Fax: (254-2) 520023
    E-mail: p.sanchez@cgnet.com

Head of Information: Michael Hailu
    E-mail: m.hailu@cgnet.com

Librarian: William Umbima
    E-mail: w.umbima@cgnet.com

Regional Offices:

Kenya
ICRAF Research Station, Machakos
P.O. Box 953
Machakos, Kenya
    Phone: (254–145) 20229/20286

Cameroon
ICRAF/IRAD Agroforestry Research Project
P.O. Box 2123
Yaoundé, Cameroon
    Phone: (237) 237560
    Telex: 1140 KN Yaounde
    Fax: (237) 237440
    E:mail: b.duguma@camnet.cm

Indonesia
ICRAF–Southeast Asia Regional Programme
Jalan Gunung Batu No. 5
P.O. Box 161
Bogor 16001, Indonesia
    Phone: (62–251) 315 234
    Fax: (62–251) 315 567
    E-mail: icraf-indonesia@cgnet.com

Kenya
KARI–KEFRI–ICRAF Regional Research Project
P.O. Box 27
Embu, Kenya
    Phone: (254–161) 20116/20873
    Fax: (254–161) 30064
    E-mail: icraf-embu@cgnet.com

KEFRI/KARI/ICRAF Agroforestry Research
  Project
P.O. Box 25199
Otonglo, Kisumu, Kenya
  Phone: (254–35) 51245, 51164, 51163
  Fax: (254–35) 51592
  E-mail: afresmaseno@form-net.com

Malawi
SADC–ICRAF Agroforestry Project
Makoka Agricultural Research Station
P.O. Box 134
Zomba, Malawi
  Phone: (265) 534277, 534209/534250
  Telex: 44017 (ICRAF Malawi)
  Fax: (265) 534283
  E-mail: fkwesiga@malawi.net

Mali
ICRAF Sahel Programme
c/o ICRISAT
B.P. 320
Bamako, Mali
  Phone: (223) 223375/227707
  Telex: ICRISAT 2681 MJ
  Fax: (223) 228683
  E-mail: e.bonkoungou@cgnet.com

Mexico
ICRAF–Mexico Programme
Km 3.5 Carretera. Chetumal–Bacalar
Apartado Postal No. 388
C.P. 77000 Chetumal
Quintana Roo, Mexico
  Phone: (52–983) 28350
  Fax: (52– 983) 28350
  E-mail: jhaggar@mpsnet.com.mx

Niger
ICRAF–Niger
c/o ICRISAT Sahelian Centre
B.P. 12 404
Niamey, Niger
  Phone: (227) 722529
  Telex: 5406 N.I.
  Fax: (227) 734329
  E-mail: icrisat.sc@cgnet.com

Peru
ICRAF Latin America Regional Programme
c/o INIA–Centro Forestal
Carretera Federico Basadre Km 4.2
Apartado Postal 558
Pucallpa, Peru
  Phone: (511) 436 6920
  Fax: (511) 435 1570
  E-mail: d.bandy@cgnet.com

Philippines
ICRAF–Philippines
2/F College of Forestry Administration
Building
P.O. Box 35024
UPLB, College
Laguna 4031, The Philippines
  Phone: (63–49) 536 2925
  Fax: (63–49) 536 2925
  E-mail: icrafphi@irri.cgnet.com

Tanzania
ICRAF–Tanzania Agroforestry Research Project
c/o HASHI
P.O. Box 797
Shinyanga, Tanzania
  Phone: (255 68) 763099
  Telex: 48102 OXMAC TZ
           (c/o OXMAC Ltd.)
  Fax: (255 68) 762172)
  E-mail: rotsyina@intafrica.com

Thailand
ICRAF–Chiang Mai
Computer Service Center
Chiang Mai University
Chiang Mai 50200, Thailand
  Phone: (66–53) 943799
  Fax: (66–53) 894133
  E-mail: icraf@loxinfo.co.th

Uganda
ICRAF–Uganda AFRENA Project
Forest Research Institute
P.O. Box 1752
Kampala, Uganda
  Phone: (256–41) 232071
  Fax: (256–41) 220268
  E-mail: aluma@starcom.co.ug

ICRAF–Uganda AFRENA Project
P O Box 311
Kabale, Uganda
    Phone: (256–486) 23931 Kabale
    Telex: 68032 KBUB PUB TLX
    Fax: (256–486) 23931 (Project Office)
    E-mail: afrenakb@starcom.co.ug

Zambia
ICRAF–Zambia AFRENA Project
c/o Provincial Agriculture Office
   (Eastern Province)
P.O. Box 510046
Chipata, Zambia
    Phone: (260–62) 21404
    Telex: ZA 63020 Chipata
    Fax: (260–62) 21404
    E-mail: zamicraf@zamnet.zm

Zimbabwe
SADC–ICRAF Agroforestry Project
c/o Department of Research and Specialist
   Services
5th Street Extension
P.O. Box CY 594, Causeway
Harare, Zimbabwe
    Phone: (263–4) 704531
    Telex: 734646 ZW
    Fax: (263–4) 728340
    E-mail   icraf-zimbabwe@cgnet.com

ICRISAT

International Crops Research Institute for the
   Semi-Arid Tropics
Corporate Office and Headquarters Asia Region
Patancheru 502 324
Andhra Pradesh, India
    Phone: (91-40) 596161
    Telex: 422203 ICRI IN
    Fax: (91-40) 241239/596182
    E-mail: ICRISAT@cgnet.com
    Internet: http://www.cgiar.org/icrisat

Chair: Ragnhild Sohlberg
Vice President, External Relations and Special
   Projects
Corporate Staff
Norsk Hydro a.s.
Bygdoy alle 2
N-0240, Oslo, Norway
    Phone: (47) 22432851
    Fax: (47) 22432615
    E-mail: ragnhild.sohlberg@chr.hydro.com

Director General: Shawki M. Barghouti

Interim Director, Information Management:
   Mark D. Winslow

Regional Offices:

India
New Delhi Liaison Office
IARI Campus, Pusa
New Delhi 110 012, India
    Phone: (91-11) 5819294
    Fax: (91-11) 5819287
    E-mail: icrisatnd@cgnet.com

Liaison Officer: P.M. Menon

Niger
ICRISAT-Niamey
BP 12404
Niamey, Niger (via Paris)
    Phone: (227) 722529/722626
    Fax: (227) 734329
    E-mail: icrisatsc@cgnet.com

ICRISAT Country Representative: K. Anand Kumar

Mali
ICRISAT-Bamako
B.P. 320
Bamako, Mali
    Phone: (223) 223375/227707
    Fax: (223) 228683
    E-mail: icrisat-w-mali@cgnet.com

ICRISAT Country Representative: F. Waliyar

Nigeria
ICRISAT-Kano
IITA Office
Sabo Bakin Zuwo Road
PMB 3491
Kano, Nigeria
    Phone: (234-64) 662050
    Fax: (234-64) 663492/669051
    E-mail: icrisat-w-nigeria@cgnet.com

ICRISAT Representative: O. Ajayi

Zimbabwe
ICRISAT-Bulawayo
SADC/ICRISAT Sorghum and Millet
   Improvement Program (SMIP)
Matopos Research Station
P.O. Box 776
Bulawayo, Zimbabwe
    Phone: (263-83) 8311/8314
    Fax: (263-83) 8253
             (263-9) 41652
    E-mail: icrisatzw@cgnet.com

ICRISAT Country Representative:
  L. K. Mughogho

Kenya
ICRISAT-Nairobi
P.O. Box 39063
Nairobi, Kenya
    Phone: (254-2) 521450 (ICRAF)
    Fax: (254-2) 521001 (ICRAF)
    E-mail: icrisat-kenya@cgnet.com

ICRISAT Country Representative: S. N. Silim

Malawi
ICRISAT-Malawi
Chitedze Agricultural Research Station
P.O. Box 1096
Lilongwe, Malawi
    Phone: (265) 720968/720906
    Fax: (265) 741872
    E-mail: icrisat-malawi@cgnet.com

ICRISAT Country Representative:
  P. Subrahmanyam

IFPRI

International Food Policy Research Institute
2033 K Street, NW
Washington, DC 20006, USA
    Phone: (1-202) 862-5600
    Telex: 440054 IFPR UI
    Cable: IFPRI
    Fax: (1-202) 467-4439
    E-mail: ifpri@cgnet.com
    Internet: http://www.cgiar.org/ifpri

Chair: Martin Pineiro
Director, Group CEO
Consultores en Economia y Organizacion
Hipolito Yrigoyen 785
Piso 5, oficina "M"
Buenos Aires (Capital Federal) 1086
Argentina
    Phone: (54-1) 342-1395
              (54-1) 331-0035
    Fax: (54-1) 342-8153

Director General: Per Pinstrup-Andersen
  E-mail: p.pinstrup-andersen@cgnet.com

Director of Information: Donald Lippincott
  E-mail: d.lippincott@cgnet.com

Librarian: Patricia Klosky
  E-mail: t.klosky@cgnet.com

IIMI

International Irrigation Management Institute
P.O. Box 2075
Colombo, Sri Lanka
    Phone: (94-1) 867404/869080/869081
    Telex: 22318, IIMIHQ CE
    Fax: (94-1) 866854
    E-mail: iimi@cgnet.com
    Internet: http://www.cgiar.org/iimi

Chair : Zafar Altaf
Chairman
Pakistan Agricultural Research Council
Plot 20, Ramna 5/1
P.O. Box 1031
Islamabad 44000, Pakistan
    Phone: (92-51) 9203966
    Fax: (92-51) 9202968

Director General: David Seckler
    E-mail: d.seckler@cgnet.com

Head of Communications and Donor Relations:
James Lenahan
    E-mail: j.lenahan@cgnet.com

Librarian: N. U. Yapa
    E-mail: n.yapa@cgnet.com

Documentalist: Ramya de Silva
    E-mail: r.desilva@cgnet.com

National Programs:

Sri Lanka
IIMI, Sri Lanka National Program
127, Sunil Mawatha
Battaramulla, Sri Lanka
    Phone: (94-1) 867404/869080/869081
    Fax: (94-1) 872185
    E-mail: iimi@cgnet.com

Burkina Faso
IIMI, Burkina Faso National Team
01 B.P. 5373
Ouagadougou 01, Burkina Faso
    Phone: (226) 308489
    Telex: 5381 SAFGRAD BF(attn: IIMI)
    Fax: (226) 310618
    E-mail: iimi-Burkina@cgnet.com

Mexico
IIMI, Mexico National Program
c/o CIMMYT
Lisboa 27, Colonia Juarez
Apdo. Postal 6-641
06600 Mexico, D.F. Mexico
    Phone: (52-595) 54400/54410
    Fax: (52-595) 54425 or (52-5) 7267558/9
    E-mail: iimi-mex@cgnet.com

Niger
IIMI, Niger National Team
BP 10883
Niamey, Niger
    Phone: (227) 73-29-53/73-23-94
    Fax: (227) 75-23-94 or, through backup
              services 44-1-491-832002
    E-mail: iimi-niger@cgnet.com

Pakistan
IIMI, Pakistan National Program
12 km, Multan Road
Chowk Thokar Niaz Baig
Lahore 53700, Pakistan
    Phone: 92-42 5410050/53 (4 lines)
    Fax: 92-42 5410054
    E-mail: iimi-pak@cgnet.com

Turkey
IIMI, Turkey National Program
c/o Director, Agrohydrology Research and
    Training Center
35600 Menemen
Izmir, Turkey
    Phone: 90-232-8310512
    Fax: 90-232-8311051
    E-mail: j.brewer@cgnet.com

IITA

International Institute of Tropical Agriculture
PMB 5320
Ibadan, Nigeria
    Phone: (234-2) 241-2626
              871-1454324 (via INMARSAT)
    Telex: (905) 31417 or 31159 TROPIB NG
    Cable: TROPFOUND, IKEJA
    Fax: 871-1454325 (via INMARSAT)
              (234-2) 2412221 Regular
    E-mail: iita@cgnet.com
    Internet: http://www.cgiar.org/iita

International Mailing Address:
IITA, Ibadan, Nigeria
c/o L.W. Lambourn & Co.
Carolyn House
26 Dingwall Road
Croydon CR9 3EE, United Kingdom
    Phone: (44-181) 686-9031
    Telex: 946979 LWL G
    Fax: (44-181) 681-8583

Chair: Enrico Porceddu
Dipartimento di Agrobiologia e Agrochimica
Universita Degli Studi Della Tuscia
Via S.C. del Lellis
01100 Viterbo, Italy
    Phone: (39-761) 25 72 31
    Telex: 614076 TUSVIT
    Fax: (39-761) 35 72 56
    E-mail: porceddu@unitus.it
             enrypo@pelagus.it

Director General: Lukas Brader
    E-mail: l.brader@cgnet.com

Deputy Director General: Robert Booth
    E-mail: r.booth@cgnet.com

Director, Corporate Services Division:
   William P. Powell
    E-mail: w.powell@cgnet.com

Director, Crop Improvement Division:
   Frances M. Quin
    E-mail: m.quin@cgnet.com

Director, International Cooperation Division:
   Michael W. Bassey
    E-mail: m.bassey@cgnet.com

Director, Plant Health Management Division:
Peter Neuenschwander
   Phone: (229) 350553/350186/3606001
   E-mail: p.neuenschwander@cgnet.com

Acting Director, Resource and Crop
   Management Division: Horst Grimme
   E-mail: h.grimme@cgnet.com

Head, Information Services: Jack Reeves
    E-mail: j.reeves@cgnet.com

Head, Library Services: Yakubu A. Adedigba
    E-mail: iita@cgnet.com

Regional Offices:

Nigeria
IITA Kano Station
Sabo Bakin Zuwa Road
PMB 3112
Kano, Nigeria
    Phone: (234-64) 645350; 645351;645353
    Telex: (905) 77330;
             77444 (box 189) TDS KN NG
    Cable: AGRISEARCH KANO
    Fax: (234-64) 645352/669051
    E-mail: icrisat-w-nigeria@cgnet.com

Contact: Bir B. Singh

IITA/High Rainfall Station Onne
PMB 008, Nchia-Eleme
Port Harcourt, Nigeria
    Phone: (234-090)501380 (cellular)
    Fax: 871-682 341882 (via INMARSAT)
    E-mail: iita-onne@cgnet.com

Contact: Piers D. Austin

République du Bénin
IITA/Benin Research Station
B.P. 08-0932 Cotonou
République du Bénin
    Phone: (229) 350553/350186/360600-1
    Telex: (972) 5329 ITA BEN
    Fax: (229) 350556
    E-mail: iita-benin@cgnet.com

Contact: Peter Neuenschwander

Cameroon
IITA Humid Forest Station
B.P. 2008 (Messa)
Yaoundé, Cameroon
    Phone: (237) 237434
    Fax: (237) 237437
    E-mail: iita-humid@cgnet.com

Contact: Stephan F. Weise

Ghana
IITA Research Liaison Office, Ghana
c/o Crops Research Institute
P.O. Box 3785
Kumasi, Ghana
  Telex: 3036 BTH 10 GH
           2630 MNJ KSI
           3014 BTH 26 GH
  Fax: (223) 5125306
  E-mail: jsuhiita@ncs.com.gh

Contact: Joseph B. Suh

Côte d'Ivoire
IITA Liaison Office, Bouaké, Côte d'Ivoire
01 B.P. 2551
Bouaké, Côte d'Ivoire
  Phone: (225) 634514/632396/
           633242
  Telex: 69138 ADRAO BOUAKE CI
  Fax: (225) 634714
  E-mail: j.fajemisin@cgnet.com

Contact: Joseph M. Fajemisin

Uganda
IITA/EARRNET Project
c/o IITA-East and Southern Africa Regional
   Center (ESARC)
P.O. Box 7878
Kampala, Uganda
  Phone: (256-41) 223460
  Telex: 61000 ESARC UGA
  Fax: (256-41) 223459
  E-mail: iita-uganda@cgnet.com
           jwhyte@imul.com

Contact: Jim B.A. Whyte

Malawi
IITA/SARRNET Project
Pagat House
P.O. Box 30258
Capital City, Lilongwe 3
Malawi
  Phone: (265) 74 02 61/74 41 39
  Telex: 45281 IITA MI
           43055 ROCKFND MI

  Fax: (265) 74 42 05
  E-mail: sarrnet@eo.wn.apc.org

Contact: James M. Teri

Mozambique
USAID/SADC/IITA/CIP-SARRNET
c/o INIA
FPLM Malvane
CP 2100
Maputo, Mozambique
  Phone: (258-1) 460097/99
  Telex: 6-166 SEEDS MO
  Fax   (258-1) 460074
  E-mail: madrade@zebra-uem.mz

Contact: Maria I. Andrade

Zambia
USAID/SADC/IITA/CIP-SARRNET
Mutanda Research Station
Luapula Reg. Research Station
PO 710129
Manza, Zambia
  Phone: (260-08) 82 12 42/82 12 30
  Telex: IRDP-LP ZA 59050
  Fax: (260-08) 82 19 13

Contact: Ambayera Muimba-Kankolongo

Tanzania
USAID/SADC/IITA/CIP SARRNET
Kibaha Research Station
P.O. Box 2066
Dar-Es-Salaam, Tanzania
  Phone: 255-811-324355
           (255-11) 700986
  Telex: c/o FAO 41320 FOODAGRI TZ
  Fax: c/o FAO (255-51) 112501
  E-mail: n.mahungu@cats-net.com

Contact: Nzola-Meso Mahungu

Zimbabwe
USAID/SADC/IITA/CIP-SARRNET
Grassland Research Station
P.O. Box 3701 Marondera
Zimbabwe
    Phone: (263-79) 23 526
    E-mail: i@kasele.icon.co.zw

Contact: Idumbo N. Kasele

ILRI

International Livestock Research Institute
P.O. Box 30709
Nairobi, Kenya
    Phone: (254-2) 630743
    Telex: 22040
    Cable: ILRI
    Fax: (254-2) 631499
    E-mail: ilri@cgnet.com
    Internet: http://www.cgiar.org/ilri

P.O. Box 5689
Addis Ababa, Ethiopia
    Phone: (251-1) 613215
    Telex: 21207 ILRI ET
    Cable: ILRI-ADDIS ABABA
    Fax: (251-1) 611892
    E-mail: ilri-ethiopia@cgnet.com

Chair: Neville P. Clarke
Centeq Research Plaza, Suite 241
The Texas A & M University System
College Station, Texas 77843-2129, USA
    Phone: (1-409) 845-2855
    Fax: (1-409) 845-6574
    E-mail: n-clarke@tamu.edu

Director General: Hank Fitzhugh
P.O. Box 30709
Nairobi, Kenya
    Phone: (254-2) 630743
    Fax: (254-2) 631259
    E-mail: h.fitzhugh@cgnet.com

Head of Publications: Paul Neate
    E-mail: p.neate@cgnet.com

Regional Sites:

Ethiopia
Debre Zeit, Ethiopia
P.O. Box 5689
Addis Ababa, Ethiopia
    Phone: (251-1) 339566
    Fax: (251-1) 338755
    E-mail: ilri-ethiopia@cgnet.com

Nigeria
ILRI/Ibadan
PMB 5320
Ibadan, Nigeria
    Phone: (234-22) 400300/14
    Telex: 31417/31159 TROPIB NG
    E-mail: ilri-ibadan@cgnet.com

Peru
ILRI/CIP
Apartado 1558
Lima 12, Peru
    Phone: (51-1) 436-6920/435-0266/
             435-9367/435-4354
    Fax: (51-1) 435-0842/435-1570
    E-mail: cip@cgnet.com
             cip@cipa.org.pe

Colombia
ILRI/CIAT
Apartado Aero 6713
Cali, Colombia
    Phone: (57-2) 4450-000
    Fax: (57-2) 4450-073
    E-mail: ciat@cgnet.com

Niger
ILRI/ICRISAT Sahelian Center
B.P. 12404
Niamey, Niger
    Phone: (227) 723071
    Telex: (ICRISAT) 5406/5560 NI
    Fax: (227) 734329
    E-mail: ilri-niamey@cgnet.com

India
ILRI/ICRISAT
Patancheru 502 324
Andhra Pradesh, India
Phone: (91-40) 596 161
Fax: (91-40) 241 239
E-mail: icrisat@cgnet.com

Burkina Faso
ILRI/CIRDES
01 B.P. 454
Bobo-Dioulasso, Burkina Faso
Phone: (226) 972-638
Fax: (226) 972-320
E-mail: toure@ouaga.orstom.bf

IPGRI

International Plant Genetic Resources Institute
Via delle Sette Chiese 142
00145 Rome, Italy
Phone: (39-6) 518921
Fax: (39-6) 575- 0309
E-mail: ipgriI@cgnet.com
Internet: http://www.cgiar.org/ipgri

Chair: Marcio de Miranda Santos
Head, Department for Research and Development
EMBRAPA
SAIN Parque Rural
Av. W3 Norte-final
70 770-901 Brasilia-DF 02138, Brazil
Phone: (55 61) 340 5518
              (55 61) 348 4451
Fax: (55 61) 347 2061
E-mail: marcio@sede.embrapa.brazil

Director General: Geoffrey C. Hawtin
Phone: (39-6) 51892247/202
Fax: (39-6) 51892405
E-mail: g.hawtin@cgnet.com

Assistant Director General: Dick van Sloten
Phone: (39-6)51892239/241
Fax: (39-6) 51892405
E-mail: d.vansloten@cgnet.com

Deputy Director General Programmes:
  Masaru Iwanaga
  Phone: (39-6) 51892200/249
  Fax: (39-6) 575-0309
  E-mail: m.iwanaga@cgnet.com

Director Finance and Administration: Koen
Geerts
  Phone: (39-6) 51892201
  Fax: (39-6) 575-0309
  E-mail: k.geerts@cgnet.com

System-Wide Genetic Resources Programme
  Secretariat (SGRP)
Coordinator: Jane Toll
c/o IPGRI
Via delle Sette Chiese 142
00145 Rome, Italy
  Phone: (39-6) 51892225/245
  Telex: 4900005332 (IBR UI) (via USA)
  Fax: (39-6) 575-0309
  E-mail: j.toll@cgnet.com

Director Documentation, Information, and
  Training: Lyndsey Withers
  Phone: (39-6) 51892237/268
  E-mail: l.withers@cgnet.com

Director Genetic Resources Science and
  Technology: Jan Engels
  Phone: (39-6) 51892222/401
  E-mail: j.engels@cgnet.com

Information/Public Awareness:
  Ruth D. Raymond
  Phone: (39-6) 51892215 (direct)
  E-mail: r.raymond@cgnet.com

Library: Julia-Anne Dearing
  Phone: (39-6) 51892216 (direct)
  E-mail: j.dearing@cgnet.com

Manager of Editorial and Publications Unit:
  Paul Stapleton
  Phone: (39-6) 51892233 (direct)
  E-mail: p.stapleton@cgnet.com

IPGRI Offices:

Kenya
Sub-Saharan Africa Regional Office
c/o ICRAF
P.O. Box 30677
Nairobi, Kenya
    Phone: (254-2) 522150/521514
    Fax: (254-2) 521209
    E-mail: ipgri-kenya@cgnet.com

Regional Director: Franck Attere

République du Bénin
West Africa Office
c/o IITA-Benin Research Station
BP 08-0932
Cotonou, Republique du Benin
    Phone: (229)350553/350189/360600-1
    Telex: (972) 5329 ITA BENIN
    Fax: (229) 350556
    E-mail: a.goli@cgnet.com

Scientist, Conservation Strategies: Ankon Goli

Malaysia
Asia, Pacific & Oceania Regional Office
P.O. Box 236
UPM Post Office
43400 Serdang
Selangor Darul Ehsan, Malaysia
    Phone: (60-3) 942-3891-4
    Fax: (60-3) 948-7655
    E-mail: ipgri-apo@cgnet.com

Regional Director: Ken Riley

China
East Asia Office
c/o CAAS
30 Bai Shi Qiao Road
Beijing 100081, China
    Phone: (86-10) 62183744
    Telex: 222720 CAAS CN
    Fax: (86-10)62174159
    E-mail: ipgri-caas@cgnet.com

Coordinator: Zhou Ming-De

India
South Asia Office
c/o NBPGR
Pusa Campus
New Delhi 110012, India
    Phone: (91-11) 578-6112
    Telex: 31-77257 NBPGR IN
    Fax: (91-11) 573-1845
    E-mail: ipgri-delhi@cgnet.com

Syria
West Asia & North Africa Regional Office
c/o ICARDA
P.O. Box 5466
Aleppo, Syria
    Phone: (963-21)231412
    Telex: (924) 331206 ICARDA SY
                  (924) 331208 ICARDA SY
                  (924) 331263 ICARDA SY
    Fax: (963-21) 225105/213490
    E-mail: ipgri-wana@cgnet.com

Regional Director: George Ayad

Colombia
Americas Regional Office
c/o CIAT
Apartado Aereo 6713
Cali, Colombia
    Phone: (57-2) 445 0048/445 0049 (IPGRI)
                  (57-2) 4450000 (CIAT)
    IVDN: 625-3329
    Telex: 05769 CIAT CO
    Cable: CINATROP
    Fax: (57-2) 445-0096 (IPGRI)
                  (57-2) 445-0073 (CIAT)
    IVDN Fax: 625-3273
    E-mail: ciat-ipgri@cgnet.com

Regional Director: Ramon Lastra

Italy
Europe Regional Office
c/o IPGRI
Via delle Sette Chiese 142
00145 Rome, Italy
    Phone: (39-6) 51892229/221
    Telex: 49900005332 (IBR UI) (via USA)
    Fax: (39-6) 575-0309
    E-mail: t.gass@cgnet.com

Regional Director: Thomas Gass

IPGRI/INIBAP Offices:

INIBAP
International Network for the Improvement
    of Banana and Plantain
Parc Scientifique Agropolis II
Montpellier Cedex 5, 34937 France
    Phone: (33) 4 67611302
    Fax: (33) 4 67610334
    E-mail: inibap@cgnet.com

Director: Emile Frison
    E-mail: e.frison@cgnet.com

Information/Communication: Claudine Picq
    E-mail: c.picq@cgnet.com

Belgium
INIBAP Transit Centre
c/o Katholieke Universiteit Leuven
Faculteit Landbouwkundige en Toegepste
Biologische Wetenschappen
Kardinaal Mercierlaan 92
B-3001 Heverlee, Belgium
    Phone: (32-16) 321417
    Telex: 25941 elekul b
    Fax: (32-16) 321993
    E-mail: lab.trop@agr.kuleuven.ac.be

Officer-in-Charge: Ines van den Houwe

Cameroon
Sub Saharan Africa Office
c/o CRBP, BO 832
Douala, Cameroon
    Phone: (237) 427129/426052
    Fax: (237) 425786

Regional Coordinator: Ekow Akyeampong

Uganda
East and Southern Africa Office
P.O. Box 24384
Kampala, Uganda
    Phone: (256-41) 223502
    Fax: (256-41) 223503
    E-mail: inibap-esa@imu.com

Regional Coordinator: Eldad Karamura

Philippines
Asia and Pacific Office
c/o PCARRD
Los Baños, Laguna 3732, Philippines
    Phone: (63-94) 536 0014
    Telex: (754) 40860 PARRS PM
    Fax: (63-94) 536 0016

Costa Rica
INIBAP Latin American and Caribbean Office
c/o CATIE
7170 Turrialba, Costa Rica
    Phone: (506) 556 62 431
    Fax: c/o (506) 556 62 431
    E-mail: lyega@catie.ac.cr

Regional Coordinator: Franklin Rosales

Honduras
INIBAP
c/o FHIA
Apartado Postal 2067
San Pedro Sula, Honduras
    Phone: (504) 682078/682470
    Fax: (504) 682313

Associate Scientist, Nematology: Nicole Viaene

IRRI

International Rice Research Institute
P.O. Box 933
Manila, The Philippines
    Phone: (63-2) 845-0563/0569/0570/0573/
               0575
               (Trunk Hunting Lines)
               762-0127 (for international calls only)
               (1-415) 833-6620
    IVDN: 620-0 IRRI Operator
               620-670 IRRI Fax

Telex: (ITT) 40890 RICE PM (Los Baños)
        CAPWIRE: 14519 IRI LB PS
        (mailbox)
Cable: RICEFOUND, Manila
Fax: (63-2) 891-1292
        (63-2) 717-8470
        (63-2) 761-2404
        (63-2) 761-2406 (for international fax
        only)
        (1-415) 833-6621
Internet:
IRRI Website: http://www.cgiar.org/irri
Information About Rice: http://www.riceweb.org
IRRI Library: http://www.ricelib.irri.cgiar.org
IRRI Rice Museum: http://www.riceworld.org

Chair: Roelof Rabbinge
Professor, Department of Theoretical
Production Ecology
Wageningen Agricultural University
Bornsesteeg 47
6708 PD Wageningen, The Netherlands
    Phone: (31-31) 748-3988
    Fax: (31-31) 748-4892
    Telex: 75209 abw nl
    E-mail: office@sec.tpe.wau.nl

Director General (interim): Robert Havener
    Phone: (63-2) 810-5337
    Fax: (63-2) 892-0354
    E-mail: r.havener@cgnet.com

Information Center: Ian M. Wallace, Head
    Phone: (63-2) 845563/0569/0570/
            0573/0575
    E-mail: i.wallace@cgnet.com

Library and Documentation Service:
Ian M. Wallace, Librarian

Communication and Publications Service:
Eugene Hettel, Head
    Phone: (63-2) 845-0563/0569/0570/
            0573/0575

Computer Services: Ian Moore, Manager
    Phone: (63-2) 845-0563/0569/0570/
            0573/0575
    E-mail: i.moore@cgnet.com

Regional Offices:

Bangladesh
IRRI Dhaka Office
House 30, Road 10B, Block H
Banani, Dhaka
Bangladesh
    Phone: (880-2) 885341; 601197
    Telex: 642671 HBP BJ
            671010 DHL BJ
    Cable: RICEFOUND DHAKA
    Fax: (880-2) 885341/883416
    E-mail: irri.dhaka@drik.bgd.toolnet.org
            irri.dhaka@driktap.tool.nl

Myanmar
IRRI Representative Office
P.O. Box 1369
Yangon, Myanmar
    Phone: (95-1) 663590
    Telex: 21311 AGRICO BM
    Fax: (95-1) 667991
    E-mail:
        garcia%remote.undp-mya@nylan.undp.org

India
IRRI-India Liaison Office
C-18 , Friends Colony (East)
New Delhi 110065, India
    Phone: (91-11) 692-4290/692-5070
    Fax: (91-11) 692-3122
    E-mail: irri@giasdl01.vsnl.net.in

Indonesia
Cooperative DEPAGRI-IRRI Program
P.O. Box 205
Bogor 16002, Indonesia
    Phone: (62-251) 334391
    Cable: IRRIAID Bogor
    Fax: (62-251) 314354
    E-mail: irri-bogor@cgnet.com

Thailand
IRRI Cooperative Project with the
Ministry of Agriculture and Cooperatives
P.O. Box 9-159
Bangkhen, Bangkok 10900, Thailand
    Phone: (66-2) 579-5249/579-9493/
            561-1581
    Telex: 84478 INTERAG TH

Fax: (66-2) 561-4894
E-mail: irri-bangkok-t@cgnet.com
         (for general administration)
         irri-bangkok@cgnet.com
         (for accomodation and travel)
         irri-bangkok-account@cgnet.com
         (for financial matters)
Japan
IRRI Japan Liaison and Library Office
c/o JIRCAS
1-2 Ohwashi, Tsukuba
Ibaraki 305, Japan
    Phone: (81-0298) 386339
    Fax: (81-0298) 386339
    Telex: 3656156 TARC JP
    Cable: MAFFTROPICAL TSUCHIURA
    E-mail: kfb03331@niftyserve.or.jp"

Madagascar-IRRI Rice Research Project
B.P. 4151
Antananarivo (101), Madagascar
    Cable: IRRIMAD, Antananarivo
    Fax: (261-2) 34883 (Attn. IRRI)
    Mahajanga Fax: (261-6) 23264
    E-mail: irrimad@dts.mg

Lao PDR
Lao-IRRI Project
P.O. Box 4195
Vientiane, Lao PDR
    Phone: (856-21) 412352/414373
    Telex: 4491 TE VTE LS (LAO IRRI Project)
             TX BOOTH LS 14491 or 14492
    Fax: (856-21) 414373 (Vientiane)
    Phone/Fax: (856-71) 212310 (Luang Prabang)
    E-mail: keithf@ksc15.th.com (Luang
Prabang)

Cambodia-IRRI Australia Project (CIAP)
P.O. Box 1
Phnom Penh, Cambodia
    Phone: (855-23) 364115, 426229, 426465
    Cable: IRRI PHNOM PENH
    Fax: (855-18) 810796
    E-mail: irri-cambodia@cgnet.com

Vietnam
IRRI Vietnam Office
Department of Science Technology and
    Product Quality
Ministry of Agriculture and Food Industries
2 Ngoc ha, Ba dinh
Hanoi, Vietnam
    Phone: (84-4) 823-4202
    Fax: (84-4) 823-4425
    E-mail: 113@remote1.msm.cgnet.com

ISNAR

International Service for National Agricultural
    Research
Laan van Nieuw Oost Indië 133
2593 BM The Hague, The Netherlands
    Phone: (31-70) 349-6100
    Telex: 33746 ISNAR NL
    Cable: ISNAR
    Fax: (31-70) 381-9677
    E-mail: isnar@cgnet.com
    Internet: http://www.cgiar.org/isnar

Mailing Address:
P.O. Box 93375
2509 AJ The Hague, The Netherlands

Chair: Amir Muhammed
President
Asianics Agro-Development International
    (Pvt) Ltd.
House 13, Street 49, F-6/4
P.O. Box 2316
Islamabad, Pakistan
    Phone: (92-51) 276424/810860/9222277
    Fax: (92-51) 276492
    Telex: 5945 CTO 5811 IBA NA
    E-mail: asianics@isb.comsats.net.pk

Director General: Stein W. Bie
    Phone: (31-70) 349-6206
    Fax: (31-70) 381-9677
    E-mail: s.bie@cgnet.com

Deputy Director General: Howard Elliott
 Phone: (31-70) 349-6210
 E-mail: h.elliott@cgnet.com

Director of Administration: Coenraad Kramer
 Phone: (31-70) 349-6227
 E-mail: c.a.kramer@cgnet.com

Program Director, Program 1. Policy and
 System Development: Helio Tollini
 Phone: (31-70) 349-6149
 E-mail: h.tollini@cgnet.com

Program Director, Program 2. Management:
 Paul Perrault
 Phone: (31-70) 349-6234
 E-mail: p.perrault@cgnet.com

Librarian: Monica Allmand
 Phone: (31-70) 349-6175
 E-mail: m.allmand@cgnet.com

Head of Publications: Kathleen Sheridan
 Phone: (31-70) 349-6107
 E-mail: k.sheridan@cgnet.com

Head, Computer Services: Paul O'Nolan
 Phone: (31-70) 349-6170
 E-mail: p.o-nolan@cgnet.com

WARDA

West Africa Rice Development Association
01 B.P. 2551
Bouaké 01, Côte d'Ivoire
 Phone: (225) 634514
 Telex: 69138 ADRAO CI, BOUAKE
 Fax: (225) 634714
 E-mail: warda@cgnet.com
 Internet: http://www.cgiar.org/warda

Chair: Just Faaland
Chr. Michelsen Institute
Development Studies and Human Rights
Fantoftvegen 38
N-5036 Fantoft, Norway
 Phone: (47-55) 574-000
 Telex: 40 006 CMIN

 Fax: (47-55) 574-166
 E-mail: JUSTF@AMADEUS.cmi.no

Director General: Kanayo F. Nwanze
 Phone: (225) 632907

Public Affairs Assistant: Lucien N'Guessan

Documentalist: Alassane Diallo

Regional Offices:

Côte d'Ivoire
WARDA Abidjan Liaison Office
01 B.P. 4029
Abidjan 01, Côte d'Ivoire
 Phone: (225) 227764
 Fax: (225) 227865

Senegal
WARDA Sahel Station
B.P. 96
St. Louis, Sénégal
 Phone: (221) 9626493/962441
 Fax: (221) 9626491/9612876
 E-mail: warda-sahel@cgnet.com

Nigeria
WARDA Ibadan Station
c/o IITA, Ibadan, Nigeria